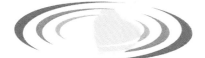

Early Diagnosis and
Treatment of Cancer:
Prostate Cancer

Early Diagnosis and Treatment of Cancer

Series Editor: Stephen C. Yang, MD

Breast Cancer
Edited by Lisa Jacobs and Christina A. Finlayson

Colorectal Cancer
Edited by Susan Lyn Gearhart and Nita Ahuja

Head and Neck Cancer
Edited by Wayne M. Koch

Ovarian Cancer
Edited by Robert E. Bristow and
Deborah K. Armstrong

Prostate Cancer
Edited by Li-Ming Su

EARLY DIAGNOSIS AND TREATMENT OF CANCER

Series Editor: Stephen C. Yang, MD

Prostate Cancer

Edited by

Li-Ming Su, MD

David A. Cofrin Professor of Urology
Associate Chairman of Clinical Affairs
Chief, Division of Robotic and Minimally Invasive Urologic Surgery
Department of Urology
University of Florida College of Medicine
Gainesville, Florida

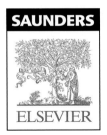

SAUNDERS

ELSEVIER

SAUNDERS
ELSEVIER

1600 John F. Kennedy Blvd.
Ste 1800
Philadelphia, PA 19103-2899

EARLY DIAGNOSIS AND TREATMENT OF CANCER: ISBN-13: 978-1-4160-4575-5
PROSTATE CANCER

Notices

Knowledge and best practice in this field are constantly changing. As new research and experience broaden our understanding, changes in research methods, professional practices, or medical treatment may become necessary.

Practitioners and researchers must always rely on their own experience and knowledge in evaluating and using any information, methods, compounds, or experiments described herein. In using such information or methods they should be mindful of their own safety and the safety of others, including parties for whom they have a professional responsibility.

With respect to any drug or pharmaceutical products identified, readers are advised to check the most current information provided (i) on procedures featured or (ii) by the manufacturer of each product to be administered, to verify the recommended dose or formula, the method and duration of administration, and contraindications. It is the responsibility of practitioners, relying on their own experience and knowledge of their patients, to make diagnoses, to determine dosages and the best treatment for each individual patient, and to take all appropriate safety precautions.

To the fullest extent of the law, neither the Publisher nor the authors, contributors, or editors, assume any liability for any injury and/or damage to persons or property as a matter of products liability, negligence or otherwise, or from any use or operation of any methods, products, instructions, or ideas contained in the material herein.

Library of Congress Cataloging-in-Publication Data

Early diagnosis and treatment of cancer : prostate cancer / edited by Li-Ming Su.
   p. ; cm.—(Early diagnosis and treatment of cancer series)
   Other title: Prostate cancer
   Includes index.
   ISBN 978-1-4160-4575-5
   1. Prostate—Cancer. I. Su, Li-Ming. II. Title: Prostate cancer. III. Series: Early diagnosis and treatment of cancer series.
   [DNLM: 1. Prostatic Neoplasms—diagnosis. 2. Prostatic Neoplasms—therapy. WJ 762 E12 2009]
   RC280.P7E27 2009
   616.99′463—dc22

                     2009009637

Acquisitions Editor: Dolores Meloni
Design Direction: Steven Stave

Printed in China.

Last digit is the print number: 9 8 7 6 5 4 3 2 1

To my loving and supportive family: Maria, Sean, and Reilly

Contents

Series Preface

Seen on a graph, the survival rate for many cancers resembles a precipice. Discovered at an early stage, most cancers are quickly treatable, and the prognosis is excellent. In late stages, however, the typical treatment protocol becomes longer, more intense, and more harrowing for the patient, and the survival rate declines steeply. No wonder, then, that one of the most important means in fighting cancer is to prevent or screen for earlier stage tumors.

Within each oncologic specialty, there is a strong push to identify new, more useful tools for early diagnosis and treatment, with an emphasis on methods amenable to an office-based or clinical setting. These efforts have brought impressive results. Advances in imaging technology, as well as the development of sophisticated molecular and biochemical tools, have led to effective, minimally invasive approaches to cancer in its early stages.

This series, *Early Diagnosis and Treatment of Cancer*, gathers state-of-the-art research and recommendations into compact, easy-to-use volumes. For each particular type of cancer, the books cover the full range of diagnostic and treatment procedures, including pathologic, radiologic, chemotherapeutic, and surgical methods, focusing on questions like these:

- What do practitioners need to know about the epidemiology of the disease and its risk factors?
- How do patients and their families wade through and interpret the many tests they face?
- What is the safest, quickest, least invasive way to reach an accurate diagnosis?
- How can the stage of the disease be determined?
- What are the best initial treatments for early-stage disease, and how should the practitioner and the patient choose among them?
- What lifestyle factors might affect the outcome of treatment?

Each volume in the series is edited by an authority within the subfield, and the contributors have been chosen for their practical skills as well as their research credentials. Key Points at the beginning of each chapter help the reader grasp the main ideas at once. Frequent illustrations make the techniques vivid and easy to visualize. Boxes and tables summarize recommended strategies, protocols, indications and contraindications, important statistics, and other essential information. Overall, the attempt is to make expert advice as accessible as possible to a wide variety of health care professionals.

For the first time since the inception of the National Cancer Institute's annual status reports, the 2008 "Annual Report to the Nation on the Status of Cancer," published in the December 3 issue of the *Journal of the National Cancer Institute*, noted a statistically significant decline in "both incidence and death rates from all cancers combined." This mark of progress encourages all of us to press forward with our efforts. I hope that the volumes in *Early Diagnosis and Treatment of Cancer* will make health care professionals and patients more familiar with the latest developments in the field, as well as more confident in applying them, so that early detection and swift, effective treatment become a reality for all our patients.

Stephen C. Yang, MD
The Arthur B. and Patricia B. Modell
Professor of Thoracic Surgery
Chief of Thoracic Surgery
The Johns Hopkins Medical Institutions
Baltimore, Maryland

Preface

According to the American Cancer Society, in 2008 an estimated 186,320 men in the United States were diagnosed with prostate cancer, with 28,660 dying of the disease. Lifetime risk estimates for prostate cancer are 17.6% for white men and 20.6% for African Americans, with a lifetime risk of death from disease of 2.8% and 4.7%, respectively. The incidence of prostate cancer increases with age more rapidly than the incidence of any other cancer. Prostate cancer is the most common cancer in men older than age 50, and more than 75% of all prostate cancers are diagnosed in men over age 65. Because prostate cancer has been the most common visceral cancer in men in the United States since 1984 and the second most common cause of cancer deaths, primary care providers should be familiar with current concepts and controversies of prostate cancer screening and treatment.

As a practicing urologist at a large tertiary referral center for prostate cancer, I continue to be amazed at the myriad questions and the degree of sophistication of these questions that patients bring to their consultation regarding treatment options for prostate cancer. Although for some patients this reflects an intelligent consumer, for many it highlights just how confused our patients have become as they face a disease with several different treatment options, including expectant management, radiation (intensity modulated radiation therapy versus brachytherapy versus proton beam), surgery (open versus laparoscopic versus robot-assisted), high-intensity frequency ultrasound, cryotherapy, and hormonal therapy. In the quest for the best treatment option for prostate cancer, patients quickly learn that there is no consensus in the medical community as to one particular treatment of choice. Although patients rely on advice from their friends, family members, internist, and ultimately their urologist, they also come to learn that the final decision on treatment is theirs and that understanding the

relative risks, cure rates, and quality of life that accompany each of these treatment modalities is essential. Expecting to gain a clear understanding of the comparative outcomes between therapies for prostate cancer, patients often turn to their immediate and "trusty" resource—the Internet. After streaming through one website after another and paging through publication after publication, patients find themselves with more questions than answers. Since many controversies exist as to the definition of cancer cure based on PSA cutoff points between surgery versus radiation, definition of potency (i.e., full versus partial erections, spontaneous erections versus successful intercourse) and continence (i.e., no pad, one precautionary pad, social continence) rates following surgical interventions, role of expectant management and focal therapy, it is no wonder that patients are bewildered, frustrated, and often discouraged.

Nevertheless, in the past two decades great strides have been made in prostate cancer diagnostics and therapeutics, especially in the fields of radiation oncology and urologic surgery, providing more effective treatments with fewer side effects and less overall morbidity than in the past. More importantly, as a result of PSA screening, approximately half of patients with newly diagnosed prostate present with early-stage, localized, and therefore potentially curable disease. In the current era of PSA screening, most patients diagnosed with localized prostate cancer, who then proceed with definitive treatment with either surgery or radiation, have a high probability of cure. It is therefore not surprising that mortality from prostate cancer has declined in the past decade due at least in part to these advances and more effective treatments. In fact, as a result of early detection and treatment, prostate cancer-specific mortality has declined from 1 in 3 men dying of their disease 20 years ago to only 1 in a 100 such deaths today.

As we in the medical profession continue to pursue new therapies and novel approaches to attacking and curing prostate cancer, it is only through constant updating and comprehensive reporting of all available treatment alternatives and their associated outcomes and risks that we will be able to better educate both patients and their treating physicians alike. Providing an up-to-date report on current treatment options for clinically localized prostate cancer, this text is written with non-urology health care professionals in mind. It is my sincere hope that this text will answer most, but perhaps not all, of the questions that patients face when given a diagnosis of prostate cancer. At the very least, it will serve to educate health care professionals and patients alike and will offer a basis for more educated and evidence-based discussions about prostate cancer treatment alternatives.

Li-Ming Su, MD

Contributors

Desiderio Avila, MD
Resident in Urology, Scott Department of Urology, Bayer College of Medicine, Houston, Texas

H. Ballentine Carter, MD
Professor of Urology, Oncology, The Johns Hopkins University School of Medicine; Director, Division of Adult Urology, Brady Urological Institute, Baltimore, Maryland

William J. Catalona, MD
Professor of Urology, Northwestern University Feinberg School of Medicine; Director, Clinical Prostate Cancer Program, Robert H. Lurie Comprehensive Cancer Center, Northwestern Memorial Hospital, Chicago, Illinois

Christian Chaussy, MD
Professor of Urology, Department of Urology, Ludwig-Maximilians-Universitat; Chairman, Department of Urology, Klinikum Harlaching, Munich, Germany

Liang Cheng, MD
Professor of Pathology and Urology, Director of Molecular Pathology Laboratory, Chief of Genitourinary Pathology Division, Department of Pathology and Laboratory Medicine and Clarian Pathology Laboratory, Indiana University School of Medicine, Indianapolis, Indiana

John Christodouleas, MD, MPH
Resident Physician, Department of Radiation Oncology and Radiation Molecular Sciences, Johns Hopkins Hospital, Baltimore, Maryland

Philipp Dahm, MD, MHSc
Associate Professor of Urology, Director of Clinical Research, University of Florida at Shands, Gainesville, Florida

Theodore DeWeese, MD
Professor and Chairman of Radiation Oncology, Professor of Oncology, Professor of Urology, Joint Appointment Department of Environmental Health Sciences, Johns Hopkins Bloomberg School of Public Health, The Johns Hopkins University School of Medicine, Baltimore, Maryland

Jana Fox, MD
Resident Physician, Department of Radiation Oncology and Radiation Molecular Sciences, Johns Hopkins Hospital, Baltimore, Maryland

Misop Han, MD, MS
Assistant Professor, James Buchanan Brady Urological Institute, The Johns Hopkins University School of Medicine, Baltimore, Maryland

Timothy D. Jones, MD
Staff Pathologist, Floyd Memorial Hospital and Health Services, New Albany, Indiana

Carol Kashefi, MD
Department of Surgery, Division of Urology, University of California, San Diego, California

Aaron Katz, MD
Associate Professor of Urology, Columbia University Medical Center, New York, New York

Mary Ann Kenneson, MD
Department of Urology, Geisinger Medical Center, Danville, Pennsylvania

Adam W. Levinson, MD, MS
Clinical Instructor, James Buchanan Brady Urological Institute, The Johns Hopkins Medical Institutions, Baltimore, Maryland

Richard E. Link, MD, PhD
Associate Professor of Urology; Director, Division of Endourology and Minimally Invasive Surgery, Scott Department of Urology, Bayer College of Medicine, Houston, Texas

Antonio Lopez-Beltran, MD, PhD
Professor of Anatomic Pathology, Faculty of Medicine, Cordoba University Medical School, Cordoba, Spain

Danil V. Makarov, MD
Instructor, Urology, The James Buchanan Brady Urological Institute, The Johns Hopkins University School of Medicine, Baltimore, Maryland

Roberta Mazzucchelli, MD, PhD
Researcher, Polytechnic University of the Marche Region, School of Medicine; Researcher, Pathology, United Hospitals, Ancona, Italy

Rodolfo Montironi, MD
Professor of Pathology, Polytechnic University of the Marche Region, School of Medicine; Director, Uropathology Program, Pathology, United Hospitals, Ancona, Italy

J. Kellogg Parsons, MD, MHS
Assistant Professor of Surgery, Division of Urologic Oncology, Moores Comprehensive Cancer Center, University of California, San Diego, California

Alan W. Partin, MD, PhD
Chairman and Director, David Hall McConnell Professor, The Brady Urological Institute, The Johns Hopkins Medical Institution, Baltimore, Maryland

Claus G. Roehrborn, MD
Professor and Chairman, Department of Urology, Southwestern Medical Center, Dallas, Texas

Daniel B. Rukstalis, MD
Director, Department of Urology, Geisinger Health System, Danville, Pennsylvania

Shahrokh F. Shariat, MD
Resident in Urology, University of Texas, Southwestern Dallas, Dallas, Texas

Danny Song, MD
Assistant Professor, Radiation Oncology and Molecular
Radiation Sciences, Joint Appointment Departments of
Urology and Oncology, The Johns Hopkins University
School of Medicine, Baltimore, Maryland

Stefan Thüroff, MD
Vice Chairman, Department of Urology, Klinikum
Harlaching; Ludwig-Maximilians-Universitat Teaching
Hospital, Munich, Germany

Timothy Y. Tseng, MD
Department of Urology, Duke University Medical Center,
Durham, North Carolina

Christopher A. Warlick, MD, PhD
Assistant Professor, University of Minnesota, Minneapolis,
Minnesota

1

Serum Markers and Screening

Carol Kashefi, Alan W. Partin, and J. Kellogg Parsons

KEY POINTS

- Prostate-specific antigen (PSA) testing has dramatically transformed the diagnosis and treatment of prostate cancer.
- Higher serum PSA concentrations are associated with prostate cancer and benign prostatic hyperplasia.
- Physicians should perform PSA testing using the same laboratory and assay to avoid spurious differences in results.
- There is insufficient evidence to recommend either for or against routine prostate cancer screening with PSA.
- The decision to screen for prostate cancer must be individualized.
- Screening for prostate cancer involves both measuring serum PSA concentration and performing a digital rectal exam.
- African-American men and men with a family history of prostate cancer should be screened annually starting at age 40. All other men should start screening at age 50.
- The decision to stop screening should take medical comorbidities into account and is reasonably made after age 75.
- The classic cut-off for recommending prostate biopsy has been 4.0 ng/mL; recently, however, a cut-off of 2.5 ng/mL has been suggested.
- 5α-Reductase inhibitors (i.e., finasteride, dutasteride) artificially lower the serum PSA concentration by 50% after 6 months of starting the medication. Therefore, the reported PSA value in these patients needs to be doubled to determine the true PSA concentration.

Introduction

Over the past 25 years, prostate specific antigen (PSA) early detection programs have transformed the diagnosis and treatment of prostate cancer. The most widely used tumor marker in clinical oncology, PSA allows for detection of prostate cancer at an early asymptomatic stage amenable to curative treatment. Early detection has resulted in a dramatic reduction in prostate cancer-specific mortality; 20 years ago, 1 in 3 men with prostate cancer died from the disease; now, only 1 in 100 does.[1]

Since prostate cancer is the most commonly diagnosed noncutaneous cancer and the second most common cause of cancer death among U.S. men,[1] primary care providers should be familiar with current concepts of prostate cancer screening and PSA testing. In this chapter, we discuss broad concepts of prostate cancer epidemiology and screening; explain clinical applications of PSA and other serum markers; and provide a practical approach to prostate cancer screening based on patient age, health status, and known risk factors.

Epidemiology of Prostate Cancer

Prostate cancer is a highly prevalent disease (Fig. 1-1) and is the second most common cause of cancer death in the United States (Fig. 1-2). In 2008, approximately 186,320 U.S. men were diagnosed with, and 28,660 men died of, prostate cancer.[1] The lifetime risk of being diagnosed with prostate cancer is now 1 in 6. As a result of PSA screening, however, 50% of newly diagnosed prostate cancer patients currently present with very early-stage, localized disease.[2] This represents a considerable stage migration over the last two decades, driven almost entirely by PSA. Indeed, in 1980, 20% of patients presented with metastases; in 2004, only 5% did.[2] Most patients diagnosed with localized prostate cancer are treated with surgery or radiation, modalities that have a high probability of cure; as a result

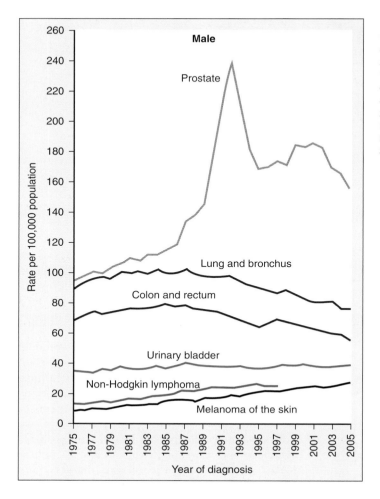

Figure 1-1. Annual age-adjusted cancer incidence rates among males for selected cancers, United States, 1975 to 2005. Rates are age-adjusted to the 2000 U.S. standard population and adjusted for delays in reporting. (Adapted from Jemal A, Siegel R, Ward E, et al: Cancer statistics, 2009. CA Cancer J Clin 59:225–249, 2009, Figure 3. © 2009 American Cancer Society. Reprinted with permission of John Wiley & Sons, Inc.)

prostate cancer mortality rates have steadily declined since the early 1990s.

There are large differences worldwide in mortality rates from prostate cancer (Fig. 1-3), and in the United States there are regional and racial discrepancies that are thought to be due to differences in rates of screening and socioeconomic factors. Washington, DC, Louisiana, Mississippi, and South Carolina had the highest rates of prostate cancer mortality in the United States between 1997 and 2001.[1] African-American men have 2.4 times greater risk of mortality from prostate cancer than do US Caucasian men. The 5-year survival rate of African Americans with prostate cancer compared with Caucasians is also slightly lower: 96% versus 100%, respectively.[1] This difference may be due in part to discrepancies in detection rates of organ-confined disease among African Americans and Caucasians—88% and 91%, respectively—and is currently under investigation.[1]

Tumor Markers

Prostate-Specific Antigen

PSA is a serine protease that liquefies the seminal coagulum after ejaculation. Produced primarily by epithelial cells that line the prostatic ducts and acini, PSA is largely confined to the prostate.[3] Although it is expressed in very small quantities in the pancreas and salivary glands, the normal concentration of PSA in serum is quite low—0.2 to 4.0 ng/mL—and a million times less than the concentration of PSA in seminal plasma.

PSA enters the serum via disruptions of the prostatic cell and basement membranes[4] (Fig. 1-4). These PSA leaks occur with both benign and cancerous prostate growths, which typically produce PSA and distort normal prostate anatomy.[4] *Thus, higher serum PSA concentrations are associated with prostate cancer and benign prostatic hyperplasia.*

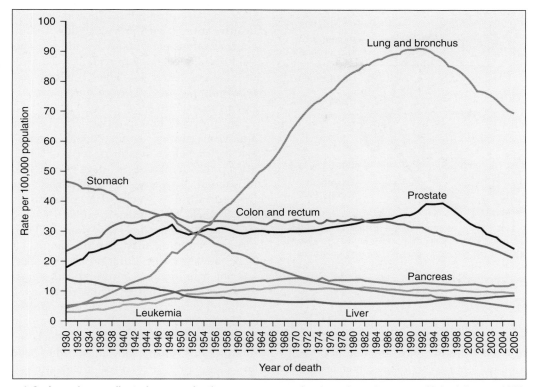

Figure 1-2. Annual age-adjusted cancer death rates among males for selected cancers, United States, 1930 to 2005.   Rates are age-adjusted to the 2000 U.S. standard population. Note that because of changes in ICD coding, numerator information has changed over time. Rates for cancers of the lung and bronchus, colon and rectum, and liver are affected by these changes. (From Jemal A, Siegel R, Ward E, et al: Cancer statistics, 2009. CA Cancer J Clin 59:225–249, 2009, Figure 4. © 2009 American Cancer Society. Reprinted with permission of John Wiley & Sons, Inc.)

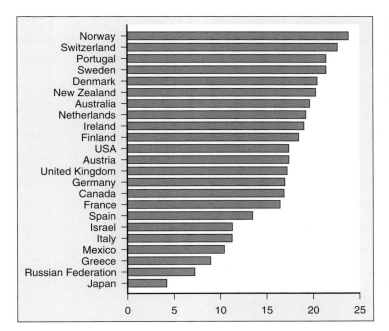

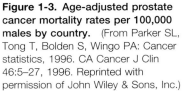

Figure 1-3. Age-adjusted prostate cancer mortality rates per 100,000 males by country.   (From Parker SL, Tong T, Bolden S, Wingo PA: Cancer statistics, 1996. CA Cancer J Clin 46:5–27, 1996. Reprinted with permission of John Wiley & Sons, Inc.)

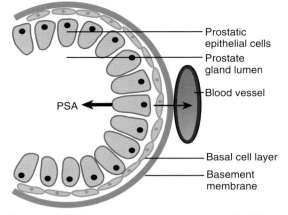

Figure 1-4. PSA is secreted by the epithelial cells of the prostatic acini. The majority of the PSA enters the lumen of prostatic acini; a minority is absorbed and enters the bloodstream. (From Kirby RS, Christmas TJ, Brawer MK: *Prostate Cancer*, 2nd ed. London: Mosby, 2001, Figure 8.2.)

Because of differences in technical performance and reference standards, PSA measurements from different labs are not necessarily comparable.[5,6] *It is therefore recommended that serial PSA assays in an individual patient be performed in the same lab with the same assay to avoid spurious differences caused by interlab and interassay variations.*

Variables Affecting Serum PSA Concentration

In addition to prostate tumors, several benign processes may also cause PSA to leak into the bloodstream (Table 1-1). Because the serum factor half-life of PSA is 3.15 days, these eleva-tions are often transient.[7] Thus, if an otherwise healthy patient with previously low serum PSA concentrations presents with a sudden, substantial PSA elevation, the provider should assess for the factors listed in Table 1-1 and *consider repeating the assay before initiating a more extensive evaluation.*

To prevent false-positive PSA elevations, approximately 48 hours should elapse after ejaculation before measuring serum PSA, 3 days after prostatic massage, 7 days after transrectal ultrasound, 4 to 6 weeks of antibiotic therapy for prostatitis, 6 weeks after prostate biopsy, and 6 weeks after prostate surgical procedures such as transurethral resection (TURP).[8-11] Urinary retention may also transiently elevate PSA; however, the duration of this elevation has not been defined. Urethral catheterization, exercise, hemodialysis, digital rectal examination, and cystoscopy have no appreciable effect on serum PSA concentration.[9-11]

The 5α-reductase inhibitors, which include finasteride (Proscar) and dutasteride (Avodart), are commonly prescribed medications used to treat benign prostatic hyperplasia (BPH). 5α-Reductase *inhibitors impede prostate growth, reduce prostate volume, and are associated with a 50% to 60% reduction in serum PSA within 6 months of initiating therapy.*[12] Therefore, in patients treated with 5α-reductase inhibitors, it is important to obtain a baseline PSA before beginning 5α-reductase inhibitor therapy and to double the reported PSA value in these patients to estimate the "true" PSA. The lower dose formulation of finasteride used as treatment for male pattern baldness

Table 1-1. Clinical Variables and Serum Prostate-Specific Antigen (PSA) Concentration	
Variable	**Effect on Serum PSA**
Catheterization	None
Exercise	None
Hemodialysis	None
Digital rectal exam (DRE)	None
Cystoscopy	None
Urinary retention	Possible short-term elevation
Ejaculation	Elevation for up to 48 hr
Prostatic massage	Elevation for up to 3 days
Transrectal ultrasound (TRUS)	Elevation for up to 7 days
Prostatitis	Elevation for up to 4–6 wk while on antibiotics
Prostate needle biopsy	Elevation for up to 6 wk
Transurethral resection (TURP)	Elevation for up to 6 wk

(Propecia) may also lower serum PSA, but to a lesser extent.

Saw palmetto (*Serenoa repens*), an herbal supplement widely used by older men to treat prostate-related symptoms, does not affect serum PSA concentrations.[13] Lycopene, vitamin E, and selenium are other popular supplements that may potentially reduce the risk of prostate cancer and are currently under study. They have no known effect on serum PSA concentrations. It is important to note, however, that unregulated supplements may contain contaminants, such as estrogen, which may potentially reduce serum PSA concentrations through hormone-related mechanisms.

PSA Velocity, Age-Specific PSA, and Free PSA

The fact that conditions such as prostatitis and BPH may increase serum PSA diminishes its specificity as a diagnostic test for cancer. Reduced specificity may lead to false-positive results, increased patient anxiety, and unnecessary prostate biopsies. Accordingly, several additional, adjuvant analyses have been developed to increase the specificity of the PSA assay for cancer. Two of the most common adjuvant PSA tests are PSA velocity and free PSA. *Routine use of these tests by primary care physicians is cautioned, and consultation with a urologic oncologist is advised.*

PSA velocity refers to the rate at which serum PSA increases over time. Faster rates of rise are associated with increased risk of prostate cancer. Studies have shown that, within a PSA range of 4.0 to 10.0 ng/mL, a rise by more than 0.75 ng/mL per year shows a specificity of cancer detection of 90% and a sensitivity of 79%.[14]

Free PSA refers to that proportion of PSA that circulates in the blood unbound to protein. The majority of PSA that circulates in the blood (65% to 95%) is complexed to one of several proteins, primarily α_1-antichymotrypsin. The remaining 5% to 35% of circulating PSA is unbound.[15,16] PSA released from prostate cancer cells tends to escape intracellular proteolytic processing, thereby leading to reduced proportions of free PSA in the serum of prostate cancer patients. This characteristic provides additional specificity for cancer detection.[17–20]

The FDA has approved the use of percent free PSA for patients with normal digital rectal exam-

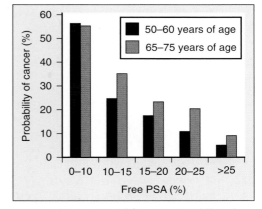

Figure 1-5. Free-to-total PSA and probability of cancer. (Data used with permission from Catalona WJ, Smith DS, Ornstein DK: Prostate cancer detection in men with serum PSA concentrations of 2.6 to 4.0 ng/mL and benign prostate examination. Enhancement of specificity with free PSA measurements. JAMA 277:1452, 1997.)

inations and total PSAs between 4 and 10 ng/mL (Fig. 1-5). Generally, a percent free PSA between 18% and 20% detects almost 50% of cancers while sparing a substantial number of men from undergoing unnecessary biopsy.[21] Since both total and free PSA concentrations decrease in men on finasteride, the percentage of free PSA is not significantly altered.[22,23]

Future Prostate Cancer Tumor Markers

Many promising tumor markers are under study, identification of which has been made possible through advances in molecular biology, genomics, and epigenetics. A close relative of PSA, human kallikrein 2 (hK2) may possibly have more specificity for cancer staging (but not detection) than PSA. This is based on studies that show dramatically more intense expression of hK2 in malignant prostate cells than in benign cells.[24-27] DNA hypermethylation has been identified in two genes involved in prostate cancer tumor suppression, with early data showing a strong positive association of DNA hypermethylation with more aggressive tumors.[28-30] Finally, the *AMACR* gene (which codes for an enzyme responsible for beta-oxidation of branched-chain fatty acids) has been found to be upregulated in most prostate cancer tissues.[31,32] Its detection in biopsy tissue has 97% sensitivity and 100% specificity rates.[32] As a potential molecular probe, it could have a great impact on prostate cancer detection by means of radiologic imaging.

A Practical Approach to Prostate Cancer Screening

Many physicians are surprised to learn that despite the widespread use of the PSA assay, there are no official recommendations governing its use. In 2003, the U.S. Preventive Services Task Force analyzed many studies and determined *that insufficient evidence existed to recommend either for or against routine prostate cancer screening with PSA.*[33]

Likewise, the American Association of Family Practitioners, the American College of Physicians, the American College of Surgeons, the American Medical Association, the American Urological Association, and the National Comprehensive Cancer Network are among the professional organizations that have *declared that the decision to screen for prostate cancer must be individualized.*

Therefore, patients—particularly older ones—should be fully informed as to the implications of prostate cancer screening. They should be made aware that an elevation in serum PSA and/or abnormal digital rectal exam may lead to prostate biopsy and diagnosis of a cancer that may or may not be clinically significant for that patient.

Within this framework, therefore, we present the following general guidelines for screening (Box 1-1):

How to Screen

Screening for prostate cancer involves both measuring serum PSA concentration and performing a digital rectal exam. This is because up to 25% of those with cancers present with "normal" PSA (i.e., less than 4.0 ng/mL; see text that follows)[34-36] and an abnormal digital rectal exam. An abnormal digital rectal exam is an indication for performing prostate biopsy, regardless of serum PSA concentration.

When to Start Screening

Although there is no consensus, *most men should begin annual screening at age 50 years.* For African Americans and men with a family history

---

Box 1-1. Recommendations for Prostate Cancer Screening

What to check:
   Serum PSA
   Digital rectal exam
When to start:
   African Americans and/or those
     with family history   40 yr
   All others   50 yr
How often:
   Annually
When to stop:
   75 yr
   Consider continuing in older men if life expectancy
     is >5–10 yr
Cut-off for abnormal serum PSA:
   ≥4.0 ng/dL
   Also consider referral to a urologist if ≥2.5 ng/dL

---

of prostate cancer (first-degree relative), screening should begin at age 40 years.

How Often to Screen

Although there is no consensus, *most men should be screened annually.* For men with consistently low PSA values and normal exams over several years, consideration may be given to extending the interval between testing.

When to Stop Screening

Because prostate cancer is generally an indolent cancer considerable debate exists as to when prostate cancer screening should be discontinued, a debate focusing on the diminishing health care benefits of prostate cancer detection and treatment in older men. A reasonable cut-off is age 75 years. However, screening may be considered in older men with life expectancy of more than 5 to 10 years. Screening in these men should be performed within the context of informed decision making and ascertainment of medical comorbidities.

What Concentration of PSA Is Abnormal?

There is also considerable debate as to what constitutes an abnormal PSA. *The classic cut-off for recommending prostate biopsy has been 4.0 ng/mL,* which is associated with a positive predictive value of 25% (i.e., a probability of 25% of detecting cancer on biopsy).[37] Recently, however, *a cut-off of 2.5 ng/mL has been suggested,* as has the use of a PSA velocity cut-off of 0.5 ng/mL for men with a PSA less than 2.5 ng/mL.[38] Given the current lack of consensus, it is reasonable to use a cut-off of 4.0 ng/mL for referral to a urologist, with consideration given to a cut-off of 2.5 ng/mL, particularly in younger men.

Conclusion

Prostate cancer early detection programs using PSA testing have altered the diagnosis and treatment of prostate cancer. Elevated serum PSA is associated with increased probability of prostate cancer; however, serum PSA may also be affected by BPH, prostate medications, and other benign clinical variables. Although evidence-based guidelines are anticipated in the near future, currently the decision to screen should be individualized to each patient.

References

1. American Cancer Society: Cancer Facts and Figures 2008, Atlanta: American Cancer Society, 2008.
2. Cooperberg MR, Lubeck DP, Meng MV, et al: The changing face of low-risk prostate cancer: trends in clinical presentation and primary management. J Clin Oncol 22:2141–2149, 2004.
3. Lilja H, Laurell CB: Liquefaction of coagulated human semen. Scand J Clin Lab Invest 44:447–452, 1984.
4. Stamey TA, Yang N, Hay AR, et al: Prostate-specific antigen as a serum marker for adenocarcinoma of the prostate. N Engl J Med 317:909–916, 1987.
5. Roth HJ, Stewart SC, Brawer MK: A comparison of three free and total PSA assays. Prostate Cancer Prostatic Dis 1:326–331, 1998.
6. Brawer MK: Prostate-specific antigen: current status. CA Cancer J Clin 49:264–281, 1999.
7. Richardson TD, Wojno KJ, Liang LW, et al: Half-life determination of serum free prostate-specific antigen following radical retropubic prostatectomy. Urology 48:40–44, 1996.
8. Tzanakis I, Kazoulis S, Girousis N, et al: Prostate-specific antigen in hemodialysis patients and the influence of dialysis in its levels. Nephron 90:230–233, 2002.
9. Klein LT, Lowe FC: The effects of prostatic manipulation on prostate-specific antigen levels. Urol Clin North Am 24:293–297, 1997.
10. Tchetgen MB, Oesterling JE: The effect of prostatitis, urinary retention, ejaculation, and ambulation on the serum prostate-specific antigen concentration. Urol Clin North Am 24:283–291, 1997.
11. Chybowski FM, Bergstralh EJ, Oesterling JE: The effect of digital rectal examination on the serum prostate specific antigen concentration: results of a randomized study. J Urol 148:83–86, 1992.
12. Guess HA, Heyse JF, Gormley GJ: The effect of finasteride on prostate-specific antigen in men with benign prostatic hyperplasia. Prostate 22:31–37, 1993.
13. Habib FK, Ross M, Ho CK, et al: *Serenoa repens* (Permixon) inhibits the 5α-reductase activity of human prostate cancer cell lines without interfering with PSA expression. Int J Cancer 114:190–194, 2005.
14. Carter HB, Pearson JD, Metter EJ, et al: Longitudinal evaluation of prostate-specific antigen levels in men with and without prostate disease. JAMA 267:2215–2220, 1992.
15. McCormack RT, Rittenhouse HG, Finlay JA, et al: Molecular forms of prostate-specific antigen and the human kallikrein gene family: a new era. Urology 45:729–744, 1995.
16. Woodrum DL, Brawer MK, Partin AW, et al: Interpretation of free prostate specific antigen clinical research studies for the detection of prostate cancer. J Urol, 159:5–12, 1998.
17. Stenman UH, Hakama M, Knekt P, et al: Serum concentrations of prostate specific antigen and its complex with alpha 1-antichymotrypsin before diagnosis of prostate cancer. Lancet 344:1594–1598, 1994.
18. Lilja H: Significance of different molecular forms of serum PSA. The free, noncomplexed form of PSA versus that complexed to alpha 1-antichymotrypsin. Urol Clin North Am 20:681–686, 1993.
19. Leinonen J, Lovgren T, Vornanen T, et al: Double-label time-resolved immunofluorometric assay of prostate-specific antigen and of its complex with alpha 1-antichymotrypsin. Clin Chem 39:2098–2103, 1993.
20. Christensson A, Bjork T, Nilsson O, et al: Serum prostate specific antigen complexed to alpha 1-antichymotrypsin as an indicator of prostate cancer. J Urol 150:100–105, 1993.
21. Haese A, Graefen M, Noldus J, et al: Prostatic volume and ratio of free-to-total prostate specific antigen in patients with prostatic cancer or benign prostatic hyperplasia. J Urol 158:2188–2192, 1997.
22. Keetch DW, Andriole GL, Ratliff TL, et al: Comparison of percent free prostate-specific antigen levels in men with benign prostatic hyperplasia treated with finasteride, terazosin, or watchful waiting. Urology 50:901–905, 1997.
23. Pannek J, Marks LS, Pearson JD, et al: Influence of finasteride on free and total serum prostate specific antigen levels in men with benign prostatic hyperplasia. J Urol 159:449–453, 1998.
24. Darson MF, Pacelli A, Roche P, et al: Human glandular kallikrein 2 (hK2) expression in prostatic intraepithelial neoplasia and adenocarcinoma: a novel prostate cancer marker. Urology 49:857–862, 1997.
25. Darson MF, Pacelli A, Roche P, et al: Human glandular kallikrein 2 expression in prostate adenocarcinoma and lymph node metastases. Urology 53:939–944, 1999.
26. Tremblay RR, Deperthes D, Tetu B, et al: Immunohistochemical study suggesting a complementary role of kallikreins hK2 and hK3 (prostate-specific antigen) in the functional analysis of human prostate tumors. Am J Pathol 150:455–459, 1997.
27. Kwiatkowski MK, Recker F, Piironen T, et al: In prostatism patients the ratio of human glandular kallikrein to free PSA improves the discrimination between prostate cancer and benign hyperplasia within the diagnostic "gray zone" of total PSA 4 to 10 ng/mL. Urology 52:360–365, 1998.
28. Gonzalgo ML, Pavlovich CP, Lee SM, et al: Prostate cancer detection by GSTP1 methylation analysis of postbiopsy urine specimens. Clin Cancer Res 9:2673–2677, 2003.
29. Kuzmin I, Gillespie JW, Protopopov A, et al: The RASSF1A tumor suppressor gene is inactivated in prostate tumors and suppresses growth of prostate carcinoma cells. Cancer Res 62:3498–3502, 2002.
30. Liu L, Yoon JH, Dammann R, et al: Frequent hypermethylation of the RASSF1A gene in prostate cancer. Oncogene 21:6835–6840, 2002.
31. Luo J, Zha S, Gage WR, et al: Alpha-methylacyl-CoA racemase: a new molecular marker for prostate cancer. Cancer Res 62:2220–2226, 2002.
32. Rubin MA, Zhou M, Dhanasekaran SM, et al: Alpha-methylacyl coenzyme A racemase as a tissue biomarker for prostate cancer. JAMA 287:1662–1670, 2002.
33. USPSTF: Screening for prostate cancer: recommendations and rationale. Am Fam Physician 67:787–792, 2003.
34. Schroder FH, Alexander FE., Bangma CH, et al: Screening and early detection of prostate cancer. Prostate 44: 255–263, 2000.
35. Thompson IM, Pauler DK, Goodman PJ, et al: Prevalence of prostate cancer among men with a prostate-specific antigen level ≤ 4.0 ng per milliliter. N Engl J Med 350:2239–2246, 2004.
36. Catalona WJ, Smith DS, Ornstein DK: Prostate cancer detection in men with serum PSA concentrations of 2.6 to 4.0 ng/mL and benign prostate examination. Enhancement of specificity with free PSA measurements. JAMA 277:1452–1455, 1997.
37. Thompson IM, Ankerst DP, Chi C, et al: Assessing prostate cancer risk: results from the Prostate Cancer Prevention Trial. J Natl Cancer Inst 98:529–534, 2006.
38. Network, N.C.C.: Prostate Cancer, 2006. Available at: http://nccn.org.

2

Biopsy, Diagnosis, and Staging of Prostate Cancer

Shahrokh F. Shariat and Claus G. Roehrborn

KEY POINTS

- An abnormal digital rectal examination (DRE) result or elevated serum prostate-specific antigen (PSA) measurement may indicate prostate cancer. The exact cutoff level of what is considered to be a normal PSA value has not been determined, but values of less than 2.5 ng/mL for younger men and slightly higher for older men are often used.
- The diagnosis of prostate cancer depends on histopathologic (or cytologic) confirmation. Biopsy and further staging investigations are indicated only if they affect the management of the patient.
- Transrectal periprostatic injection with a local anesthetic may be offered to patients as effective analgesia when undergoing prostate biopsies. Several types of local anesthesia are now available, but periprostatic nerve block with 1% or 2% lidocaine is the recommended form of pain control and comfort management during transrectal ultrasound (TRUS)-guided prostate biopsy.
- TRUS-guided systemic biopsy is the recommended method in most cases in which there is suspicion of prostate cancer. Transperineal biopsy is an up-to-standard alternative.
- Initial biopsy:
  - A minimum of 10 systemic, laterally directed cores are recommended, eventually with more cores in larger glands.
  - Extended prostate biopsy schemes that require cores weighted more laterally at the base (lateral horn) and medially to the apex show better cancer detection rates without increasing adverse events.
  - Transition zone biopsies are not recommended in the first set of biopsies because of low detection rates.
- One set of repeat biopsies is warranted in cases with persistent indication (abnormal DRE, elevated PSA, abnormal PSA derivatives, and/or histopathologic find-

ings suggestive of malignancy at the initial biopsy). Biopsy of the transition zone of the prostate should be considered for men undergoing a repeat biopsy for whom a suspicion of a missed cancer anteriorly is high. Overall recommendations for further (third or more) sets of biopsies cannot be made; the decision must be made based on the individual patient.
- A repeat biopsy is not indicated for men with high-grade prostatic intraepithelial neoplasia (PIN) if the original biopsy technique was adequate. A prostate biopsy that reveals atypical glands that are suspicious for but not diagnostic of cancer should be repeated.
- Saturation biopsy (20 cores) should be reserved for repeat biopsy in patients who have a negative initial biopsy but are still strongly suspected to have prostate cancer. Complications and risk of diagnosing clinically insignificant cancer using saturation biopsy following a prior negative biopsy are reported to be no higher than with routine sextant or extended core biopsy unless general or regional anesthesia is used, whereas the detection of clinically significant cancer is higher.
- Local staging (T staging) of prostate cancer is based on findings from DRE and possibly MRI. Further information is provided by the number and sites of positive prostate biopsies, tumor grade, and level of serum PSA.
- Lymph node status (N staging) is important only when potentially curative treatment is planned for. Patients with stage T2 or less, PSA less than 20 ng/mL, and a Gleason score lower than 6 have a less than 10% likelihood of having node metastases and may be spared nodal evaluation. Accurate lymph node staging can be determined only by operative lymphadenectomy.
- Skeletal metastasis (M staging) is best assessed by bone scan. This may not be indicated in asymptomatic patients if the serum PSA level is less than 20 ng/mL in the presence of well- or moderately differentiated tumors.

Introduction

Prostate cancer rarely causes symptoms unless it is advanced. Thus, suspicion of prostate cancer resulting in a recommendation for prostatic

biopsy is most often raised by abnormalities found on digital rectal examination (DRE) or by serum prostate-specific antigen (PSA) elevations. Although there is controversy regarding the benefits of early diagnosis, it has been demonstrated that an early diagnosis of prostate cancer is best achieved with a combination of DRE and PSA.

A virtually non-negotiable requirement before initiating treatment for prostate cancer is the establishment of a tissue diagnosis, since at the present time there are no serum- or urine-based markers with sufficient specificity to allow a provider to confidently start treatment. There are some legitimate exceptions to this rule, such as a patient presenting with a very high serum PSA and obvious evidence of metastatic cancer of unknown origin (but presumed to be prostatic). In such patients, when time is of the essence (e.g., pending paraplegia due to spine metastases), reversible hormonal ablation may be initiated awaiting tissue diagnosis. In all other patients, however, as with most other solid organ cancers, the first goal is to obtain sufficient amounts of tissue to allow a histopathologic assessment and a confident diagnosis of cancer if present. Transrectal ultrasound (TRUS)-guided, systematic needle biopsy is the most reliable method of ensuring accurate sampling of prostatic tissue in men considered at high risk for harboring prostatic cancer on the basis of DRE and PSA findings.

The goal of cancer staging is to determine the extent of disease as precisely as possible to assess prognosis and guide management recommendations. The local extent of disease determined by DRE (tumor [T] stage), serum PSA level before prostatic biopsy, and tumor grade correlates directly with the pathologic extent of disease and is useful in the staging evaluation of men with adenocarcinoma of the prostate. MRI and nuclear medicine imaging have been investigated as modalities for identifying early local extra-prostatic and lymphatic spread of disease.

Prostate Biopsy

General Procedures

TRUS-guided prostate biopsies are recommended for men who have a DRE that is suspicious for cancer of the prostate or who have an elevated or rising PSA level, suggesting the presence of prostate cancer. Prostate tissue sampling is done almost universally by transrectal needle biopsy (Fig. 2-1), although in very rare

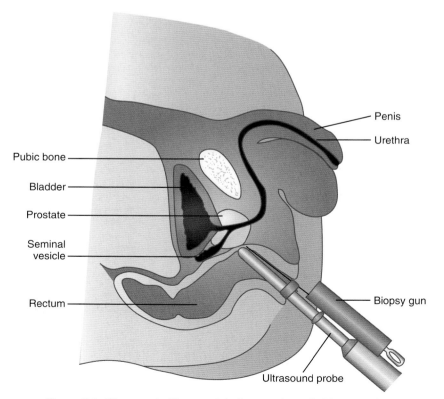

Figure 2-1. Placement of transrectal ultrasound needle biopsy probe.

circumstances, a biopsy of a metastatic site (bone lesion) or a suspicious lymph node may be easier and more advantageous. There are also circumstances in which the usual transrectal route is not feasible (e.g., after anterior-posterior resection of the rectosigmoid; see discussion in text that follows). As nearly universal as is the approach, as nearly universal is the technique, namely, a TRUS-guided biopsy using an 18G needle to obtain a tissue core. To be certain, the same biopsy device and needle may be used to perform a finger-guided biopsy, but this is reserved for some unusual circumstances as well (e.g., when TRUS imaging is not available or finger-guided directed biopsy of suspicious nodule is not seen on TRUS). Lastly, in decades past physicians in many countries performed fine-needle aspiration (FNA) of the prostate, but this technique is used less and less often, although advocates claim that it is cheaper, faster, and easier to perform and that it results in lower morbidity than any other technique developed so far. Appropriate training in performing transrectal FNA of the prostate and in interpreting the smears is, of course, essential.[1] FNA plays a major role in the aforementioned situations in which the diagnosis is established from nonprostatic tissue sources, such as lymph nodes and others.[2,3]

Since the landmark paper by Hodge et al.[4] demonstrated the superiority of TRUS guidance compared with digitally guided biopsy, the so-called TRUS-guided biopsy technique has become the worldwide accepted standard in prostate cancer diagnosis. Statistical performance (sensitivity, specificity, positive and neg-

ative predictive values) of all other diagnostic tests (e.g., DRE, PSA) is calculated based on the assignment (cancer present versus absent) made by prostate biopsy. Recognizing the fact that all sampling procedures including prostate biopsies incur the risk of being false-negative (i.e., cancer is present but missed by the biopsies), calculation of the statistical performance characteristics of all other tests using biopsy outcomes as gold standard are inherently incorrect and biased. Similarly, when comparing the statistical performance of various biopsy strategies, usually the most extensive strategy is chosen as the gold standard to define disease presence or absence. Moreover, the performance of all other strategies are calculated based on that particular strategy, again incurring a significant bias owing to the remaining false-negative rate of even the most extensive sampling strategy.

Likelihood of Missing Cancer

The question of how often a prostate biopsy will turn out to be false-negative is of clinical as well as statistical importance (Fig. 2-2). Computed biopsy simulations on a series of mapped whole-mount sections of radical prostatectomy specimens showed that the chance of missing a cancer by sextant biopsy is estimated at about 25%.[5] A repeat sextant biopsy of the prostate performed in 118 men with biopsy-proven cancer failed to identify cancer in 27 men, or 23%.[6] Although these patients with repeat negative biopsies tended to have lower PSAs and larger glands, none of the differences in clinical or pathologic parameters or PSA relapse rates were

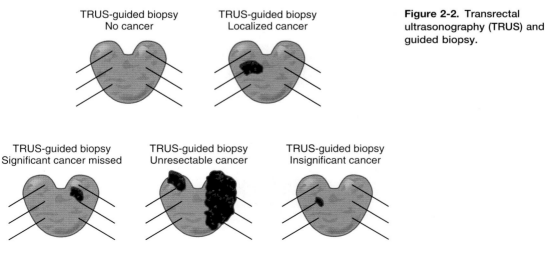

TRUS-guided biopsy
No cancer

TRUS-guided biopsy
Localized cancer

Figure 2-2. Transrectal ultrasonography (TRUS) and guided biopsy.

TRUS-guided biopsy
Significant cancer missed

TRUS-guided biopsy
Unresectable cancer

TRUS-guided biopsy
Insignificant cancer

significant. Svetec et al.[7] performed an ex vivo sextant biopsy on 90 prostates removed for biopsy-proven cancer, which was negative in 41 prostates (46%). Depending on the presenting characteristics, such as age and serum PSA, the risk of a false-negative re-biopsy varied widely. Although one might argue that the ex vivo biopsy of a removed prostate significantly differs from an in vivo TRUS biopsy, the results clearly validate the concept of false-negative biopsies and their impact on detection and statistical performance characteristics.

A similar but more extensive study was performed by Fink et al.,[8] who did ex vivo sextant and 10-core biopsies on 91 radical prostatectomy specimens. The first sextant set found 60% and the second sextant set 75% of all cancer, whereas the 10-core biopsy sets found 78% and 90% of the cancers, respectively. Thus, even using two 10-core biopsies, approximately 10% of the cancers were missed, of which eight were significant based on a tumor volume of larger than 0.5 mL.

Equipment for TRUS-Guided Prostate Biopsy

Many ultrasound manufacturers have produced devices designed for the practicing urologist (Fig. 2-3). Key to the successful performance of a TRUS biopsy is a dedicated TRUS probe. Given that the prostate rests directly on the rectum, that is, in close proximity to the ultra-sound probe, either the transducer must have excellent near-field resolution or a water balloon must be inflated to achieve the necessary distance from the rectal wall.

Axial resolution is a direct reflection of increase in frequency. Therefore, ideally one would use a very high-frequency transducer. The commonly used transrectal transducers have frequencies ranging from 5.0 to 8.5 MHz. To achieve good lateral resolution, the sound wave beam must be focused, resulting in a focal point of best resolution and a focal range of adequate lateral resolution. Considering the average size of the prostate, the focal range of the probe should extend at least 4 cm away from the rectal wall.

Aside from the transducer, there are fundamental design differences in the TRUS probes, namely, endfire and sidefire probes, referring to the way in which the biopsy needle is passed either alongside or through the transducer to reach the prostate. Imaging and specific measurements of prostates with these two different designs differ as a result of the differing angles in which the sound waves are aimed at the prostate. The endfire probes never achieve a strict transverse image of the prostate, but rather a diagonal image, which may impact volume calculations. However, in both cases the needle enters the prostate in an oblique or flat angle, and thus the peripheral zone of the prostate is preferentially sampled. The choice of the

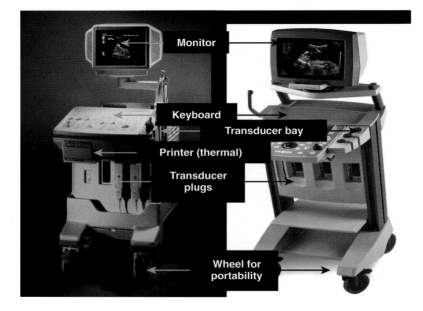

Figure 2-3. Equipment for transrectal ultrasound-guided prostate biopsy. (Reproduced with permission from Claus G. Roehrborn.)

Monitor

Keyboard

Transducer bay

Printer (thermal)

Transducer plugs

Wheel for portability

transducer design for the purpose of TRUS biopsies is largely the physician's preference.

An indispensable part of the TRUS equipment is the so-called biopsy gun, a spring-loaded device that has immensely simplified the performance of prostate biopsies compared with the old-style finger-guided Vim-Silverman or Tru-cut needles. The standard needles for the biopsy guns are 18G in diameter, and the maximal length of the core is 15 mm.

Patient Preparation

To prevent the presence of fecal material in the rectal vault, the administration of enemas before the biopsy is commonly recommended and is practiced by about 80% (n = 6) of participants in a survey,[9] although others dispute their benefit.[10] To prevent air from collecting in front of the ultrasound probe and interfering with sound wave penetration and resolution, the patient is ideally positioned in the left lateral decubitus position, although some physicians prefer the lithotomy position.

The issue of antibiotic prophylaxis has been settled by controlled trials. Two hundred thirty-one patients were randomized into three groups: one group receiving placebo, another group receiving a single dose of ciprofloxacin 500 mg and tinidazole 600 mg, and another group receiving the same combination twice a day for 3 days. Among the three groups, no significant differences were seen in noninfective complications (27, 29, and 31 in groups 1 to 3, respectively), but the incidence of infective complications (19, 6, and 8, respectively) was significantly higher in group 1 (P = .003).[11] Isen et al.[12] investigated the efficacy of prophylactic use of single-dose oral ofloxacin and trimethoprim-sulfamethoxazole regimens in 110 men. In the ofloxacin, trimethoprim-sulfamethoxazole, and control groups, urinary infection was found in two (4.76%), three (6.66%), and six (26.08%) patients, respectively. Both of these antibiotic regimens produced a statistically significant reduction in urinary infection (P < .02, P < .05). Kapoor et al.[13] randomized 537 patients to receive either oral ciprofloxacin 500 mg or placebo before transrectal needle biopsy of the prostate. Six ciprofloxacin-treated (3%) and 19 placebo-treated (8%) patients had bacteriuria (more than 10^4 CFU/mL) after the procedure (P = .009). Six ciprofloxacin recipients (3%) and 12 placebo recipients (5%) had clinical signs and symptoms of a urinary tract infection (UTI) (P = .15). Bacteriuria was reduced in patients with single-dose oral ciprofloxacin after biopsy compared with that with placebo in patients undergoing transrectal prostatic biopsy, which also provided an economic advantage. In addition, this study established the actual rate of bacteriuria after transrectal needle biopsy of the prostate without antibiotic prophylaxis to be 8%, with a clinical rate of UTI of 5% and a hospitalization rate of 2%.

Anesthesia Issues

The traditional finger-guided biopsy of the prostate was performed either with no anesthesia or with spinal or general anesthesia, depending on physician preferences. With the introduction of the TRUS-guided biopsy, most practitioners used either no analgesia/anesthesia and/or oral pain medications. With the recognition that more than six biopsies might be advantageous in the diagnosis of cancer, more and more practitioners have explored the use of various methods of achieving analgesia/anesthesia during the biopsy.

The results of intrarectal lidocaine gel (2%) have been controversial when compared with placebo. Some investigators such as Desgrandchamps et al.[14] found no improved pain control when comparing intrarectal lidocaine gel with simple hydrophilic gel in a randomized study of 109 patients. In contrast, Issa et al.[15] found a significantly lower median pain score in patients using intrarectal lidocaine compared with placebo in 50 randomized patients. In a recent meta-analysis of five studies involving 466 patients, Tiong et al.[16] found that intrarectal local anesthesia was associated with pain reduction compared with placebo, but the effect size was not statistically significant.

Several randomized studies have recently shown that intrarectal local anesthesia is inferior to periprostatic nerve block with lidocaine injection.[17–22] Alavi et al.,[23] for example, randomized 150 patients undergoing TRUS biopsy to either 2% lidocaine gel intrarectally or periprostatic infiltration with 1% aqueous lidocaine. The mean pain scores were 3.7 versus 2.4 (P < .001) in favor of the infiltration.

The results of periprostatic nerve block with aqueous lidocaine have been positive in randomized controlled trials. Bulbul et al.[24] performed 12-core biopsies in 47 patients with 2% lidocaine periprostatic infiltration and 25 matched patients without lidocaine. The researchers found no discomfort in 70% of the lidocaine patients compared with 48% of the control patients ($P < .05$). Moderate to severe discomfort was reported by 32% of the control patients compared with 11% of the lidocaine patients. Randomized and sham controlled studies performed in series of 152,[25] 90,[26] 132,[27] and 157 patients[28] all found less discomfort and pain with the infiltration of lidocaine. Given these data, the periprostatic infiltration with 1% or 2% lidocaine is the recommended form of pain control and comfort management during TRUS-guided prostate biopsy.

Although the efficacy of periprostatic nerve block is established, the optimal dosage and technique remain controversial. Various infiltration sites have been described, including the apex only, the bilateral neurovascular bundle regions only (defined variously as basolateral, posterolateral, periprostatic nerve plexus, prostate-vesicular junction injections), the apex and neurovascular bundle, and three locations (base, mid, and apex) posterolaterally and lateral to the tip of the seminal vesicles. A study using a placebo and groups of escalating doses of 1% lidocaine infiltration (2.5, 5, and 10 mL) demonstrated that the best pain relief was obtained with 10 mL of lidocaine infiltrated solely at the neurovascular bundle region (single site) or at the neurovascular bundle and apical regions (double site).[29] Therefore, the authors recommended single-site, 10-mL infiltration in the region of the neurovascular bundle. Even if infiltration of the neurovascular bundle region seems essential for effective anesthesia, apical infiltration alone has been reported to provide significant pain relief.[30] However, the combination of neurovascular bundle and peri-apical local anesthesia is not superior to neurovascular bundle block alone in reducing pain during prostate biopsy.[31]

The issue of whether periprostatic nerve block should be associated with intrarectal lidocaine or oral medication remains an open question. Pendleton et al.[32] recently reported that oral administration of 75 mg tramadol/650 mg acetaminophen 3 hours before periprostatic nerve block appears to provide more effective pain control than periprostatic nerve

block alone without causing any additional complications.

The introduction of periprostatic nerve block has allowed extended prostate biopsy to be performed easily in the office and furthermore for the number of biopsies taken to be increased without increasing the discomfort and pain of the patients. Despite the variability of location and dosage of infiltration, the periprostatic nerve block is presently the most effective method of reducing pain during TRUS biopsy. It remains controversial whether periprostatic nerve block should be associated with intrarectal lidocaine or oral medication.

Complications of TRUS Biopsies

TRUS-guided prostate biopsy in general is a safe procedure. Aside from infectious complications and pain, most complaints center on the issues of urethral and rectal bleeding as well as hematospermia. In a contemporary series, the morbidity of 1000 patients undergoing a TRUS-guided biopsy was compared with the morbidity of 820 of these patients with a second biopsy in whom the initial biopsy was negative for cancer.[23] Immediate morbidity was minor and included rectal bleeding (2.1% and 2.4% for first and second biopsy, respectively, $P = .13$), mild hematuria (62% and 57%, respectively, $P = .06$), severe hematuria (0.7% and 0.5%, respectively, $P = .09$), and moderate to severe vasovagal episodes (2.8% and 1.4%, respectively, $P = .03$). Delayed morbidity of first and re-biopsy comprised fever (2.9% versus 2.3%, $P = .08$), hematospermia (9.8% versus 10.2%, $P = .1$), recurrent mild hematuria (15.9% versus 16.6%, $P = .06$), persistent dysuria (7.2% versus 6.8%, $P = .12$), and urinary tract infection (10.9% versus 11.3%, respectively, $P = .07$). Major complications were rare and included urosepsis (0.1% versus 0%) and rectal bleeding that required intervention (0% versus 0.1%, respectively). Roberts et al.[33] reviewed 2258 biopsies performed in Olmsted County, Minnesota, from 1980 to 1997 and found overall a 16.7% complication rate, which was remarkably constant from the first period (1980–1986; 16.9%) to the last period (1993–1997; 16.5%). Gross hematuria was by far the most common complication in the last period (12.8%), and major complication occurred in only 1.9% of cases.

Clinically Significant Cancer

The original TRUS-guided technique was described as a sextant biopsy done both in a randomized and systematic fashion.[4] The term "random" implies that the needle is inserted into the tissue without aiming at a specific target, whereas "systematic" implies that six specific sectors of the prostate are sampled. Many modifications have been proposed to this scheme, and generally the more cores that are taken, the greater the diagnostic yield of cancer is. Given these considerations, we must assume that more cores will find more cancer, and that we will never be able to find all cancer. The key therefore is to determine the most appropriate number of biopsies for an individual patient that ensures with the greatest statistical probability that all clinically significant cancers are found (Fig. 2-4).

The term "clinically significant cancer," however, is the crux of the matter, since little information is available to determine what constitutes clinical significance. Stamey et al.[34] examined prostates after 139 consecutive unselected cystoprostatectomies from patients with bladder cancers in whom it was unknown whether they had prostate cancer.[34] Prostate cancer was found in 55 patients (40%); the volume of the largest cancer in each specimen was determined using morphometry. The largest 11 of the 55 cancers represented 7.9% of the total 139 samples. These cancers ranged in volume from 0.5 to 6.1 mL, representing only 20% of all patients with prostate cancer. Prostate cancers larger than 0.5 mL appear to correspond to the 8% of men who will be diagnosed with a clinically significant carcinoma, and the authors concluded that these represent "clinically significant" cancer. In a series of prostatectomy patients, Epstein et al.[35] found that tumors smaller than 0.2 mL had no capsular penetration or progression over 5 years, whereas tumors 0.2 to 0.5 mL had extracapsular penetration or progression in 13% of cases, suggesting that the smallest tumors were clinically insignificant. Crawford et al.[36] defined insignificant cancers as smaller than 0.25 mL with a Gleason score of 7 or less based on computer modeling.

Vashi et al.[37] determined significance by the tumor size at time of diagnosis, taking into consideration the age of the patient as well as the doubling time of the cancer. This is an intuitively appealing process, although it confounds the calculation with the uncertainty of the doubling time as well as the patient's life expectancy. A doubling time of 3 to 6 years was assumed for the calculations.[38] A study by Bostwick et al.[39] demonstrated a 10% probability of metastasis for tumors at 5 mL, 50% at 13 mL, and 87% at 20 mL. Using these assumptions and life tables from the US Department of Health and Human Services, the following formula can be used to determine life-threatening tumor volume at time of diagnosis:

$$V_0 = V_D/2 \ LE/DT = 20 \ mL/2 \ LE/DT$$

where V_0 = life-threatening volume at time of diagnosis, V_D = critical tumor volume at time of death, LE = life expectancy, and DT = doubling time.

Based on these assumptions, a life-threatening tumor volume may range from 0.05 mL in a 50-year-old man assuming a doubling time of 3 years to 6.7 mL in a 75-year-old man assuming a doubling time of 6 years. Depending on prostate size, the authors then calculated the number of cores needed to ensure 90% certainty of cancer detection stratified by tumor volume. Finally, the number of cores was recommended, stratified by prostate gland volume and age of patients, taking into consideration the volume of life-threatening tumor for each age group. The number of cores needed ranges from 2 (75-year-old man with a 10-mL prostate) to 23 (50-year-old man with a 30-mL prostate).

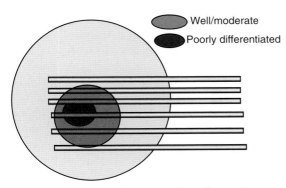

Well/moderate

Poorly differentiated

Figure 2-4. Transrectal ultrasound grading and staging limitations.

Initial Prostatic Biopsy

Results of Biopsy Strategies (Number and Location of Cores)

Over the last few years, there has been increasing interest in defining more efficient biopsy schemes for prostate cancer detection. Adding more biopsies to prostatic areas not sampled by standard sextant schemes should increase the detection rate for prostate cancer. However, it is not clear whether the increased detection rate is simply due to the additional biopsies or to the location from which the cores are taken. Moreover, the number of biopsies required for the optimal detection of clinically significant prostate cancer remains controversial. One thing, however, is established: Biopsies of the transitional zone add little to cancer detection and should therefore not be sampled during the initial biopsy.[40] Moreover, the necessity of biopsy of single hypoechoic lesions seems to be no longer necessary, because a visible lesion itself is as likely to be the source of cancer as the next adjacent area.[41]

Although the diagnostic yield of sextant biopsies varies according to the population studied, in general between 20% and 35% of patients are found to have cancer using the original description by Hodge et al.[4] Several researchers have evaluated the diagnostic yield of lateral biopsies within an extended prostate biopsy scheme. Most of the studies have demonstrated that extended prostate biopsy is superior to the sextant protocol in cancer detection, without significant morbidity and without increasing the number of insignificant cancer cases.[42] Addition of laterally directed biopsies, which are aimed at also sampling the lateral horn, have been shown to yield an approximately 5% to 35% increased sensitivity.[40,43-46] Most extra cancers were detected in the far lateral midlobar region, an area well sampled by the technique of laterally directed sextant biopsy.

In addition to the number of cores, the direction of the biopsies may well be as important. The apex and the base of the peripheral gland are the sites at which prostate cancer is most likely located and at which the biopsies should be directed, whereas the midline biopsies have been demonstrated to have the lowest probability of being positive.[40,43-46]

Eskew and coworkers[46] demonstrated that the five-region biopsy protocol with 13 to 18 cores increased the detection rate of prostate cancer by 35% when compared with standard, midlobar sextant biopsies. Ravery et al.[47] performed TRUS biopsies in 303 men who had DRE and PSA abnormalities using either 10 or 12 cores (if total prostate volume was more than 50 mL) and found cancer in 38%, which represents a 6.6% increase in the cancer detection rate compared with sextant biopsy. The increase was particularly pronounced in patients with a PSA of less than 10 ng/mL and/or a total prostate volume of greater than 50 mL.

Presti et al.[48] performed sextant biopsies in 483 men who had abnormal DRE or PSA and added four lateral cores at the base and midgland. If total prostate volume was over 50 mL, two additional midlobar, parasagittal transition zone biopsies were performed. The overall cancer detection rate was 42%, and the sextant technique missed 20%.

Babaian and coworkers evaluated an 11-core multisite-directed biopsy scheme incorporating the anterior transition zone, midline peripheral zone, and inferior portions of the anterior horn in the peripheral zone in 362 patients and compared it with the sextant biopsy.[49-51] The additional sites were identified based on computer simulations. Overall, a 33% increase (36 of 110 patients) in cancer detection was observed when biopsy technique included the alternate areas (P = .0021). The anterior horn was the most frequently positive biopsy site, followed by the transition zone and midline sites. The 11-core technique had significantly better cancer detection rates when DRE and TRUS were normal in men with serum PSA between 4.1 and 10 ng/mL.

Gore et al.[40] studied 396 consecutive patients who underwent biopsy of the lateral peripheral zone in addition to standard sextant biopsy. The cancer detection rate for each biopsy core was calculated. The sensitivity of different combinations of biopsy cores was compared with those of standard sextant biopsies and with a 12-core biopsy protocol that combined the standard sextant biopsy with a complete set of laterally directed cores. Cancer was detected in 160 of 396 (40.3%) patients. Of the possible combinations of biopsy cores, a strategy that included laterally directed cores at the base, midgland, and apex of the prostate with midlobar base and apical cores detected 98.5% of cancers. The detection rate of this 10-core biopsy regimen was significantly better than that of the standard sextant protocol ($P = .001$) and was equivalent to that of the 12-core biopsy. The authors recommend using a 10-core biopsy regimen that combined laterally directed cores at the base, midgland, and apex of the prostate with midlobar biopsy cores at the base and apex.

Despite the use of an extended protocol, sampling error can still occur in some patients, especially those with large prostate glands. Prostate volume is well known to be one of the factors that may influence the prediction of cancer at first biopsy, and a significant inverse relation exists between the cancer detection rate and prostate volume. Therefore, some investigators have advocated even more aggressive biopsy schemes with more than 12 cores up to a saturation biopsy (i.e., 20 cores) and reported even higher cancer detection rates.[44,46] A recent study demonstrated that a scheme with 8 cores is appropriate only in patients with prostate volumes smaller than 30 mL.[52] On the other hand, with prostate volumes larger than 50 mL, an extended procedure with more than 12 to 14 cores was necessary to detect cancer.

In accordance with these findings, Inahara et al.[53] have shown that a 14-core protocol is superior to an 8-core protocol for patients with prostate volumes of 30 to 40 mL. In a study of 303 patients comparing 6-, 12-, 18- and 21-core protocols in the same patient, de la Taille et al.[44] found that a 21-sample needle biopsy scheme increases the prostate cancer detection rate. The authors have reported a prostate cancer detection improvement of about 25% and 11% when 12- versus 6-core and 21- versus 12-core protocols were compared. It is interesting that they have demonstrated that the improvement was most marked in patients with a prostate volume greater than 40 mL.

On the other hand, in a recent meta-analysis, Eichler et al.[54] studied the efficacy and adverse effects of various biopsy schemes and concluded that a 12-core extended biopsy scheme strikes a balance between adequate cancer detection and an acceptable level of adverse effects. There seemed to be no significant benefit in taking more than 12 cores, and methods requiring 18 cores had a poor side-effect profile. In agreement with these findings, Jones et al.[55] demonstrated that the saturation technique with over 20 cores as an initial prostate biopsy strategy does not improve cancer detection. They sug-

---

Box 2-1. Recommended Biopsy Strategy (Number and Location of Cores)

- Take at least 10 biopsy cores.
- Focus the biopsies laterally and the areas listed above.
- Adjust the number of cores taken according to prostate volume.

---

gested that saturation biopsy should be reserved for repeat biopsy in patients who have a negative initial biopsy but are still strongly suspected to have prostate cancer. Recognizing the findings of these and other authors, as well as the various computer simulation and mathematical models, we recommend the steps listed in Box 2-1.

Repeat Biopsy

For men whose prostate biopsy shows only benign tissue but for whom there is continued suspicion of prostate cancer on the basis of DRE findings, repeat PSA measurements or other PSA derivatives (i.e., percentage of free PSA, complexed PSA, PSA density, PSA velocity), a repeat prostate biopsy should be considered.[56] Clearly, the yield of the repeat biopsy depends on the population studied, the particular features of a given patient (PSA, DRE, prostate volume, and so on), the type of prior biopsy, and the type of biopsy performed during the repeat biopsy. In the second set of biopsies, a cancer detection rate of about 10% to 35% has been reported in patients with a negative first set of biopsies.[57–67]

Even patients who have undergone more extensive biopsies may still have a significant detection rate at repeat biopsy.[57,68,69] Moreover, a third biopsy has been shown to identify nearly 10% of cancers.[58] Today, there is no proven biopsy scheme that omits the need for re-biopsy in the case of a persistent indication. However, more than 90% of prostate cancers are detected by performing two sextant biopsies.[70] Therefore, with the biopsy approaches preferred today, it is unlikely that two extended biopsies would miss a life-threatening cancer. Indeed, two sets of biopsies have been shown to detect most clinically significant cancers.[58]

Biopsy of the transition zone of the prostate, though not recommended at initial biopsy, should be considered for men undergoing a repeat biopsy for whom a suspicion of a missed cancer anteriorly is high.[56]

For men with high-grade prostatic intraepithelial neoplasia (PIN) found at the time of an extended prostate biopsy, the risk of cancer on a repeat biopsy is similar to the risk of cancer on repeat biopsy if the initial biopsy is negative.[66,71] Thus, a repeat biopsy is not indicated for men with high-grade PIN if the original biopsy technique was adequate.[56] A prostate biopsy that reveals atypical glands that are suspicious but not diagnostic of cancer should be repeated because the chance of finding prostate cancer on a repeat biopsy is 40% to 50%.[56,72,73]

Recent studies have suggested that treatment with 5α-reductase inhibitors may unmask prostate cancer by preferential suppression of benign prostate hyperplasia-derived PSA. Kaplan et al.[74] have suggested that after 1 year of finasteride treatment, prostate cancer detection is more likely in men with a smaller decrease in PSA. This hypothesis is supported by a meticulous analysis of the Prostate Cancer Prevention Trial (PCPT), which found that accuracy for detecting prostate cancer was greater in the finasteride group compared with the placebo group.[75]

Saturation Biopsy

The concept of increasing the number of cores and/or repeating the biopsy can be taken further by using the idea of saturation or mapping biopsy, in which 20 or more cores are obtained in a systematic fashion. Jones et al.[55] have demonstrated that saturation biopsy does not offer benefit as an initial biopsy technique. However, saturation biopsy may serve as a follow-up strategy in men with negative initial office biopsy.[76,77] The results of saturation biopsy studies are shown in Table 2-1. For example, Stewart et al.[67] performed TRUS-guided saturation biopsy (mean number of cores 23, range 15 to 45) in 224 men with negative previous biopsies (mean 1.8) in an outpatient surgical setting. They detected cancer in 77 patients (34%). The number of previous negative sextant biopsies was not predictive of subsequent cancer detection by saturation biopsy. At prostatectomy, median cancer volume was 1.04 mL, and 85.7% of removed tumors were clinically significant, assuming a 3-year doubling time. Complications and risk of diagnosing clinically insignificant cancer using saturation biopsy after a prior negative biopsy are reported to be no higher than with routine sextant or extended-core biopsy unless general or regional anesthesia is used, whereas the detection of clinically significant cancer is higher.[78]

Although initial investigators used regional or general anesthesia, periprostatic block has allowed several authors to now report this to be performed routinely in the office setting. This appears to overcome the increased risk of urinary retention related to systemic anesthesia. One useful application of saturation biopsy is to predict the likelihood of finding insignificant cancer at the time of prostatectomy, thus allow-

Table 2-1. Prostate Cancer Detection Rates Using Saturation Scheme in a Re-biopsy Setting

Reference	Route	No. of Patients	Cancer Detection Rate (%)	No. of Previous Cores	Pts with Initial Biopsy	No. of Cores	Clinically Insignifiant Cancer
de la Taille et al.[44]	TR	303	31.3	NR	188	21	NR
Rabets et al.[76]	TR	116	29	Mixed	0	20–24, mean 22.8	0
Walz et al.[171]	TR	161	41	8+	0	24.2	15.6
Jones et al.[55]	TR	139	44.6	NA	139	24	15.8
Pryor et al.[172]	TR	35	20	6	0	14–28, median 21	0
Stewart et al.[67]	TR	224	34	6	0	14–45, mean 23	14.3
Borboroglu et al.[64]	TR	57	30	6	0	22.5 mean	7
Fleshner et al.[173]	TR	37	13.5	Mixed	0	32–38	NR
Pinkstaff et al.[174]	TP	210	37	NR	0	21 mean	0
Bott et al.[175]	TP	60	38	8	0	24 mean	
Satoh et al.[176]	TP	128	22.7	8-Jun	0	22	NR
Moran et al.[177]	TP	180	38	12 median	0	41 median	NR

NA, not applicable; NR, not reported; TP, transperineal; TR, transrectal.

ing the selection of men for a watchful waiting or surveillance strategy.[79] The role and appropriate number of cores for saturation biopsy continue to be defined, but a threshold of 20 cores with emphasis on the lateral areas and apex is supported by the literature.

Tissue Diagnosis in Patients with No Rectal Access

In patients with no rectal access (e.g., anterior-posterior resection), there are several ways to obtain a tissue diagnosis. The most commonly used route is a transperineal biopsy. We have found that this often results in cores obtaining no prostate tissue, but rather fibromuscular or adipose tissue only, and we have resorted to performing such biopsy under cystoscopic guidance. The cystoscope with a 0- or 12-degree lens is situated at the verumontanum, and an assistant advances the needle through the perineum until the needle tip hits the prostate capsule. This is clearly noted as a movement of the prostate cystoscopically. The biopsy gun is then fired, and again a motion and sometimes even the needle becomes visible. In our hands, this has resulted in a relevant tissue diagnosis in 100% of cases with the majority of all cores containing prostate tissue.

Other options include image-guided biopsy through the perineum (MRI, CT, or ultrasound; see the following section) or transurethral resection of the prostate, with its inherent limitation of obtaining mostly transition zone tissue.

Transrectal versus Transperineal Biopsy

In the United States, transperineal biopsy is seldom performed. In contrast, in some European and Asian centers, it is the standard technique. Theoretically, the direction of the transperineal biopsies might be better than with the transrectal route because of the longitudinal sampling of the peripheral zone. Initially, the transperineal route was demonstrated to be less accurate than the transrectal route in identifying hypoechoic lesions[80] and systematic sextant-directed detected cancer.[81] However, in a simulation experiment, Vis et al.[82] have shown that the two approaches did not differ in prostate cancer detection. Moreover, Emiliozzi et al.[83] reported that sextant transperineal biopsy is superior to transrectal biopsy for detecting prostate cancer

in humans. On the other hand, two studies have shown that the overall cancer detection rate did not differ between the two approaches when the same number of cores was used.[84,85]

Indeed, 12-core transperineal prostate biopsy is superior to 6-core biopsy, and the number of cores may have a greater impact on cancer detection than does the route of the prostate biopsy.[83,86] In the last few years, the concept of extended biopsies has been applied equally to the transperineal approach, with results similar to those achieved with the transrectal approach.[84,85]

Doppler Imaging as an Aid for Cancer Detection

Standard gray-scale TRUS technology has limited specificity and sensitivity for prostate cancer detection because of its inability to detect isoechoic neoplasms. To increase its accuracy and usefulness, researchers have investigated a number of alternatives, including color Doppler TRUS, power Doppler imaging with and without intravenous contrast administration, and recently elastography. Increased microvascularity accompanies cancer growth, and neovascularity may be detectable by color Doppler TRUS and power Doppler TRUS because of abnormal blood flow patterns in larger feeding vessels.

However, several studies have, shown that color Doppler TRUS does not add significant information to gray-scale TRUS in detecting early stages of prostate cancer.[87,88] Overall, the sensitivity of color Doppler TRUS for the diagnosis of prostate cancer ranges between 49% and 87%, and specificity ranges between 38% and 93%.[87,88]

Power Doppler TRUS is considered the next generation of color Doppler imaging because it has the advantage of increased sensitivity for detecting small, low-flow blood vessels. Halpern et al.[89] have shown that power Doppler TRUS may be useful for targeted biopsies when the number of biopsy passes must be limited but that there is no substantial advantage of power Doppler over color Doppler. Remzi et al.[90] have recently reported a reduction in the number of unnecessary biopsies because a normal power Doppler TRUS signal might exclude the presence of a prostate cancer.

Contrast-enhanced color Doppler is an ultrasound-based technology for imaging of the prostate that is used after intravenous administration of gas-encapsulated microbubbles. This methodology allows for better prostate cancer visualization and for targeted biopsies to iso-echoic areas that generally become hypervascular after contrast infusion. Halpern et al.[91] have reported significantly improved sensitivity—from 38% to 65%—for detecting prostate cancer with preserved specificity at approximately 80%. Recently, different authors have demonstrated that targeted biopsy with contrast-enhanced color Doppler detects a number of tumors equal to that of systematic biopsies with less than half the number of cores.[91–94] Unfortunately, the poor discrimination of benign from malignant tissue, which is due to the contrast-enhanced color Doppler ultrasound signal arising from areas of benign disease such as benign prostatic hyperplasia, has diminished the specificity of this technology. Thus, contrast-enhanced color Doppler has not yet gained popularity because of its low specificity, complexity, and high cost.

Some investigators reported the use of sonography with manual compression of the prostate gland with the transrectal probe to generate elastograms.[88] The basis for improved detection of cancer is that the elasticity of the neoplastic tissue is less than the normal prostate. There is only limited amount of data available on the ability of elastography to detect prostate cancer. Investigators have shown that a targeted biopsy detects as many cancers as a systematic biopsy with less than half the number of biopsy cores.[88] However, more clinical trials are needed to determine this technology before widespread use.

Overdiagnosis and Insignificant Cancer

The critical question clearly is whether or not the cancers detected in sequential biopsies or saturation biopsies with increasing numbers of cores are clinically significant. There is mounting evidence that a substantial proportion of men with screen-detected prostate cancer would otherwise not have known about the disease during their lifetime in the absence of screening. In these men, cancer treatment is not beneficial. Identifying the patients with newly diagnosed prostate cancer who have indolent disease for which surveillance or expectant management may be an appropriate alternative to immediate curative intervention is a timely and important

issue. There is currently no marker for biologically indolent cancer. Although life expectancy and comorbidity are as important as pathologic characteristics of the cancer, most authors define indolent disease based on pathologic stage, tumor volume, and cancer grade (organ-confined tumor less than 0.5 mL with no Gleason pattern 4 or 5) (Table 2-2).

The issue of nonsignificant prostate cancer is becoming even more important with the advent of extended biopsy schemes. Indeed, several studies have shown that extended biopsy increases the likelihood of detecting smaller volume tumors of little clinical relevance. There is no doubt that the recent stage migration of prostate cancer has been witnessed by regular increases in the proportion of patients with moderately differentiated low-volume tumor and a significant decrease in the volume of the cancers removed at surgery.[95] Recently, Master et al.[96] demonstrated that a higher number of biopsy cores was associated with smaller tumor volumes at radical prostatectomy. Boccon-Gibod et al.[97] reported that 30% of patients with microfocal prostate cancer on extended biopsy have the risk of having insignificant tumor and of being overtreated. Unfortunately, no parameter was able to identify on an individual basis the patients harboring a prostate cancer potentially amenable to surveillance with delayed therapy. In contrast to these studies, Siu et al.[42] have demonstrated that it is possible not only to enhance tumor detection using an initial extended biopsy scheme but also to ultimately lead to the finding of clinically significant disease. Similarly, several authors reported no association between more-extensive biopsy schemes and the number of lower-risk tumors identified.[98,99]

Even if extended biopsy is recommended, the risk of detecting insignificant tumor should not be neglected. Saturation biopsies/re-biopsies, which are now used as part of active surveillance protocols, have recently proved to provide helpful information about quantitative and qualitative histology to predict the clinical significance of prostate cancer.[79,100] The concern of overdetection must be weighed against the risk of missing clinically significant malignancy. Cancer detection does not need to immediately trigger a treatment since men with low-volume and low-grade diseases may also be managed expectantly. Avoiding undertreatment of men

Table 2-2. Preoperative Parameters Predicting the Presence of Insignificant Prostate Cancer Defined as Tumor <0.58 mL and No Gleason 4 and 5 on Final Pathology

Reference	Continent of Origin	Insignificant Cancer (%)	Biopsy Protocol	Preoperative Variables Predicting Insignificant Cancer
Epstein et al.[35]	United States	26	Sextant	Gleason sum ≤6 Adenocarcinoma present in <3 of 6 cores No more than 50% malignancy involvement in each positive biopsy core PSA density <0.15 ng/mL/g
Goto et al.[178]	United States	10	Sextant	Quantitative analysis of the extent of cancer PSA, PSA density and grade
Carter et al.[179]	United States	17	Sextant	PSA density Quantitative histology (number of cores involved with cancer and percentage of cancer within the core)
Epstein et al.[180]	United States	30	Sextant	Needle biopsy findings Free/total PSA levels
Kattan et al.[161]	United States	20	≥6	Nomogram incorporating pretreatment variables (clinical stage, Gleason grade, PSA and the amount of cancer in a systematic biopsy specimen)
Ochiai et al.[181]	United States	22	10–11 cores	Combination of tumor length <2 mm, Gleason score 3 + 4 or less and prostate volume >50 mL
Augustin et al.[182]	Europe	6	Sextant	PSA density % Cancer per biopsy core
Chun et al.[183]	Europe	6	≥6	Preoperative nomograms (predictor variables: PSA, clinical stage, biopsy Gleason scores, core cancer length and percent of positive biopsy cores)
Steyerberg et al.[162]	Europe	49	Sextant	Updated Kattan nomogram[162] in screening setting
Miyake H et al.[184]	Japan	14	8	Gleason score <7 % Positive biopsy core <15%

PSA, prostate-specific antigen.

with larger-volume, higher-grade cancer requires treatment in a large proportion (50% or more) of those with small-volume, low-grade disease. In time, our methods of assessing the biologic behavior of prostate cancer based on needle biopsy may be augmented or replaced by molecular profiles or panels of biomarkers that predict life-threatening prostate cancer.

Role of Nomograms as Decision Tools for Prediction of Biopsy Outcome
(Box 2-2 and Fig. 2-5)

Traditionally, physician judgment has formed the basis for risk estimation, patient counseling, and decision making. However, humans have difficulty predicting outcomes because of the biases that exist at all stages of the prediction process.[101–104] First, clinicians do not recall all cases equally; certain cases can stand out and exert an unsuitably large influence when predicting future outcomes. Second, clinicians tend to be inconsistent when processing their memory and tend to resort to heuristics (rules of thumb) when processing becomes difficult.[105] When it is time to make a prediction, they tend to predict the preferred outcome rather than the outcome with the highest probability.[103] Third, it is difficult to integrate the multitude of predictive variables that have been shown to be of importance in clinical judgment.[106,107] Finally, clinicians have difficulty weighing the relative importance of each of these factors when formulating predictions of outcome. Therefore, to obtain more accurate predictions, researchers have developed decision aids based on statistical models.[108]

Decision aids consist of the Kattan-type nomograms,[109] risk groupings, artificial neural networks (ANNs), probability tables, and clas-

---

Box 2-2. Case Study: Risk of Prostate Cancer Before and After Initial Biopsy

A 60-year-old Caucasian patient with a family history of prostate cancer undergoes prostate cancer screening. Tests indicate a PSA level of 8.0 ng/mL. An abnormal DRE is also detected. Based on the prediction model developed in the study by Thompson and associates,[227] the patient's estimated risk of biopsy-detected prostate cancer based on a minimum of 6 cores is 75%.

In particular, if 100 patients exactly like this patient were seen, it is expected that 75 of these patients would have biopsy-detected prostate cancer based on a minimum of 6 cores. Based on the clinical results and the predicted risk of prostate cancer, the patient undergoes a prostate biopsy.

Results from the prostate biopsy taken from the patient in this case study indicate no presence of prostate cancer. During routine follow-up, the patient again has an abnormal DRE and a PSA level of 8.0 ng/mL.

Given an initial negative biopsy, the prediction model developed by Thompson and associates[227] now indicates that the patient's estimated risk of biopsy-detected prostate cancer based on a minimum of 6 cores has decreased from 75% to 67%.

From Thompson IM, Ankerst DP, Chi C, et al.: Assessing prostate cancer risk: results from the Prostate Cancer Prevention Trial. J Natl Cancer Inst 98: 529, 2006. Reprinted with permission.

sification and regression tree (CART) analyses. In general, these predictive models have been shown to perform as well as or better than clinical judgment when predicting probabilities of outcome.[107] Even so, physician input is obviously essential and crucial for the measurement of variables that are used in the prediction process and for the entire decision-making process.

Tables 2-3 and 2-4 show the multitude of models for prediction of prostate cancer presence on initial and repeat biopsy, respectively. A nomogram developed by Eastham et al.[110] for prediction of the probability of prostate cancer on initial biopsy in men with suspicious DRE and serum PSA less than 4.0 ng/mL yielded a predictive accuracy of 75%. Despite good accuracy, this nomogram suffers from limited generalizability. Unfortunately, the nomogram cannot be applied to men with unremarkable DRE findings and does not apply to patients with a PSA level greater than 4.0 ng/mL.

Garzotto et al.[111] developed a nomogram predicting prostate cancer on needle biopsy using

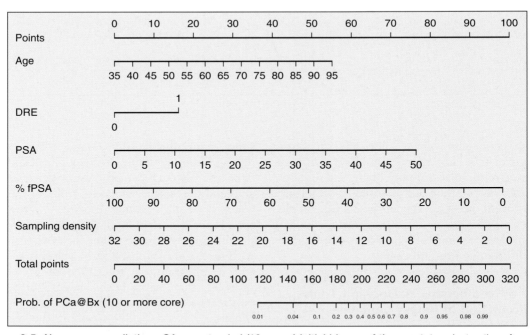

Figure 2-5. Nomogram predicting pCA on extended (10+-core) initial biopsy of the prostate. Instructions for physicians: To obtain nomogram predicted probability of prostate cancer on initial extended 10-core biopsy, locate patient values at each axis. Draw a vertical line to the "Points" axis to determine how many points are attributed for each variable value. Sum the points for all variables. Locate the sum on the "Total points" line to be able to assess the individual probability of prostate cancer on extended 10-core biopsy on the "Prob. of PCa@Bx" line. DRE, digital rectal examination (1 = suspicious, 0 = normal); %fPSA, % free prostate-specific antigen; PSA, prostate-specific antigen; Sampling Density: ratio between prostate volume and number of planned biopsy cores. (Reprinted with permission from Chun FK, Briganti A, Graefen M, et al: Development and external validation of an extended 10-core biopsy nomogram. Eur Urol 52:436, 2007.)

Table 2-3. Prostate Biopsy Nomograms for Prediction of Prostate Cancer Presence in Initial Biopsy Setting

Reference	Prediction Form	No. of Patients	Variables	Mean No. of Cores	Cancer Detection (%)	Accuracy (%)	Validation
Babaian et al.[185]	Risk group	151	Age, creatinine phosphokinase isoenzyme activity, prostatic acid phosphatase, PSA	6	24	74	Not performed
Eastham et al.[110]	Probability nomogram development	700	Age, race, DRE, PSA (0–4 ng/mL)	6	9	75	Internal
Virtanen et al.[186]	Neural network	212	% free PSA, DRE, heredity	Not available	25	81	Not performed
Finne et al.[187]	Neural network	656	% free PSA, PSA, DRE, TRUS	Not available	23	Not available	Not performed
Horninger et al.[188]	Neural network	3474	Age, PSA, % free PSA, DRE, TRUS, PSA density, PSA density of transition zone, transition zone volume	Not available	Not available	Not available	Not performed
Kalra et al.[189]	Neural network	348	Age, ethnicity, heredity, IPSS, DRE, PSA, complexed PSA	6	Not available	83	Not performed
Garzotto et al.[111]	Probability nomogram development	1239	Age, race, family history, referral indications, prior vasectomy, DRE, PSA (≤10 ng/mL), PSA density, TRUS findings	6.7 (6–13)	24	73	Not performed
Finne et al.[190]	Neural network	1775	DRE, % free PSA, TRUS, PSA	Not available	22	76	Not performed
Karakiewicz et al.[112]	Probability nomogram development	6469	Age, DRE, PSA, % free PSA	6	35–42	77	Internal and external
Suzuki et al.[191]	Probability nomogram development	834	Age, PSA, % free PSA, prostate volume, DRE	≥6	29	82	Internal
Chun et al.[183]	Probability nomogram validation[112] and development	2900	Age, DRE, PSA, % free PSA, sampling density*	11 (10–20)	41	77	Internal and external
Porter et al.[192]	Neural network	3814	Age, PSA, gland volume, PSA density, DRE, TRUS	6	27–42	72–75	Internal and external

*Sampling density is the ratio of TRUS-derived total gland volume by the number of cores at biopsy.
ASAP, atypical small acinar proliferation of prostate; DRE, digital rectal examination; HGPIN, high-grade intraepithelial neoplasia; IPSS, International Prostate Symptom Score; PSA, prostate-specific antigen; TRUS, transrectal ultrasound.

Table 2-4. Prostate Biopsy Nomograms for Prediction of Prostate Cancer in Other Than Initial Biopsy Setting

Reference	Prediction Form	Design	No. of Patients	Variables	Median No. Previous Biopsies	Mean No. of Cores	Cancer Detection (%)	Accuracy (%)	Validation
Repeat Biopsy									
O'Dowd et al.[66]	Probability nomogram development	Repeat biopsy	813	Age, initial biopsy diagnosis, PSA, % free PSA	Not available	Not available	29	70	Not performed
Lopez-Corona et al.[113]	Probability nomogram development	Repeat biopsy	343	Age, DRE, number previous negative biopsies, HGPIN history, ASAP history, PSA, PSA slope, family history, months from initial negative biopsy	2.9 (2-12)	9.2 (6-22)	20	70	Internal
Remzi et al.[193]	Neural network	Repeat biopsy	820	PSA, % free PSA, TRUS, PSA density, PSA density of the transition zone, transition zone volume	Not available	8	10	83	Not performed
Yanke et al.[194]	Probability nomogram validation[114]	Repeat biopsy	230 (356 biopsies)	Age, DRE, number previous negative biopsies, HGPIN history, ASAP history, PSA, PSA slope, family history, months from initial negative biopsy, months from previous negative biopsy	2.6 (2-7)	17.9 (12-54)	34	71	Internal
Chun et al.[114]	Probability nomogram development	Repeat biopsy	2393	Age, DRE, PSA, % free PSA, number previous negative biopsies, sampling density*	1.5 (1-7)	11 (10-24)	30	76	Internal and external

Saturation Biopsy

Walz et al.[171]	Probability nomogram development	Repeat saturation biopsy	161	Age, PSA, % free PSA, prostate and BPH volume, PSA doubling time, PSA density of the transition zone, number of previous biopsy sessions, number of cores at saturation biopsy	2.5 (2–5)	24.5 (20–32)	41	75	Internal

Mixed—Initial and Repeat Biopsy

Snow et al.[195]	Neural network	Initial and repeat biopsy	1787	Age, change on PSA, DRE, PSA, TRUS	Not available	6	34	87	Not performed
Carlson et al.[196]	Probability table	Initial and repeat biopsy	3773	Age, PSA, % free PSA	Not available	6	33	Not available	Internal
Djavan et al.[197]	Neural network	Initial and repeat biopsy	272	PSA density of the transition zone, % free PSA, PSA density, TRUS (PSA: 2.5–4.0 ng/mL)	Not available	8	24	88	Not performed
			974	PSA density of the transition zone, % free PSA, PSA velocity, transition zone volume, PSA density (PSA: 4.0–10.0 ng/mL)	Not available	8	35	91	Not performed
Stephan et al.[198]	Neural network	Initial and repeat biopsy	1188	Age, DRE, PSA, % free PSA, TRUS	Not available	Not available	61	86	Not performed
Porter et al.[199]	Neural network	Initial and repeat biopsy	319	Age, PSA, gland volume, TRUS, DRE, previous negative biopsy, African-American race	Not available	9.7 (6–10)	39	76	Not performed
Matsui et al.[200]	Neural network	Initial and repeat biopsy	228	PSA density, DRE, age, TRUS	Not available	10–12	26	73	Not performed
Benecchi[201]	Neural network	Initial and repeat biopsy	1030	Age, PSA, % free PSA	Not available	6–12	19	80	Not performed
Yanke et al.[202]	Probability nomogram development	Initial and repeat biopsy	8851	Age, race, PSA, DRE, number of cores	Not available	6–13	27–38	75	Internal

*Sampling density is the ratio of TRUS-derived total gland volume by the number of cores at biopsy.
ASAP, atypical small acinar proliferation of prostate; DRE, digital rectal examination; HGPIN, high-grade intraepithelial neoplasia; PSA, prostate-specific antigen; TRUS, transrectal ultrasound.

routinely available clinical and transrectal ultrasound variables. Their model yielded a predictive accuracy of 73%. This model has two limitations: (1) use of ultrasound-based input is highly impractical because men who undergo TRUS are also likely to undergo ultrasound-guided needle biopsy, and (2) the predictions of this nomogram are applicable only after TRUS, since TRUS variables are necessary for risk estimation. Predictions based on input that does not require ultrasound findings are more practical and may be interpreted before planned ultrasound-guided biopsy.

Karakiewicz et al.[112] developed two nomograms for prediction of the probability of having prostate cancer. The first nomogram was based on patient age, DRE, and serum PSA. Percent of free PSA was added as a predictor in the second nomogram. External validation of the nomograms with and without % free PSA yielded predictive accuracies of 77% and 69%, respectively. Unfortunately, these predictive models were based on sextant biopsy regimens limiting their transportability to current biopsy strategies. Therefore, Chun et al.[113] updated these nomograms in 2900 men who underwent extended prostate biopsy. Moreover, they complemented the variables with sampling density (i.e., ratio of gland volume and the number of planned biopsy cores). Internal validation of the new nomogram demonstrated 77% accuracy, and validation in external cohorts demonstrated 73% to 76% accuracy.

Accurate prediction of repeat biopsy would be helpful to spare men who don't have prostate cancer a negative repeat biopsy and to identify patients who need a re-biopsy to detect prostate cancer. O'Dowd et al.[66] used age, previous histologic findings, % free PSA, and total PSA to predict repeat biopsy results in 813 men. Their multivariate logistic regression model yielded 70% accuracy, but it was neither internally nor externally validated.

Lopez-Corona et al.[114] developed a nomogram that predicts the probability of a positive repeat biopsy following one or more negative biopsies. The input variables of the nomogram were patient age, DRE, cumulative number of negative cores previously taken, histories of high-grade PIN and/or atypical small acinar proliferations, PSA, PSA slope, and family history of prostate cancer. The nomogram yielded a predictive accuracy of 71%. However, the complexity of the nomogram makes it impractical in the clinical setting.

Finally, Chun et al.[113] developed and validated a nomogram for prediction of repeat biopsy outcome based on systematic 10 or more cores. The model comprised patient age, DRE, PSA, % free PSA, number of previous negative biopsy sessions, and sampling density (i.e., ratio between prostate volume assessed at initial biopsy and the planned number of cores at repeat biopsy). Using three cohorts of men, they reported predictive accuracies of 68% to 78% after external validation.

Interpretation of Biopsy Material

The most important task for the pathologist is to make the dichotomous determination whether or not the biopsy material obtained contains any prostate cancer. Once this is established, some relevant qualitative and quantitative assessments are of great use to the clinicians ultimately counseling patients regarding treatment options. Table 2-5 shows the variables that help clinical decision making. (See also Chapter 3, The Pathology of Prostate Cancer.)

Tumor Grade

Most pathologists use the classification system originally described in 1966 by Donald

---

Table 2-5. Prostate Biopsy Parameters That Should Be Reported for Optimal Decision Making

1. Number and total length of the cores (exclude those <1 cm and those without epithelial component)
2. Number of cores with cancer (percentage of cores involved)
3. Longest single length of tumor and location
4. Total tumor length in all cores
5. Mean tumor length in all cores (reported as a percentage): total tumor length divided by total length of cores multiplied by 100 (i.e., overall percentage of cancer in all biopsies)
6. Number of cores with perineural invasion (extent: focal, multifocal) and caliber of nerve bundles
7. Number of cores with vascular invasion
8. Gleason score for each core
9. Number and location of cores with atypical glands, suspicious for cancer
10. High-grade prostatic intraepithelial neoplasia (extent: focal or multifocal; number of cores involved; laterality: unilateral or bilateral)
11. Each core reported individually

Gleason.[115] In this system, there are five grades (1–5) in increasing order of aggressiveness. Because prostate cancer is usually heterogeneous, the most common and second most common grades are combined for the so-called Gleason score, which theoretically can run from 2 to 10. Practically, however, a grade of 2 or less is rarely ever assigned, and thus, the score runs from 6 to 10.

There is agreement that a pattern of 4 carries a significantly worse prognosis than a pattern of 3; thus, it is important to correctly identify the most and second most common pattern if grades 3 and 4 are most common (i.e., 3 + 4 = 7 versus 4 + 3 = 7, which has a worse prognosis).[116–119]

Because the prognosis is predicated on the worst pattern or grade, it has recently been advocated to also report a higher tertiary pattern, since a systematic review established the association of a tertiary grade with poorer outcome than that associated with no tertiary grade.[120]

Number of Cores and Percent of Cores Involved with Cancer

Many investigators have used multivariate analyses to determine the importance of factors other than the Gleason grade/score in the prognosis of men with prostate cancer. The literature is replete with examples of such analyses in which a variety of factors are found to be significantly related to outcomes such as biochemical recurrence-free survival and overall or cancer-specific survival.[121–123] These factors are listed in Box 2-3.

Other Histologic Findings

Multivariate analyses have also demonstrated the prognostic significance of findings such as perineural invasion,[124] lymphovascular inva-

sion[125] in terms of biochemical recurrence-free survival and overall or cancer-specific survival. Topics such as high-grade PIN,[126] atypical small acinar proliferation (ASAP)[127,128] and inflammation are discussed in Chapter 3.

Staging of Prostate Cancer

Importance and Goals

Clinical staging of prostate cancer aims to use pretreatment parameters to predict the true extent of disease. The goals of cancer staging are to allow the assessment of prognosis and facilitate educated decision making regarding available treatment options. An accurate assessment of disease extent is critical for men with newly diagnosed prostate cancer because pathologic stage is the most reliable means of predicting the outcome of definitive treatment in men with clinically localized cancer. Available pretreatment modalities that can help predict true disease extent in men with prostate cancer include DRE, serum PSA, tumor grade, radiologic imaging, and pelvic lymphadenectomy. The local extent of disease can be predicted by a combination of DRE, serum PSA, and tumor grade. Although in unique circumstances, imaging modalities may assist in the detection of extraprostatic spread of cancer, in most cases these tests are not yet reliable. Pelvic lymphadenectomy remains the gold standard for the detection of lymph node spread in men at high risk for harboring occult lymph node metastases. Ultimately, clinical staging may provide the patient and the urologist with valuable information regarding whether newly diagnosed prostate cancer is localized, locally advanced, or metastatic. This information helps guide management decisions.

Clinical Staging Classification Systems

Two main classification systems for clinical staging exist today: the Whitmore-Jewett and the tumor, node, metastases (TNM) classification systems. Whitmore introduced the first clinical staging classification system for prostate cancer in 1956, and Jewett modified it in 1975.[129,130] The TNM system was first adopted in 1975 by the American Joint Committee for Cancer Staging and End Results Reporting (AJCC) (Fig. 2-6).

Box 2-3. Biospy Factors Associated with Prostate Cancer Outcomes

- Number of biopsy cores involved with cancer
- Percent of biopsy cores involved with cancer (number of involved cores/total cores as percentage)
- Total length of biopsy cores involved with cancer (sum of the mm of cancer in each individual core)
- Percent of biopsy core involved with cancer (mm involved with cancer/total length of core in mm as percentage)

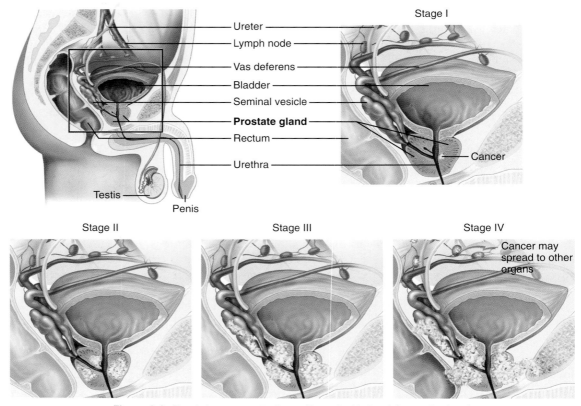

Figure 2-6. Prostate cancer staging.   (From the National Cancer Institute.)

Historically, tumor (T) classification, lymph node (N) status, and the presence of metastases (M) have been the cornerstones of staging for solid tumors. Unfortunately, the exclusive use of the current TNM staging system has limited relevance for predicting outcome and directing therapy for men with clinically localized prostate cancer. In part, this limitation is because nearly 75% of men who currently are diagnosed with clinically localized prostate cancer have nonpalpable disease, and the incidence of lymph node involvement is less than 4% in men who undergo radical prostatectomy.

T Stage

Prostate cancer found incidentally during removal of prostate tissue for presumed benign disease is given a clinical T stage of cT1a or T1b, depending on the amount of cancer found (less than 5% or more than 5%) and the prevailing grade (Table 2-6). By far the most common clinical stage is cT1c, indicating that the diagno-sis was made by a needle biopsy triggered by a suspiciously elevated serum PSA. The clinical stages cT2a-c are reserved for the rarer event of a palpable nodule involving more or less than 50% of both lobes of the prostate. This leads to an unusual and prognostically very heteroge-neous grouping of patients into the stage cate-gory cT1c, who may have only a small portion of one core positive for cancer or who may have cancer in all cores obtained. A clinical stage cT3 is rarely assigned based on DRE and/or imaging studies. The pathologic T stage does not have a category pT1, but rather only pT2 and T3. As previously discussed, the number and percent of cores involved are very important prognostic parameters that are ignored in the current T stage entirely. Similarly, the other important prognostic factors—serum PSA and Gleason score—are also ignored, although virtually every major recent series that has reported prostate cancer outcomes used a risk-classification scheme based on PSA and Gleason score in addition to clinical T classification.[131]

Table 2-6. TNM and AUA Staging Systems

TNM Staging System

Primary Tumor (T)

TX	Primary tumor cannot be assessed
T0	No evidence of primary tumor
T1	Clinically inapparent tumor neither palpable nor visible by imaging
	T1a Tumor incidental histologic finding in ≤5% of tissue resected
	T1b Tumor incidental histologic finding in >5% of tissue resected
	T1c Tumor identified by needle biopsy (e.g., because of elevated PSA)
T2	Tumor confined within prostate*
	T2a Tumor involves one half of a lobe or less
	T2b Tumor involves more than one half of lobe, but not both lobes
	T2c Tumor involves both lobes†
T3	Tumor extends through the prostate capsule
	T3a Unilateral extracapsular extension
	T3b Bilateral extracapsular extension
	T3c Tumor invades seminal vesicle(s)
T4	Tumor is fixed or invades adjacent structures other than seminal vesicles
	T4a Tumor invades bladder neck, external sphincter, or rectum
	T4b Tumor invades levator muscles or is fixed to pelvic wall, or both

Node (N)

NX	Regional lymph nodes cannot be assessed
N0	No regional node metastasis
N1	Metastasis in single lymph node, ≤ 2 cm
N2	Metastasis in a single node, >2 cm but ≤5 cm
N3	Metastasis in a node >5 cm

Metastasis (M)

MX	Presence of metastasis cannot be assessed
M0	No distant metastasis
M1	Distant metastasis
	M1a Nonregional lymph node(s)
	M1b Metastasis in bone(s)
	M1c Metastasis in other site(s)

AUA Staging System

Stage A	Clinically unsuspected disease
A1	Focal carcinoma, well differentiated
A2	Diffuse carcinoma, usually poorly differentiated
Stage B	Tumor confined to prostate gland
B1	Small, discrete nodule of one lobe of gland
B2	Large or multiple nodules or areas of involvement
Stage C	Tumor localized to periprostatic area
C1	Tumor outside prostate capsule, estimated weight ≤ 70 g, seminal vesicles uninvolved
C2	Tumor outside prostate capsule, estimated weight > 70 g, seminal vesicles involved
Stage D	Metastatic prostate cancer
D1	Pelvic lymph node metastases or ureteral obstruction causing hydronephrosis, or both
D2	Bone, soft tissue, organ, or distant lymph node metastases

*Invasion into the prostatic apex or into (but not beyond) the prostatic capsule is not classified as T3, but as T2.
†Tumor found in one or both lobes by needle biopsy but not palpable or visible by imaging is classified T1c.
AUA, American Urological Association; PSA, prostate-specific antigen; TNM, tumor-node-metastasis.

N Stage

The clinical and pathologic N stages are identical and differentiate between no assessment made (Nx), no lymph node involvement (N0), and involvement of regional lymph nodes (N1). Although they appear reasonably straightfor-ward, there are problems with both the clinical and the pathologic N stage.

Clinical assessment of regional and thus pelvic lymph nodes relies almost entirely on imaging. It is well known that imaging of pelvic lymph nodes by either computed scanning (CT) or magnetic resonance imaging (MRI) has notoriously poor sensitivity and specificity. This is because the criterion for detection of positive nodal disease at CT is based on node size (larger than 1-cm diameter), and nodal enlargement due to metastases occurs relatively late in the progression of prostate cancer. Since nodal metastases are often microscopic, neither CT nor standard MRI can be used to reliably rule them out. Reported CT sensitivity for the detection of lymph node metastases varies, but it is typically in the range of 36%.[132,133]

In the evaluation of lymph node metastases, unenhanced MRI has no advantage over CT. However, promising results have been reported with ultrasmall superparamagnetic iron oxide particles as an aid for diagnosing lymph node metastasis at MRI. The nanoparticles are taken up by circulating macrophages, which then traffic to the normal nodal tissue. The inability of malignant nodes to take up the agent provides tissue contrast within the lymph node and allows detection of metastases, even in nodes that do not meet the standard size criteria for metastasis.[134,135] Current guidelines suggest the use of CT and/or MRI, depending on the clinical presentation and the level of presumed risk for lymph node involvement.[132]

Imaging

The selection of an imaging modality for prostate cancer should be based on the questions that need to be answered for a particular patient (Box 2-4). The menu of available imaging options is continuously evolving in response to changes in clinical care, scientific discoveries, and technologic innovations. TRUS, MRI, CT, radionuclide bone scanning, and positron emission tomography (PET) each have advantages, disadvantages, and specific indications. Table 2-7 summarizes the recommendations for imaging test utilization published in reports supported by the American Urological Association, the American Joint Committee on Cancer, and the American College of Radiology.

TRUS is an insensitive method for detecting local extension of tumor. Intravenous urography is rarely obtained to stage prostate cancer, but it can evaluate the upper urinary tract in cases of hematuria or suspected obstruction. A chest radiograph is generally a low-yield examination in the staging of prostate cancer because lung metastases are exceedingly

---

Box 2-4. Essentials of Prostate Cancer Imaging

- The use of imaging tests should be guided according to the patient's risk category, which is determined by the patient's age, PSA level, Gleason score, and number of positive biopsy cores.
- Transrectal US is primarily used to guide prostate biopsies, but new developments in microbubble contrast agents offer the possibility of improving prostate cancer detection by detecting tumor angiogenesis.
- MR imaging, with high-resolution T2-weighted scans, MR spectroscopy, and dynamic contrast enhancement, is increasingly seen as a method that can improve prostate cancer detection, characterization, staging, and treatment follow-up.
- Although early reports with ^{18}F fluorodeoxyglucose PET in prostate cancer were disappointing, newer reconstruction techniques and new PET agents, including ^{11}C methionine, ^{11}C acetate, ^{11}C choline, and ^{18}F fluorodihydrotestosterone, hold great promise for the metabolic evaluation of prostate cancer and the improvement of our understanding of tumor biology.

From Hricak H, et al.: Imaging prostate cancer: a multidisciplinary perspective. Radiology 243: 28–83, 2007. Reprinted with permission.

Table 2-7. Use of Imaging in Staging Prostate Cancer

Source	Recommendation
American College of Radiology[224]	Bone scanning, CT, or MR imaging; PSA level > 10.0 ng/mL; Gleason score > 6
American Urological Association[225]	Bone scanning, PSA level > 20 ng/mL unless prostate cancer is poorly differentiated or high grade (stage T3 or higher). CT or MR imaging, PSA level > 25.0 ng/mL. Utility of endorectal MR and MR spectroscopic imaging not determined.
American Joint Committee on Cancer, 2002[226]	Bone scanning or cross-sectional imaging, PSA level > 20.0 ng/mL, Gleason score > 7–8

From Hricak H, et al.: Imaging prostate cancer: a multidisciplinary perspective. Radiology 243: 28–83, 2007. Reprinted with permission.

---

rare in the absence of widespread metastatic disease.

Radionuclide bone scanning (bone scintigraphy) is the most sensitive modality for the detection of skeletal metastases (Fig. 2-7). This is in contrast to bone survey films (skeletal radiography), which require more than 50% of the bone density to be replaced with tumor before

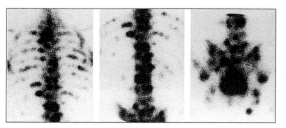

Figure 2-7. Positive bone scan. Thorax (*left*); lumbar spine (*center*); pelvis (*right*). (From Kirby RS, Christmas TJ, Brawer MK: Prostate Cancer, 2nd ed. London: Mosby, 2001, Figure 8.20. Reprinted with permission.)

they can identify distant spread. Today, skeletal radiography is obtained only to confirm a positive bone scan in men at low risk for bone metastases. Radionuclide bone scan can also screen for upper urinary tract obstruction and thus can obviate the need for further evaluation of the urinary tract in men with prostate cancer.[136] Because bone metastases at diagnosis are rare in men without bone pain in the PSA screening era, the routine use of bone scans in this population may not be useful and can create needless stress by detecting benign conditions that require further tests to rule out occult malignant disease.

In addition, a strategy of using bone scintigraphy in the staging evaluation of all PSA-screened men may not be cost-effective.[137] Radionuclide bone scans detect metastatic prostate cancer in less than 1% of men with a serum PSA value of 20 ng/mL or less and are not recommended for the initial evaluation of men with low- or intermediate-risk prostate cancer.[138] Bone scans are not routinely obtained for patients with PSA levels less than 10 ng/mL and no bone pain. When a bone scan is performed, however, it provides a baseline evaluation for comparison in men who later may complain of bone pain.

Although CT scanning is used routinely by radiation oncologists for prostate cancer treatment planning, no imaging technique available today has proved to add additional useful information when used to evaluate the extent of prostate cancer in men with low- and intermediate-risk disease.[139] CT and MRI to evaluate the local extent of disease and the possibility of nodal involvement are not routinely recommended because of the low sensitivity of these modalities. Such tests may be appropriately reserved for high-risk patients, such as those with locally advanced disease by DRE,

those with a PSA greater than 20 ng/mL, or those with poorly differentiated cancer on needle biopsy. Furthermore, the cost-effectiveness of these tests in populations with probabilities of lymph node involvement less than 30% has been questioned.[133,140] Given the rarity of lymph node involvement in screened populations, it appears that these imaging modalities are being overused in the staging of prostate cancer. Thus, cross-sectional imaging of the pelvis, by CT scan or MRI, for the purpose of detecting lymph node metastases, and radionuclide bone scans for the detection of bony metastases, should be reserved for men with high-risk prostate cancer.

[111In]Capromab penditide, a radioimmunoconjugate featuring a monoclonal antibody to an intracellular domain of prostate-specific membrane antigen (PSMA; ProstaScint, Cytogen Corporation) has been approved by the U.S. FDA for use in the evaluation of men for treatment of clinically localized prostate cancer. Some evidence indicates that when [111In]capromab pendetide immunoscintigraphy is used in combination with other pretreatment prostate cancer staging tools, the predictive value for the presence of lymph node metastases increases.[141] However, this scan is not being used routinely today for assessment of prostate cancer extent, in large part because of frequent difficulties in scan interpretation and because of the lack of scan sensitivity, even among men with fairly high-risk prostate cancer.[142,143]

Positron emission tomography has not yet been found to be useful in the evaluation of men with prostate cancer.[144] New imaging technologies, including three-dimensional color Doppler, contrast-enhanced color Doppler, magnetic resonance spectroscopy, and high-resolution MRI with magnetic nanoparticles have great potential for improving the assessment of local and distant prostate cancer extent.[135,139]

Prediction of Tumor Extent

Combined Use of Pretreatment Parameters in Staging Nomograms

Several multivariate statistical models have been proposed to estimate pathologic stage at radical prostatectomy with the intent of facilitating intraoperative decision making (Tables 2-8 and 2-9). Of these methods, the Partin tables, rep-

Table 2-8. Prediction of Pathologic Stage in Men Treated with Radical Prostatectomy for Clinically Localized Prostate Cancer

Reference	Prediction Form	Outcome	No. of Patients	Variables	Accuracy (%)	Validation
Narayan et al.[203]	Probability graph	Pathologic stage	813	Biopsy based stage, biopsy Gleason sum, PSA	Not available	Not performed
Partin et al.[204]	Probability table	Pathologic stage	703	Biopsy Gleason sum, clinical stage, PSA	Not available	External[205]
Partin et al.[145]	Probability table	Pathologic stage	4133	Biopsy Gleason sum, clinical stage, PSA	72	Internal and external[148,149,206]
Makarov et al.[148]	Probability table	Pathologic stage	5730	Biopsy Gleason sum, clinical stage, PSA	Not available	Not performed

resent the most widely used tool. This look-up table categorizes clinical stage, pretreatment PSA, and prostate biopsy Gleason grade to predict pathologic stage at radical prostatectomy[145] (see Table 2-8). After its introduction in 1997, the validity of the Partin tables was confirmed,[146,147] and the tables have been continuously updated to remain contemporaneous.[148,149]

Ohori et al.[150] developed three nomograms to predict the presence of extracapsular extension specific to either side of the prostate (see Table 2-9). The most basic model relies on preoperative PSA, side-specific clinical stage, and side-specific biopsy Gleason grade. The intermediate model uses these variables plus the side-specific percent of positive cores. The enhanced model uses the ingredients from the intermediate model plus the side-specific percent of cancer. The predictive accuracies of these three models were 79%, 80%, and 81%, respectively. These models predict the side-specific probability of extracapsular extension, which is more helpful in surgical planning than knowledge of the overall probability of extracapsular extension. Another advantage of these models compared with the Partin tables[145,148,149] is that they predict the probability of extracapsular extension without regard to whether the seminal vesicles or lymph nodes are involved. Partin tables predict the probability of extracapsular extension assuming negative seminal vesicles and lymph nodes. Steuber et al.[151] validated these nomograms (predictive accuracy 83.1% for the base nomogram and 84.0% for the full nomogram) and demonstrated that these models were more accurate than the CART analysis.[152]

Using the same cohort as Ohori et al.,[150] Koh et al.[153] derived a nomogram to predict the probability of seminal vesicle invasion. The predictors in this nomogram are preoperative PSA, clinical stage, primary and secondary biopsy Gleason grade, and percent of cancer at the base of the prostate. The c-index of this nomogram is 0.88. Similar to the extracapsular extension nomogram, the seminal vesicle invasion nomogram differs from the Partin tables in that it does not make any assumptions about the status of the lymph nodes.

Recently, Gallina et al.[154] developed a new nomogram for prediction of seminal vesicle invasion in a contemporary series of European patients. They then compared head-to-head the performance of their model to that of the nomogram of Koh et al.[153] and the Partin tables.[145,148,149] The nomogram of Gallina et al.[154] was more accurate and better calibrated than that of Koh et al.[153] and the Partin tables.

Cagiannos et al.[155] pooled the data from 5510 patients from six institutions to construct a nomogram for predicting lymph node status. The predictors are preoperative PSA, biopsy Gleason sum, and clinical stage. This nomogram had a predictive accuracy of 76%, which was higher than that of the Partin tables (0.74) when applied to the same population. This nomogram might help with the surgical decision of whether to avoid performing lymph node dissections, which are associated with cost and possible morbidity. Although this nomogram is a useful tool, it was developed in a population of men who underwent a limited or standard lymphadenectomy. Lymph node invasion prevalence is, however, directly related to the extent of pelvic

Table 2-9. Prediction of Specific Pathologic Features in Men Treated with Radical Prostatectomy for Clinically Localized Prostate Cancer

Reference	Prediction form	Outcome	No. of Patients	Variables	Accuracy (%)	Validation
Epstein et al.[35]	Risk group	Clinically indolent cancer defined as pathologically organ confined, tumor volume ≤ 0.2 mL, Gleason score < 7	157	Biopsy Gleason sum, millimeter core with cancer, PSA density, no adverse pathologic findings on needle biopsy	Not available	External[182]
Goto et al.[178]	Risk group	Clinically indolent cancer defined as pathologically organ confined, tumor volume ≤ 0.5 mL, Gleason score < 7	569	PSA density, maximal millimeter cancer in any core	Not available	Not performed
Kattan et al.[161]	Probability nomogram development	Clinically indolent cancer defined as pathologically organ confined, tumor volume ≤ 0.5 mL, no Gleason grade 4 or 5	409	PSA, primary and secondary biopsy Gleason score	64	Internal
				PSA, primary and secondary biopsy Gleason score, percent positive cores, TRUS volume	74	Internal
				PSA, clinical stage, primary and secondary biopsy Gleason score, TRUS volume, millimeter core with cancer, millimeter core without cancer	79	Internal
Steyerberg et al.[162]	Nomogram validation[162]	Clinically indolent cancer defined as pathologically organ confined, tumor volume ≤ 0.5 mL, no Gleason grade 4 or 5	247	PSA, primary and secondary biopsy Gleason score	61	—
				PSA, primary and secondary biopsy Gleason score, percent positive cores, TRUS volume	72	—
				PSA, clinical stage, primary and secondary biopsy Gleason score, TRUS volume, millimeter core with cancer, millimeter core without cancer	76	—
Chun et al.[164]	Probability nomogram development	Gleason upgrading between biopsy and radical prostatectomy	2982	PSA, clinical stage, primary and secondary biopsy Gleason score	80	Internal

Table continued on following page

Table 2-9. Prediction of Specific Pathologic Features in Men Treated with Radical Prostatectomy for Clinically Localized Prostate Cancer—cont'd

Reference	Prediction form	Outcome	No. of Patients	Variables	Accuracy (%)	Validation
Chun et al.[170]	Probability nomogram development	Significant Gleason upgrading between biopsy and radical prostatectomy	4789	PSA, clinical stage, biopsy Gleason sum	76	Internal
Steuber et al.[165]	Probability nomogram development	Tumor location: transition versus peripheral zone	945	PSA, biopsy Gleason sum, positive biopsy cores at mid-prostate only, number of positive biopsy cores at base, cumulative percent biopsy tumor volume	77	Internal
Peller et al.[207]	Probability table	Tumor volume	102	Biopsy Gleason sum, number positive sextant cores, PSA	Not available	Not performed
Ackerman et al.[208]	Probability formula	Surgical margin positivity	107	Number positive sextant cores, PSA density	70	Not performed
Rabbani et al.[209]	Probability graph	Surgical margin positivity	242	Androgen deprivation, number ipsilateral positive cores, PSA	Not available	Not performed
Bostwick et al.[210]	Probability graph	Capsular penetration	314	Biopsy Gleason sum, percent cancer in biopsy cores, PSA	78	Not performed
Garnito et al.[211]	Neural network	Capsular penetration	4133	Age, race, PSA, PSA velocity, Gleason sum, and clinical stage	30–76	External
Gilliland et al.[212]	Probability graph	Extracapsular extension	3826	Age, biopsy Gleason sum, PSA	63	Not performed
Ohori et al.[150]	Probability nomogram development	Side-specific extracapsular extension	763	PSA, clinical stage, side-specific biopsy Gleason sum, side-specific percent positive cores, side-specific percent of cancer in cores	81	External[152]
Steuber et al.[151]	Probability nomogram development	Side-specific extracapsular extension	1118	PSA, clinical stage, biopsy Gleason sum, percent positive cores, percent of cancer in positive cores	84	Internal
Badalament et al.[213]	Probability formula	Organ confined disease	192	Biopsy Gleason sum, involvement of greater than 5% of base with or without apex biopsy, nuclear grade, PSA, total percent tumor involvement	86	Not performed

Study	Method	Endpoint	N	Variables	Accuracy (%)	Validation
Bostwick et al.[210]	Probability graph	Seminal vesicle invasion	314	Biopsy Gleason sum, percent cancer in cores, PSA	76	Not performed
Pisansky et al.[214]	Probability graph	Seminal vesicle invasion	2953	Biopsy Gleason primary grade, clinical stage, PSA	80	Internal
Koh et al.[153]	Probability nomogram development	Seminal vesicle invasion	763	PSA, clinical stage, primary and secondary Gleason score, and percent of cancer at the base	88	Internal
Baccala et al.[215]	Probability nomogram development	Seminal vesicle invasion	6740	Age, PSA, biopsy Gleason sum, clinical stage	80	Internal
Gallina et al.[154]	Probability nomogram development	Seminal vesicle invasion	896	PSA, clinical stage, biopsy Gleason sum, percent positive biopsy cores	79	Internal and external
Ackerman et al.[208]	Probability formula	Lymph node invasion assessed with limited pelvic lymphadenectomy	107	Number positive sextant cores, PSA	94	Not performed
Bluestein et al.[216]	Probability graph	Lymph node invasion assessed with limited pelvic lymphadenectomy	816	Biopsy Gleason sum, clinical stage, PSA	82	Internal
Batuello et al.[217]	Neural network	Lymph node invasion assessed with limited pelvic lymphadenectomy	6454	Biopsy Gleason sum, clinical stage, PSA	77–81	Internal and external
Roach et al.[218]	Probability graph	Lymph node invasion assessed with limited pelvic lymphadenectomy	212	Biopsy Gleason sum, PSA	Not available	Not performed
Cagiannos et al.[155]	Probability nomogram development	Lymph node invasion assessed with limited pelvic lymphadenectomy	5510	PSA, clinical stage, biopsy Gleason sum / PSA, clinical stage, biopsy Gleason sum, institution	76 / 78	Internal / Internal
Briganti et al.[123,158,219]	Probability nomogram development	Lymph node invasion assessed with extended pelvic lymphadenectomy (≥10 nodes)	602[158] / 781[219] / 278[123]	PSA, clinical stage, biopsy Gleason sum / PSA, clinical stage, biopsy Gleason sum, number of lymph nodes / PSA, clinical stage, biopsy Gleason sum, percentage positive biopsy cores	76 / 79 / 83	Internal / Internal / Internal

PSA, prostate-specific antigen; TRUS, transrectal ultrasound.

lymph node dissection.[156,157] Thus, extended lymph node dissection might be necessary to detect clinically occult lymph node metastases that would not otherwise be detected by a more limited lymph node dissection. It is more important that prostate cancer nodal metastases do not follow a predefined pathway of metastatic spread.

Therefore, Briganti et al.[158] developed a nomogram predicting the probability of lymph node invasion among patients undergoing radical prostatectomy and an extended pelvic lymphadenectomy (Fig. 2-8). In addition, the authors considered landing zones of positive lymph nodes and, based on the assumption to be able to spare extended lymph node dissection in low-risk patients, developed a second highly accurate nomogram to predict presence of extraobturator lymph node involvement.[159]

PSA screening leads to the early detection of cancers, of which some are so small, low-grade and noninvasive that they may be assumed to pose little risk to the patient (indolent cancer).[160] Kattan et al.[161] developed nomograms that predict the probability of harboring indolent prostate cancer (pathologically organ confined cancer, 0.5 mL or less in volume and without poorly differentiated elements). The authors developed three models: the first model included preoperative PSA and primary and secondary biopsy Gleason grade; the second added ultrasound volume and percent of positive cores as predictors to the predictors of the first model; and the third model further added millimeters of cancerous and noncancerous tissue found in biopsy cores. The predictive accuracies for these three models were 64%, 74%, and 79%, respectively. The models might help in deciding when aggressive therapy can be delayed or avoided. Steyerberg et al.[162] evaluated transportability of these nomograms to the screening setting, where overdiagnosis and overtreatment are of key concern.[163] They found that the percentage of patients with indolent cancer was higher in the setting of a screening trial[162] than in the non-screened setting in which the models were created (49% versus 20%). They concluded that models predicting indolent prostate cancer in

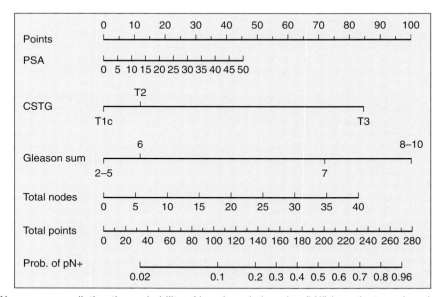

Figure 2-8. Nomogram predicting the probability of lymph node invasion (LNI) in patients undergoing pelvic lymph node dissection of various extents, based on pretreatment PSA level, clinical stage, biopsy Gleason sum, and number of lymph nodes removed.   Instructions: Locate the patient's pretreatment PSA level on the PSA axis. Draw a line straight upward to the point axis to determine how many points toward the probability of positive lymph nodes the patient receives for his PSA value. Repeat the process for each additional variable. Total the points for each of the predictors. Locate the final sum on the total point axis. Draw a line straight down to find the patient's probability of having LNI. CSTG, clinical stage; Gleason sum, biopsy Gleason sum; total nodes, total number of nodes removed and examined; Prob. of pN+, probability of LNI. (Reprinted with permission from Briganti A, Chun FK-H, Salonia A, et al: Validation of a nomogram predicting the probability of lymph node invasion based on the extent of pelvic lymphadenectomy in patients with clinically localized prostate cancer. BJU Int 98[4]:788–793, 2006.)

the clinical setting provide probabilities that are too low for cancers identified in a screening setting. Therefore, they developed an updated model that predicts the probability of indolent disease in patients with screen-detected prostate cancer.

Beyond pathologic features, nomograms predicting Gleason upgrading between biopsy and radical prostatectomy[164] and of tumor location[165] have been developed. For example, Chun et al.[164] developed and internally validated a nomogram for predicting the probability of biopsy Gleason sum upgrading in a cohort of 2982 patients treated with radical prostatectomy. Using preoperative PSA, clinical stage, and primary and secondary biopsy Gleason grade, their model achieved an accuracy of 80.4%, and its predictions closely approximated the observed rate of Gleason sum upgrading between biopsy and final pathology.

Tumor Upgrading Between Biopsy and Prostatectomy

Various studies have demonstrated that the ability to predict the final Gleason score by means of standard sextant biopsy is poor with a concordance rate between the biopsy and prostatectomy Gleason scores of only 28% to 48% (Table 2-10). On average, the Gleason score is undergraded in 43% of cases. Extended prostate biopsy schemes have proved to be beneficial in the pretreatment decision-making process because an increased number of biopsies increase the Gleason concordance. San Francisco et al.[166] have reported an improvement in the concordance rate from 63% to 72%. Mian et al.[167] reported that the rate of upgrading to a worsening risk category was significantly reduced with extended prostate biopsy. Numao et al.[168] recently reported that a 26-core systematic biopsy can more accurately predict the presence of Gleason pattern 4/5 on surgical specimen compared with transrectal 12-core prostate biopsy. King et al.[169] distinguished between any upgrading and significant upgrading (Gleason sum increases either from 6 to 7 or from 7 to 8).

These and other authors[168,169] have demonstrated that the risk of significant upgrading decreases with increasing biopsy cores taken because of higher sampling density and more accurate pathologic biopsy evaluation. The two largest published cohorts[122,123] showed a rate of overall Gleason sum upgrading of 29.3% and 32.6%, and a rate of significant upgrading of 32% and 28.2%, respectively. Because significant Gleason sum upgrading between biopsy and final pathology may have an impact on treatment decision making, predictive nomograms

Table 2-10. Degree of Gleason Grade Discordance (i.e., Biopsy Upgrading and Downgrading) Between Biopsy and Radical Prostatectomy

Reference	Year	No. of Cores Taken	Grade Discordance (%)	Upgrading (%)	Downgrading (%)
San Francisco IF et al.[166]	2003	≤9	37	12	25
		≥10	24	10	4
King CR et al.[220]	2004	6	38	25	12
		10	37	12	25
Emiliozzi P et al.[221]	2004	6	51	11	39
		12	30	6	24
Coogan CL et al.[222]	2005	6	59	20	39
		8	60	23	37
		10	43	11	32
Mian BM et al.[167]	2006	6	52	41	NR
		12	32	17	NR
Numao N et al.[168]	2006	TP14	15	NR	51
		TR12	17	NR	48
		3D26	8	2	26
Elabbady A et al.[223]	2006	6	50	NR	NR
		12	25	NR	NR

NR, not reported; TP, transperineal; TR, transrectal; 3D, three-dimensional.

have been developed as prognostic models capable of predicting the probability of significant upgrading.[164,170]

References

1. Perez-Guillermo M, Acosta-Ortega J, Garcia-Solano J: The continuing role of fine-needle aspiration of the prostate gland into the 21st century: a tribute to Torsten Lowhagen. Diagn Cytopathol 32:315–320, 2005.
2. Rosa M, Chopra HK, Sahoo S: Fine needle aspiration biopsy diagnosis of metastatic prostate carcinoma to inguinal lymph node. Diagn Cytopathol 35:565–567, 2007.
3. Mai KT, Roustan Delatour NL, Assiri A, et al: Secondary prostatic adenocarcinoma: a cytopathological study of 50 cases. Diagn Cytopathol 35:91–95, 2007.
4. Hodge KK, McNeal JE, Terris MK, et al: Random systematic versus directed ultrasound guided transrectal core biopsies of the prostate. J Urol 142:71–74; discussion 74–75, 1989.
5. Daneshgari F, Taylor GD, Miller GJ, et al: Computer simulation of the probability of detecting low volume carcinoma of the prostate with six random systematic core biopsies. Urology 45:604–609, 1995.
6. Rabbani F, Stroumbakis N, Kava BR, et al: Incidence and clinical significance of false-negative sextant prostate biopsies. J Urol 159:1247–1250, 1998,
7. Svetec D, McCabe K, Peretsman S, et al: Prostate rebiopsy is a poor surrogate of treatment efficacy in localized prostate cancer. J Urol 159:1606–1608, 1998.
8. Fink KG, Hutarew G, Lumper W, et al: Prostate cancer detection with two sets of ten-core compared with two sets of sextant biopsies. Urology 58:735–739, 2001.
9. Davis M, Sofer M, Kim SS, et al: The procedure of transrectal ultrasound guided biopsy of the prostate: a survey of patient preparation and biopsy technique. J Urol 167:566–570, 2002.
10. Carey JM, Korman HJ: Transrectal ultrasound guided biopsy of the prostate. Do enemas decrease clinically significant complications? J Urol 166:82–85, 2001.
11. Aron M, Rajeev TP, Gupta NP: Antibiotic prophylaxis for transrectal needle biopsy of the prostate: a randomized controlled study. BJU Int 85:682–685, 2000.
12. Isen K, Kupeli B, Sinik Z, et al: Antibiotic prophylaxis for transrectal biopsy of the prostate: a prospective randomized study of the prophylactic use of single dose oral fluoroquinolone versus trimethoprim-sulfamethoxazole. Int Urol Nephrol 31:491–495, 1999.
13. Kapoor DA, Klimberg IW, Malek GH, et al: Single-dose oral ciprofloxacin versus placebo for prophylaxis during transrectal prostate biopsy. Urology 52:552–558, 1998.
14. Desgrandchamps F, Meria P, Irani J, et al: The rectal administration of lidocaine gel and tolerance of transrectal ultrasonography-guided biopsy of the prostate: a prospective randomized placebo-controlled study. J Urol 83:1007–1009, 1999.
15. Issa MM, Bux S, Chun T, et al: A randomized prospective trial of intrarectal lidocaine for pain control during transrectal prostate biopsy: the Emory University experience. J Urol 164:397–399, 2000.
16. Tiong HY, Liew LC, Samuel M, et al: A meta-analysis of local anesthesia for transrectal ultrasound-guided biopsy of the prostate. Prostate Cancer Prostatic Dis 10:127–136, 2007.
17. Alavi AS, Soloway MS, Vaidya A, et al: Local anesthesia for ultrasound guided prostate biopsy: a prospective randomized trial comparing 2 methods. J Urol 166:1343–1345, 2001.
18. Lynn NN, Collins GN, Brown SC, et al: Periprostatic nerve block gives better analgesia for prostatic biopsy. BJU Int 90:424–426, 2002.
19. Matlaga BR, Lovato JF, Hall MC: Randomized prospective trial of a novel local anesthetic technique for extensive prostate biopsy. Urology 61:972–976, 2003.
20. Obek C, Ozkan B, Tunc B, et al: Comparison of 3 different methods of anesthesia before transrectal prostate biopsy: a prospective randomized trial. J Urol 172:502–505, 2004.
21. Rodriguez A, Kyriakou G, Leray E, et al: Prospective study comparing two methods of anaesthesia for prostate biopsies: apex periprostatic nerve block versus intrarectal lidocaine gel: review of the literature. Eur Urol 44:195–200, 2003.
22. Stirling BN, Shockley KF, Carothers GG, et al: Comparison of local anesthesia techniques during transrectal ultrasound-guided biopsies. Urology 60:89–92, 2002.
23. Alavi AS, Soloway MS, Vaidya A, et al: Local anesthesia for ultrasound guided biopsy: a prospective randomized trial comparing 2 methods. J Urol 166:1343–1345, 2001.
24. Bulbul MA, Haddad MC, Khauli RB, et al: Periprostatic infiltration with local anesthesia during transrectal ultrasound-guided prostate biopsy is safe, simple, and effective: a pilot study. Clin Imaging 26:129–132, 2002.
25. Kaver I, Mabjeesh NJ, Matzkin H: Randomized prospective study of periprostatic local anesthesia during transrectal ultrasound-guided prostate biopsy. Urology 59:405–408, 2002.
26. Leibovici D, Zisman A, Siegel YI, et al: Local anesthesia for prostate biopsy by periprostatic lidocaine injection: a double-blind placebo controlled study. J Urol 167:563–565, 2002.
27. Pareek G, Armenakas NA, Fracchia JA: Periprostatic nerve blockade for transrectal ultrasound guided biopsy of the prostate: a randomized, double-blind, placebo controlled study. J Urol 166:894–897, 2001.
28. Seymour H, Perry MJ, Lee-Elliot C, et al: Pain after transrectal ultrasonography-guided prostate biopsy: the advantages of periprostatic local anaesthesia. BJU Int 88:540–544, 2001.
29. Ozden E, Yaman O, Gogus C, et al: The optimum doses of and injection locations for periprostatic nerve blockade for transrectal ultrasound guided biopsy of the prostate: a prospective, randomized, placebo controlled study. J Urol 170:2319–2322, 2003.
30. Schostak M, Christoph F, Muller M, et al: Optimizing local anesthesia during 10-core biopsy of the prostate. Urology 60:253–257, 2002.
31. Cevik I, Dillioglugil O, Zisman A, et al: Combined "periprostatic and periapical" local anesthesia is not superior to "periprostatic" anesthesia alone in reducing pain during Tru-Cut prostate biopsy. Urology 68:1215–1219, 2006.
32. Pendleton J, Costa J, Wludyka P, et al: Combination of oral tramadol, acetaminophen and 1% lidocaine induced periprostatic nerve block for pain control during transrectal ultrasound guided biopsy of the prostate: a prospective, randomized, controlled trial. J Urol 176:1372–1375, 2006.
33. Roberts RO, Bergstralh EJ, Besse JA, et al: Trends and risk factors for prostate biopsy complications in the pre-PSA and PSA eras, 1980 to 1997. Urology 59:79–84, 2002.
34. Stamey TA, Freiha FS, McNeal JE, et al: Localized prostate cancer. Relationship of tumor volume to clinical significance for treatment of prostate cancer. Cancer 71:933–938, 1993.
35. Epstein JI, Walsh PC, Carmichael M, et al: Pathologic and clinical findings to predict tumor extent of nonpalpable (stage T1c) prostate cancer [see comments]. JAMA 271:368–374, 1994.
36. Crawford ED, Hirano D, Werahera PN, et al: Computer modeling of prostate biopsy: tumor size and location—not clinical significance—determine cancer detection. J Urol 159:1260–1264, 1998.
37. Vashi AR, Wojno KJ, Gillespie B, et al: A model for the number of cores per prostate biopsy based on patient age and prostate gland volume. J Urol 159:920–924, 1998.
38. Schmid HP, McNeal JE, Stamey TA: Observations on the doubling time of prostate cancer. The use of serial prostate-specific antigen in patients with untreated disease as a measure of increasing cancer volume. Cancer 71:2031–2040, 1993.
39. Bostwick DG, Graham SDJ, Napalkov P, et al: Staging of early prostate cancer: a proposed tumor volume-based prognostic index. Urology 41:403–411, 1993.
40. Gore JL, Shariat SF, Miles BJ, et al: Optimal combinations of systematic sextant and laterally directed biopsies for the detection of prostate cancer. J Urol 165:1554–1559, 2001.
41. Onur R, Littrup PJ, Pontes JE, et al: Contemporary impact of transrectal ultrasound lesions for prostate cancer detection. J Urol 172:512–514, 2004.
42. Siu W, Dunn RL, Shah RB, et al: Use of extended pattern technique for initial prostate biopsy. J Urol 174:505–509, 2005.
43. Singh H, Canto EI, Shariat SF, et al: Six additional systematic lateral cores enhance sextant biopsy prediction of pathological features at radical prostatectomy. J Urol 171:204–209, 2004.
44. de la Taille A, Antiphon P, Salomon L, et al: Prospective evaluation of a 21-sample needle biopsy procedure designed to

improve the prostate cancer detection rate. Urology 61:1181–1186, 2003.

45. Presti JC, Jr, O'Dowd GJ, Miller MC, et al: Extended peripheral zone biopsy schemes increase cancer detection rates and minimize variance in prostate specific antigen and age related cancer rates: results of a community multi-practice study. J Urol 169:125–129, 2003.

46. Eskew LA, Bare RL, McCullough DL: Systematic 5 region prostate biopsy is superior to sextant method for diagnosing carcinoma of the prostate. J Urol 157:199–202; discussion 202–203, 1997.

47. Ravery V, Goldblatt L, Royer B, et al: Extensive biopsy protocol improves the detection rate of prostate cancer. J Urol 164:393–396, 2000.

48. Presti JC, Jr, Chang JJ, Bhargava V, et al: The optimal systematic prostate biopsy scheme should include 8 rather than 6 biopsies: results of a prospective clinical trial. J Urol 163:163–166; discussion 166–167, 2000.

49. Babaian RJ: Extended field prostate biopsy enhances cancer detection. Urology 55:453–456, 2000.

50. Babaian RJ, Toi A, Kamoi K, et al: A comparative analysis of sextant and an extended 11-core multisite directed biopsy strategy. J Urol 163:152–157, 2000.

51. Chen ME, Troncoso P, Tang K, et al: Comparison of prostate biopsy schemes by computer simulation. Urology 53:951–960, 1999.

52. Ficarra V, Novella G, Novara G, et al: The potential impact of prostate volume in the planning of optimal number of cores in the systematic transperineal prostate biopsy. Eur Urol 48:932–937, 2005.

53. Inahara M, Suzuki H, Kojima S, et al: Improved prostate cancer detection using systematic 14-core biopsy for large prostate glands with normal digital rectal examination findings. Urology 68:815–819, 2006.

54. Eichler K, Hempel S, Wilby J, et al: Diagnostic value of systematic biopsy methods in the investigation of prostate cancer: a systematic review. J Urol 175:1605–1612, 2006.

55. Jones JS, Patel A, Schoenfield L, et al: Saturation technique does not improve cancer detection as an initial prostate biopsy strategy. J Urol 175:485–488, 2006.

56. National Comprehensive Cancer Network: National Comprehensive, 2004. http://www.nccn.org/professionals/physician_gls/PDF/prostate_detection.pdf. 2004.

57. Applewhite JC, Matlaga BR, McCullough DL: Results of the 5 region prostate biopsy method: the repeat biopsy population. J Urol 168:500–503, 2002.

58. Djavan B, Ravery V, Zlotta A, et al: Prospective evaluation of prostate cancer detected on biopsies 1, 2, 3 and 4: when should we stop? J Urol 166:1679–1683, 2001.

59. Roehrborn CG, Pickens GJ, Sanders JS: Diagnostic yield of repeated transrectal ultrasound-guided biopsies stratified by specific histopathologic diagnoses and prostate specific antigen levels. Urology 47:347–352, 1996.

60. Keetch DW, Catalona WJ, Smith DS: Serial prostatic biopsies in men with persistently elevated serum prostate specific antigen values. J Urol 151:1571–1574, 1994.

61. Fleshner NE, O'Sullivan M, Fair WR: Prevalence and predictors of a positive repeat transrectal ultrasound guided needle biopsy of the prostate. J Urol 158:505–508; discussion 508–509, 1997.

62. Rietbergen JB, Kruger AE, Hoedemaeker RF, et al: Repeat screening for prostate cancer after 1-year followup in 984 biopsied men: clinical and pathological features of detected cancer. J Urol 160:2121–2125, 1998.

63. Letran JL, Blase AB, Loberiza FR, et al: Repeat ultrasound guided prostate needle biopsy: use of free-to-total prostate specific antigen ratio in predicting prostatic carcinoma. J Urol 160:426–429, 1998.

64. Borboroglu PG, Comer SW, Riffenburgh RH, et al: Extensive repeat transrectal ultrasound guided prostate biopsy in patients with previous benign sextant biopsies. J Urol 163:158–162, 2000.

65. Djavan B, Zlotta A, Remzi M, et al: Optimal predictors of prostate cancer on repeat prostate biopsy: a prospective study of 1,051 men. J Urol 163:1144–1148; discussion 1148–1149, 2000.

66. O'Dowd GJ, Miller MC, Orozco R, et al: Analysis of repeated biopsy results within 1 year after a noncancer diagnosis. Urology 55:553–559, 2000.

67. Stewart CS, Leibovich BC, Weaver AL, et al: Prostate cancer diagnosis using a saturation needle biopsy technique after previous negative sextant biopsies. J Urol 166:86–91; discussion 91–92, 2001.

68. Hong YM, Lai FC, Chon CH, et al: Impact of prior biopsy scheme on pathologic features of cancers detected on repeat biopsies. Urol Oncol 22:7–10, 2004.

69. Singh H, Canto EI, Shariat SF, et al: Predictors of prostate cancer after initial negative systematic 12 core biopsy. J Urol 171:1850–1854, 2004.

70. Roehl KA, Antenor JA, Catalona WJ: Serial biopsy results in prostate cancer screening study. J Urol 167:2435–2439, 2002.

71. Lefkowitz GK, Sidhu GS, Torre P, et al: Is repeat prostate biopsy for high-grade prostatic intraepithelial neoplasia necessary after routine 12-core sampling? Urology 58:999–1003, 2001.

72. Chan TY, Epstein JI: Follow-up of atypical prostate needle biopsies suspicious for cancer. Urology 53:351–355, 1999.

73. Iczkowski KA, Bassler TJ, Schwob VS, et al: Diagnosis of "suspicious for malignancy" in prostate biopsies: predictive value for cancer. Urology 51:749–757; discussion 757–758, 1998.

74. Kaplan SA, Ghafar MA, Volpe MA, et al: PSA response to finasteride challenge in men with a serum PSA greater than 4 ng/ml and previous negative prostate biopsy: preliminary study. Urology 60:464–468, 2002.

75. Thompson IM, Pauler DK, Goodman PJ, et al: Prevalence of prostate cancer among men with a prostate-specific antigen level < or = 4.0 ng per milliliter. N Engl J Med 350:2239–2246, 2004.

76. Rabets JC, Jones JS, Patel A, et al: Prostate cancer detection with office based saturation biopsy in a repeat biopsy population. J Urol 172:94–97, 2004.

77. Chrouser KL, Lieber MM: Extended and saturation needle biopsy for the diagnosis of prostate cancer. Curr Urol Rep 5:226–230, 2004.

78. Jones JS: Saturation biopsy for detecting and characterizing prostate cancer. BJU Int 99:1340–1344, 2007.

79. Epstein JI, Sanderson H, Carter HB, et al: Utility of saturation biopsy to predict insignificant cancer at radical prostatectomy. Urology 66:356–360, 2005.

80. Terris MK, Hammerer PG, Nickas ME: Comparison of ultrasound imaging in patients undergoing transperineal and transrectal prostate ultrasound. Urology 52:1070–1072, 1998.

81. Shinghal R, Terris MK: Limitations of transperineal ultrasound-guided prostate biopsies. Urology 54:706–708, 1999.

82. Vis AN, Boerma MO, Ciatto S, et al: Detection of prostate cancer: a comparative study of the diagnostic efficacy of sextant transrectal versus sextant transperineal biopsy. Urology 56:617–621, 2000.

83. Emiliozzi P, Corsetti A, Tassi B, et al: Best approach for prostate cancer detection: a prospective study on transperineal versus transrectal six-core prostate biopsy. Urology 61:961–966, 2003.

84. Watanabe M, Hayashi T, Tsushima T, et al: Extensive biopsy using a combined transperineal and transrectal approach to improve prostate cancer detection. Int J Urol 12:959–963, 2005.

85. Kawakami S, Okuno T, Yonese J, et al: Optimal sampling sites for repeat prostate biopsy: a recursive partitioning analysis of three-dimensional 26-core systematic biopsy. Eur Urol 51:675–682; discussion 682–683, 2007.

86. Takenaka A, Hara R, Hyodo Y, et al: Transperineal extended biopsy improves the clinically significant prostate cancer detection rate: a comparative study of 6 and 12 biopsy cores. Int J Urol 13:10–14, 2006.

87. Amiel GE, Slawin KM: Newer modalities of ultrasound imaging and treatment of the prostate. Urol Clin North Am 33:329–337, 2006.

88. Pallwein L, Mitterberger M, Gradl J, et al: Value of contrast-enhanced ultrasound and elastography in imaging of prostate cancer. Curr Opin Urol 17:39–47, 2007.

89. Halpern EJ, Strup SE: Using gray-scale and color and power Doppler sonography to detect prostatic cancer. AJR Am J Roentgenol 174:623–627, 2000.

90. Remzi M, Dobrovits M, Reissigl A, et al: Can Power Doppler enhanced transrectal ultrasound guided biopsy improve prostate cancer detection on first and repeat prostate biopsy? Eur Urol 46:451–456, 2004.

91. Halpern EJ, Ramey JR, Strup SE, et al: Detection of prostate carcinoma with contrast-enhanced sonography using intermittent harmonic imaging. Cancer 104:2373–2383, 2005.

92. Frauscher F, Klauser A, Volgger H, et al: Comparison of contrast enhanced color Doppler targeted biopsy with conventional systematic biopsy: impact on prostate cancer detection. J Urol 167:1648–1652, 2002.

93. Mitterberger M, Pinggera GM, Horninger W, et al: Comparison of contrast enhanced color Doppler targeted biopsy to conventional systematic biopsy: impact on Gleason score. J Urol 178:464–468; discussion 468, 2007.

94. Pelzer A, Bektic J, Berger AP, et al: Prostate cancer detection in men with prostate specific antigen 4 to 10 ng/ml using a combined approach of contrast enhanced color Doppler targeted and systematic biopsy. J Urol 173:1926–1929, 2005.

95. Cooperberg MR, Lubeck DP, Meng MV, et al: The changing face of low-risk prostate cancer: trends in clinical presentation and primary management. J Clin Oncol 22:2141–2149, 2004.

96. Master VA, Chi T, Shariat SF, et al: The independent impact of extended pattern biopsy on prostate cancer stage migration. J Urol 174:1789–1793; discussion 1793, 2005.

97. Boccon-Gibod LM, Dumonceau O, Toublanc M, et al: Microfocal prostate cancer: a comparison of biopsy and radical prostatectomy specimen features. Eur Urol 48:895–899, 2005.

98. Singh H, Canto EI, Shariat SF, et al: Improved detection of clinically significant, curable prostate cancer with systematic 12-core biopsy. J Urol 171:1089–1092, 2004.

99. Meng MV, Elkin EP, DuChane J, et al: Impact of increased number of biopsies on the nature of prostate cancer identified. J Urol 176:63–68; discussion 69, 2006.

100. Boccon-Gibod LM, de Longchamps NB, Toublanc M, et al: Prostate saturation biopsy in the reevaluation of microfocal prostate cancer. J Urol 176:961–963; discussion 963–964, 2006.

101. Elstein AS: Heuristics and biases: selected errors in clinical reasoning. Acad Med 74:791–794, 1999.

102. Vlaev I, Chater N: Game relativity: how context influences strategic decision making. J Exp Psychol Learn Mem Cogn 32:131–149, 2006.

103. Kattan M: Expert systems in medicine. In Smelser NJ, Baltes PB (eds): International Encyclopedia of the Social and Behavioral Sciences. Oxford: Pergamon, 2001, pp 5135–5139.

104. Hogarth RM, Karelaia N: Heuristic and linear models of judgment: matching rules and environments. Psychol Rev 114:733–758, 2007.

105. Kattan MW: Nomograms. Introduction. Semin Urol Oncol 20:79–81, 2002.

106. Rabbani F, Stapleton AM, Kattan MW, et al: Factors predicting recovery of erections after radical prostatectomy. J Urol 164:1929–1934, 2000.

107. Ross PL, Gerigk C, Gonen M, et al: Comparisons of nomograms and urologists' predictions in prostate cancer. Semin Urol Oncol 20:82–88, 2002.

108. Ross PL, Scardino PT, Kattan MW: A catalog of prostate cancer nomograms. J Urol 165:1562–1568, 2001.

109. Kattan MW, Eastham JA, Stapleton AM, et al: A preoperative nomogram for disease recurrence following radical prostatectomy for prostate cancer. J Natl Cancer Inst 90:766–771, 1998.

110. Eastham JA, May R, Robertson JL, et al: Development of a nomogram that predicts the probability of a positive prostate biopsy in men with an abnormal digital rectal examination and a prostate-specific antigen between 0 and 4 ng/mL. Urology 54:709–713, 1999.

111. Garzotto M, Hudson RG, Peters L, et al: Predictive modeling for the presence of prostate carcinoma using clinical, laboratory, and ultrasound parameters in patients with prostate specific antigen levels < or = 10 ng/mL. Cancer 98:1417–1422, 2003.

112. Karakiewicz PI, Benayoun S, Kattan MW, et al: Development and validation of a nomogram predicting the outcome of prostate biopsy based on patient age, digital rectal examination and serum prostate specific antigen. J Urol 173:1930–1934, 2005.

113. Lopez-Corona E, Ohori M, Scardino PT, et al: A nomogram for predicting a positive repeat prostate biopsy in patients with a previous negative biopsy session. J Urol 170:1184–1188; discussion 1188, 2003.

114. Chun FK, Briganti A, Graefen M, et al: Development and external validation of an extended repeat biopsy nomogram. J Urol 177:510–515, 2007.

115. Gleason DF: Classification of prostatic carcinomas. Cancer Chemotherapy Reports—Part 1 50:125–128, 1966.

116. Chan TY, Partin AW, Walsh PC, et al: Prognostic significance of Gleason score 3 + 4 versus Gleason score 4 + 3 tumor at radical prostatectomy. Urology 56:823–827, 2000.

117. Sakr WA, Tefilli MV, Grignon DJ, et al: Gleason score 7 prostate cancer: a heterogeneous entity? Correlation with pathologic parameters and disease-free survival. Urology 56:730–734, 2000.

118. Makarov DV, Sanderson H, Partin AW, et al: Gleason score 7 prostate cancer on needle biopsy: is the prognostic difference in Gleason scores 4 + 3 and 3 + 4 independent of the number of involved cores? J Urol 167:2440–2442, 2002.

119. Khoddami SM, Shariat SF, Lotan Y, et al: Predictive value of primary Gleason pattern 4 in patients with Gleason score 7 tumours treated with radical prostatectomy. BJU Int 94:42–46, 2004.

120. Harnden P, Shelley MD, Coles B, et al: Should the Gleason grading system for prostate cancer be modified to account for high-grade tertiary components? A systematic review and meta-analysis. Lancet Oncol 8:411–419, 2007.

121. Lotan Y, Shariat SF, Khoddami SM, et al: The percent of biopsy cores positive for cancer is a predictor of advanced pathological stage and poor clinical outcomes in patients treated with radical prostatectomy. J Urol 171:2209–2214, 2004.

122. Briganti A, Chun FK, Hutterer GC, et al: Systematic assessment of the ability of the number and percentage of positive biopsy cores to predict pathologic stage and biochemical recurrence after radical prostatectomy. Eur Urol 52:733–745, 2007.

123. Briganti A, Karakiewicz PI, Chun FK, et al: Percentage of positive biopsy cores can improve the ability to predict lymph node invasion in patients undergoing radical prostatectomy and extended pelvic lymph node dissection. Eur Urol 51:1573–1581, 2007.

124. Harnden P, Shelley MD, Clements H, et al: The prognostic significance of perineural invasion in prostatic cancer biopsies: a systematic review. Cancer 109:13–24, 2007.

125. Shariat SF, Khoddami SM, Saboorian H, et al: Lymphovascular invasion is a pathological feature of biologically aggressive disease in patients treated with radical prostatectomy. J Urol 171:1122–1127, 2004.

126. Schoenfield L, Jones JS, Zippe CD, et al: The incidence of high-grade prostatic intraepithelial neoplasia and atypical glands suspicious for carcinoma on first-time saturation needle biopsy, and the subsequent risk of cancer. BJU Int 99:770–774, 2007.

127. Flury SC, Galgano MT, Mills SE, et al: Atypical small acinar proliferation: biopsy artefact or distinct pathological entity? BJU Int 99:780–785, 2007.

128. Mancuso PA, Chabert C, Chin P, et al: Prostate cancer detection in men with an initial diagnosis of atypical small acinar proliferation. BJU Int 99:49–52, 2007.

129. Whitmore WF, Jr: Hormone therapy in prostate cancer. Am J Med 21:697–713, 1956.

130. Jewett HJ: Significance of the palpable prostatic nodule. JAMA 160:838–839, 1956.

131. Roach M, III, Weinberg V, Sandler H, et al: Staging for prostate cancer: time to incorporate pretreatment prostate-specific antigen and Gleason score? Cancer 109:213–220, 2007.

132. Hricak H, Choyke PL, Eberhardt SC, et al: Imaging prostate cancer: a multidisciplinary perspective. Radiology 243:28–53, 2007.

133. Wolf JS, Jr, Cher M, Dall'era M, et al: The use and accuracy of cross-sectional imaging and fine needle aspiration cytology for detection of pelvic lymph node metastases before radical prostatectomy. J Urol 153:993–999, 1995.

134. Bellin MF, Roy C, Kinkel K, et al: Lymph node metastases: safety and effectiveness of MR imaging with ultrasmall superparamagnetic iron oxide particles—initial clinical experience. Radiology 207:799–808, 1998.

135. Harisinghani MG, Barentsz J, Hahn PF, et al: Noninvasive detection of clinically occult lymph-node metastases in prostate cancer. N Engl J Med 348:2491–2499, 2003.

136. Narayan P, Lillian D, Hellstrom W, et al: The benefits of combining early radionuclide renal scintigraphy with routine

bone scans in patients with prostate cancer. J Urol 140:1448–1451, 1988.

137. Chybowski FM, Keller JJ, Bergstralh EJ, et al: Predicting radionuclide bone scan findings in patients with newly diagnosed, untreated prostate cancer: prostate specific antigen is superior to all other clinical parameters. J Urol 145:313–318, 1991.

138. Oesterling JE: Using PSA to eliminate the staging radionuclide bone scan. Significant economic implications. Urol Clin North Am 20:705–711, 1993.

139. Purohit RS, Shinohara K, Meng MV, et al: Imaging clinically localized prostate cancer. Urol Clin North Am 30:279–293, 2003.

140. Tempany CM, Zhou X, Zerhouni EA, et al: Staging of prostate cancer: results of Radiology Diagnostic Oncology Group project comparison of three MR imaging techniques. Radiology 192:47–54, 1994.

141. Polascik TJ, Manyak MJ, Haseman MK, et al: Comparison of clinical staging algorithms and 111indium-capromab pendetide immunoscintigraphy in the prediction of lymph node involvement in high risk prostate carcinoma patients. Cancer 85:1586–1592, 1999.

142. Elgamal AA, Troychak MJ, Murphy GP: ProstaScint scan may enhance identification of prostate cancer recurrences after prostatectomy, radiation, or hormone therapy: analysis of 136 scans of 100 patients. Prostate 37:261–269, 1998.

143. Ponsky LE, Cherullo EE, Starkey R, et al: Evaluation of preoperative ProstaScint scans in the prediction of nodal disease. Prostate Cancer Prostatic Dis 5:132–135, 2002.

144. Hofer C, Kubler H, Hartung R, et al: Diagnosis and monitoring of urological tumors using positron emission tomography. Eur Urol 40:481–487, 2001.

145. Partin AW, Kattan MW, Subong EN, et al: Combination of prostate-specific antigen, clinical stage, and Gleason score to predict pathological stage of localized prostate cancer. A multi-institutional update [see comments] [published erratum appears in JAMA 278:118, 1997]. JAMA 277:1445–1451, 1997.

146. Penson DF, Grossfeld GD, Li YP, et al: How well does the Partin nomogram predict pathological stage after radical prostatectomy in a community based population? Results of the cancer of the prostate strategic urological research endeavor. J Urol 167:1653–1657; discussion 1657–1658, 2002.

147. Augustin H, Eggert T, Wenske S, et al: Comparison of accuracy between the Partin tables of 1997 and 2001 to predict final pathological stage in clinically localized prostate cancer. J Urol 171:177–181, 2004.

148. Makarov DV, Trock BJ, Humphreys EB, et al: Updated nomogram to predict pathologic stage of prostate cancer given prostate-specific antigen level, clinical stage, and biopsy Gleason score (Partin tables) based on cases from 2000 to 2005. Urology 69:1095–1101, 2007.

149. Partin AW, Mangold LA, Lamm DM, et al: Contemporary update of prostate cancer staging nomograms (Partin tables) for the new millennium. Urology 58:843–848, 2001.

150. Ohori M, Kattan MW, Koh H, et al: Predicting the presence and side of extracapsular extension: a nomogram for staging prostate cancer. J Urol 171:1844–1849; discussion 1849, 2004.

151. Steuber T, Graefen M, Haese A, et al: Validation of a nomogram for prediction of side specific extracapsular extension at radical prostatectomy. J Urol 175:939–944; discussion 944, 2006.

152. Graefen M, Haese A, Pichlmeier U, et al: A validated strategy for side specific prediction of organ confined prostate cancer: a tool to select for nerve sparing radical prostatectomy. J Urol 165:857–863, 2001.

153. Koh H, Kattan MW, Scardino PT, et al: A nomogram to predict seminal vesicle invasion by the extent and location of cancer in systematic biopsy results. J Urol 170:1203–1208, 2003.

154. Gallina A, Chun FK, Briganti A, et al: Development and split-sample validation of a nomogram predicting the probability of seminal vesicle invasion at radical prostatectomy. Eur Urol 52:98–105, 2007.

155. Cagiannos I, Karakiewicz P, Eastham JA, et al: A preoperative nomogram identifying decreased risk of positive pelvic lymph nodes in patients with prostate cancer. J Urol 170:1798–1803, 2003.

156. Heidenreich A, Varga Z, Von Knobloch R: Extended pelvic lymphadenectomy in patients undergoing radical prostatec-

tomy: high incidence of lymph node metastasis. J Urol 167:1681–1686, 2002.

157. Bader P, Burkhard FC, Markwalder R, et al: Is a limited lymph node dissection an adequate staging procedure for prostate cancer? J Urol 168:514–518; discussion 518, 2002.

158. Briganti A, Chun FK, Salonia A, et al: Validation of a nomogram predicting the probability of lymph node invasion among patients undergoing radical prostatectomy and an extended pelvic lymphadenectomy. Eur Urol 49:1019–1026; discussion 1026–1027, 2006.

159. Briganti A, Chun FK, Salonia A, et al: A nomogram for staging of exclusive nonobturator lymph node metastases in men with localized prostate cancer. Eur Urol 51:112–119; discussion 119–120, 2007.

160. Johansson JE, Andren O, Andersson SO, et al: Natural history of early, localized prostate cancer. JAMA 291:2713–2719, 2004.

161. Kattan MW, Eastham JA, Wheeler TM, et al: Counseling men with prostate cancer: a nomogram for predicting the presence of small, moderately differentiated, confined tumors. J Urol 170:1792–1797, 2003.

162. Steyerberg EW, Roobol MJ, Kattan MW, et al: Prediction of indolent prostate cancer: validation and updating of a prognostic nomogram. J Urol 177:107–112; discussion 112, 2007.

163. Schroder FH: Prostate cancer: to screen or not to screen? BMJ 306:407–408, 1993.

164. Chun FK, Steuber T, Erbersdobler A, et al: Development and internal validation of a nomogram predicting the probability of prostate cancer Gleason sum upgrading between biopsy and radical prostatectomy pathology. Eur Urol 49:820–826, 2006.

165. Steuber T, Chun FK, Erbersdobler A, et al: Development and internal validation of a preoperative transition zone prostate cancer nomogram. Urology 68:1295–1300, 2006.

166. San Francisco IF, DeWolf WC, Rosen S, et al: Extended prostate needle biopsy improves concordance of Gleason grading between prostate needle biopsy and radical prostatectomy. J Urol 169:136–140, 2003.

167. Mian BM, Lehr DJ, Moore CK, et al: Role of prostate biopsy schemes in accurate prediction of Gleason scores. Urology 67:379–383, 2006.

168. Numao N, Kawakami S, Yokoyama M, et al: Improved accuracy in predicting the presence of Gleason pattern 4/5 prostate cancer by three-dimensional 26-core systematic biopsy. Eur Urol 52:1663–1668, 2007.

169. King CR, Patel DA, Terris MK: Prostate biopsy volume indices do not predict for significant Gleason upgrading. Am J Clin Oncol 28:125–129, 2005.

170. Chun FK, Briganti A, Shariat SF, et al: Significant upgrading affects a third of men diagnosed with prostate cancer: predictive nomogram and internal validation. BJU Int 98:329–334, 2006.

171. Walz J, Graefen M, Chun FK, et al: High incidence of prostate cancer detected by saturation biopsy after previous negative biopsy series. Eur Urol 50:498–505, 2006.

172. Pryor MB, Schellhammer PF: The pursuit of prostate cancer in patients with a rising prostate-specific antigen and multiple negative transrectal ultrasound-guided prostate biopsies. Clin Prostate Cancer 1:172–176, 2002.

173. Fleshner N, Klotz L: Role of "saturation biopsy" in the detection of prostate cancer among difficult diagnostic cases. Urology 60:93–97, 2002.

174. Pinkstaff DM, Igel TC, Petrou SP, et al: Systematic transperineal ultrasound-guided template biopsy of the prostate: three-year experience. Urology 65:735–739, 2005.

175. Bott SR, Henderson A, Halls JE, et al: Extensive transperineal template biopsies of prostate: modified technique and results. Urology 68:1037–1041, 2006.

176. Satoh T, Matsumoto K, Fujita T, et al: Cancer core distribution in patients diagnosed by extended transperineal prostate biopsy. Urology 66:114–118, 2005.

177. Moran BJ, Braccioforte MH, Conterato DJ: Re-biopsy of the prostate using a stereotactic transperineal technique. J Urol 176:1376–1381; discussion 1381, 2006.

178. Goto Y, Ohori M, Arakawa A, et al: Distinguishing clinically important from unimportant prostate cancers before treatment: value of systematic biopsies. J Urol 156:1059–1063, 1996.

179. Carter HB, Epstein JI: Prediction of significant cancer in men with stage T1c adenocarcinoma of the prostate. World J Urol 15:359–363, 1997.
180. Epstein JI, Chan DW, Sokoll LJ, et al: Nonpalpable stage T1c prostate cancer: prediction of insignificant disease using free/total prostate specific antigen levels and needle biopsy findings. J Urol 160:2407–2411, 1998.
181. Ochiai A, Troncoso P, Chen ME, et al: The relationship between tumor volume and the number of positive cores in men undergoing multisite extended biopsy: implication for expectant management. J Urol 174:2164–2168; discussion 2168, 2005.
182. Augustin H, Hammerer PG, Graefen M, et al: Insignificant prostate cancer in radical prostatectomy specimen: time trends and preoperative prediction. Eur Urol 43:455–460, 2003.
183. Chun FK, Briganti A, Graefen M, et al: Development and external validation of an extended 10-core biopsy nomogram. Eur Urol 52:436–445, 2007.
184. Miyake H, Sakai I, Harada K, et al: Prediction of potentially insignificant prostate cancer in men undergoing radical prostatectomy for clinically organ-confined disease. Int J Urol 12:270–274, 2005.
185. Babaian RJ, Fritsche HA, Zhang Z, et al: Evaluation of prostAsure index in the detection of prostate cancer: a preliminary report. Urology 51:132–136, 1998.
186. Virtanen A, Gomari M, Kranse R, et al: Estimation of prostate cancer probability by logistic regression: free and total prostate-specific antigen, digital rectal examination, and heredity are significant variables. Clin Chem 45:987–994, 1999.
187. Finne P, Finne R, Auvinen A, et al: Predicting the outcome of prostate biopsy in screen-positive men by a multilayer perceptron network. Urology 56:418–422, 2000.
188. Horninger W, Bartsch G, Snow PB, et al: The problem of cutoff levels in a screened population: appropriateness of informing screenees about their risk of having prostate carcinoma. Cancer 91:1667–1672, 2001.
189. Kalra P, Togami J, Bansal BSG, et al: A neurocomputational model for prostate carcinoma detection. Cancer 98:1849–1854, 2003.
190. Finne P, Finne R, Bangma C, et al: Algorithms based on prostate-specific antigen (PSA), free PSA, digital rectal examination and prostate volume reduce false-positive PSA results in prostate cancer screening. Int J Cancer 111:310–315, 2004.
191. Suzuki H, Komiya A, Kamiya N, et al: Development of a nomogram to predict probability of positive initial prostate biopsy among Japanese patients. Urology 67:131–136, 2006.
192. Porter CR, Gamito EJ, Crawford ED, et al: Model to predict prostate biopsy outcome in large screening population with independent validation in referral setting. Urology 65:937–941, 2005.
193. Remzi M, Anagnostou T, Ravery V, et al: An artificial neural network to predict the outcome of repeat prostate biopsies. Urology 62:456–460, 2003.
194. Yanke BV, Gonen M, Scardino PT, et al: Validation of a nomogram for predicting positive repeat biopsy for prostate cancer. J Urol 173:421–424, 2005.
195. Snow PB, Smith DS, Catalona WJ: Artificial neural networks in the diagnosis and prognosis of prostate cancer: a pilot study. J Urol 152:1923–1926, 1994.
196. Carlson GD, Calvanese CB, Partin AW: An algorithm combining age, total prostate-specific antigen (PSA), and percent free PSA to predict prostate cancer: results on 4298 cases. Urology 52:455–461, 1998.
197. Djavan B, Remzi M, Zlotta A, et al: Novel artificial neural network for early detection of prostate cancer. J Clin Oncol 20:921–929, 2002.
198. Stephan C, Cammann H, Semjonow A, et al: Multicenter evaluation of an artificial neural network to increase the prostate cancer detection rate and reduce unnecessary biopsies. Clin Chem 48:1279–1287, 2002.
199. Porter CR, O'Donnell C, Crawford ED, et al: Predicting the outcome of prostate biopsy in a racially diverse population: a prospective study. Urology 60:831–835, 2002.
200. Matsui Y, Utsunomiya N, Ichioka K, et al: The use of artificial neural network analysis to improve the predictive accuracy of prostate biopsy in the Japanese population. Jpn J Clin Oncol 34:602–607, 2004.
201. Benecchi L: Neuro-fuzzy system for prostate cancer diagnosis. Urology 68:357–361, 2006.
202. Yanke BV, Carver BS, Bianco FJ, Jr, et al: African-American race is a predictor of prostate cancer detection: incorporation into a pre-biopsy nomogram. BJU Int 98:783–787, 2006.
203. Narayan P, Gajendran V, Taylor SP, et al: The role of transrectal ultrasound-guided biopsy-based staging, preoperative serum prostate-specific antigen, and biopsy Gleason score in prediction of final pathologic diagnosis in prostate cancer. Urology 46:205–212, 1995.
204. Partin AW, Yoo J, Carter HB, et al: The use of prostate specific antigen, clinical stage and Gleason score to predict pathological stage in men with localized prostate cancer [see comments]. J Urol 150:110–114, 1993.
205. Kattan MW, Stapleton AM, Wheeler TM, et al: Evaluation of a nomogram used to predict the pathologic stage of clinically localized prostate carcinoma. Cancer 79:528–537, 1997.
206. Blute ML, Bergstralh EJ, Partin AW, et al: Validation of Partin tables for predicting pathological stage of clinically localized prostate cancer. J Urol 164:1591–1595, 2000.
207. Peller PA, Young DC, Marmaduke DP, et al: Sextant prostate biopsies. A histopathologic correlation with radical prostatectomy specimens. Cancer 75:530–538, 1995.
208. Ackerman DA, Barry JM, Wicklund RA, et al: Analysis of risk factors associated with prostate cancer extension to the surgical margin and pelvic node metastasis at radical prostatectomy. J Urol 150:1845–1850, 1993.
209. Rabbani F, Bastar A, Fair WR: Site specific predictors of positive margins at radical prostatectomy: an argument for risk based modification of technique. J Urol 160:1727–1733, 1998.
210. Bostwick DG, Qian J, Bergstralh E, et al: Prediction of capsular perforation and seminal vesicle invasion in prostate cancer. J Urol 155:1361–1367, 1996.
211. Gamito EJ, Stone NN, Batuello JT, et al: Use of artificial neural networks in the clinical staging of prostate cancer: implications for prostate brachytherapy. Tech Urol 6:60–63, 2000.
212. Gilliland FD, Hoffman RM, Hamilton A, et al: Predicting extracapsular extension of prostate cancer in men treated with radical prostatectomy: results from the population based prostate cancer outcomes study. J Urol 162:1341–1345, 1999.
213. Badalament RA, Miller MC, Peller PA, et al: An algorithm for predicting nonorgan confined prostate cancer using the results obtained from sextant core biopsies with prostate specific antigen level. J Urol 156:1375–1380, 1996.
214. Pisansky TM, Blute ML, Suman VJ, et al: Correlation of pre-therapy prostate cancer characteristics with seminal vesicle invasion in radical prostatectomy specimens. Int J Radiat Oncol Biol Phys 36:585–591, 1996.
215. Baccala A, Jr, Reuther AM, Bianco FJ, Jr, et al: Complete resection of seminal vesicles at radical prostatectomy results in substantial long-term disease-free survival: multi-institutional study of 6740 patients. Urology 69:536–540, 2007.
216. Bluestein DL, Bostwick DG, Bergstralh EJ, et al: Eliminating the need for bilateral pelvic lymphadenectomy in select patients with prostate cancer. J Urol 151:1315–1320, 1994.
217. Batuello JT, Gamito EJ, Crawford ED, et al: Artificial neural network model for the assessment of lymph node spread in patients with clinically localized prostate cancer. Urology 57:481–485, 2001.
218. Roach M, 3rd, Marquez C, Yuo HS, et al: Predicting the risk of lymph node involvement using the pre-treatment prostate specific antigen and Gleason score in men with clinically localized prostate cancer. Int J Radiat Oncol Biol Phys 28:33–37, 1994.
219. Briganti A, Chun FK, Salonia A, et al: Validation of a nomogram predicting the probability of lymph node invasion based on the extent of pelvic lymphadenectomy in patients with clinically localized prostate cancer. BJU Int 98:788–793, 2006.
220. King CR, McNeal JE, Gill H, et al: Extended prostate biopsy scheme improves reliability of Gleason grading: implications for radiotherapy patients. Int J Radiat Oncol Biol Phys 59:386–391, 2004.
221. Emiliozzi P, Maymone S, Paterno A, et al: Increased accuracy of biopsy Gleason score obtained by extended needle biopsy. J Urol 172:2224–2226, 2004.
222. Coogan CL, Latchamsetty KC, Greenfield J, et al: Increasing the number of biopsy cores improves the concordance of biopsy

Gleason score to prostatectomy Gleason score. BJU Int 96:324–327, 2005.

223. Elabbady AA, Khedr MM: Extended 12-core prostate biopsy increases both the detection of prostate cancer and the accuracy of Gleason score. Eur Urol 49:49–53; discussion 53, 2006.

224. Amis ES, Jr, Bigongiari LH, Bluth EI, et al: Pretreatment staging of clinically localized prostate cancer. Radiology 215(S):703–708, 2000.

225. Carroll P, Coley C, McLeod D, et al: Prostate-specific antigen best practice policy. II. Prostate cancer staging and post-treatment follow-up. Urology 57:225–229, 2001.

226. Green FL, Page DL, Fleming ID, et al (eds): AJCC Cancer Staging Manual. New York: Springer-Verlag, 2002.

227. Thompson IM, Ankerst DP, Chi C, et al: Assessing prostate cancer risk: results from the Prostate Cancer Prevention Trial. J Natl Cancer Inst 98:529, 2006.

3

The Pathology of Prostate Cancer

Liang Cheng, Roberta Mazzucchelli, Timothy D. Jones, Antonio Lopez-Beltran, and Rodolfo Montironi

KEY POINTS

- Accurate pathologic evaluation of prostate biopsy and radical prostatectomy specimens is critical for patient management.
- A wealth of clinically important information may be gleaned from even the smallest tissue specimens of the prostate, such as from needle biopsies.
- Both pathologists and urologists should be aware of morphologic diversity and histologic variants of prostate cancer, treatment effect, and their prognostic implications.
- This chapter also provides a comprehensive review of prostate cancer pathology, high-grade prostatic intraepithelial neoplasia (HGPIN), and "atypical small acinar proliferation [ASAP] suspicious for but not diagnostic of malignancy."

Introduction

The incidence of prostate cancer has tripled during the past decade mainly because of increased detection secondary to the widespread use of serum prostate-specific antigen (PSA) testing, digital rectal examination, and transrectal ultrasound. Needle biopsy of the prostate plays a central role in the morphologic and clinical evaluation of prostate cancer.[1-3] The increase in prostate cancer detection has induced a sharp increase in the number of radical prostatectomies. The pathologist has an important and challenging task in evaluating tissue specimens for the presence or absence of lesions such as cancer and its well-known precursor high-grade prostatic intraepithelial neoplasia (HGPIN).[4,5] In difficult cases in which a definite diagnosis of cancer may not be feasible, a term indicating diagnostic uncertainty needs to be used.[6]

Substantial effort has been expended in recent years in describing available clinical and

pathologic factors and determining whether such factors may be used for staging or for predicting patient outcome.[7] Clinically important information may be gleaned from even the smallest tissue specimens of the prostate, as from needle biopsies. This includes information regarding the histologic type of prostate cancer, the Gleason score, the extent of involvement by tumor, the location and distribution of tumor, and the presence or absence of local invasion (extraprostatic extension and seminal vesicle involvement), perineural invasion, and lymphovascular invasion.[3,8-14] Molecular analyses of prostate cancer may eventually generate knowledge which improves prognostication.[3,15-26]

Diagnostic Criteria for Prostate Cancer

Most clinically palpable prostate cancers that are diagnosed on needle biopsy are located predominantly in the posterior and posterolateral prostate.[27,28] Less commonly, large transition zone tumors may extend into the peripheral zone and become palpable. Cancers detected on transurethral resection of the prostate (TURP) are predominantly located within the transition zone. Nonpalpable cancers detected on needle biopsy are most often located peripherally, although 15% to 25% have tumor predominantly within the transition zone.[29] Large tumors may extend into the central zone, although cancers do not commonly arise in this region. Multifocal adenocarcinoma of the prostate is present in more than 85% of radical prostatectomy specimens from prostate cancer patients.[25,30-33] In countries with widespread PSA testing, grossly evident prostate cancer has become relatively uncommon. Grossly evident

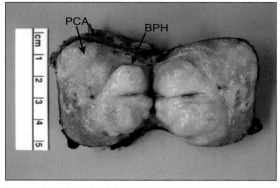

Figure 3-1. Grossly visible prostatic cancer (PCA) is typically located in the peripheral zone, whereas benign prostatic hyperplasia (BPH) shows transitional zone location.

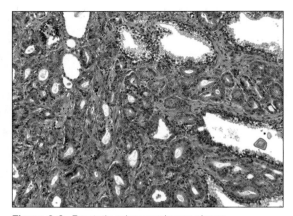

Figure 3-2. Prostatic adenocarcinoma shows architectural distortion and variation in acinar size.

cancers are firm and solid and range in color from white-gray to yellow-orange, with the latter having increased concentrations of cytoplasmic lipid. The tumors contrast with the adjacent benign parenchyma, which is typically tan and spongy (Fig. 3-1).

Morphology of Untreated Prostate Cancer

The diagnosis of carcinoma relies on a combination of architectural and cytologic findings. The light microscopic features are usually sufficient, but cases with small suspicious foci may benefit from immunohistochemical studies. Causes of false-positive diagnoses include but are not limited to atrophy, basal cell hyperplasia, postatrophic hyperplasia, inadequate sample preparation, treatment effect, inflammation, and other benign mimickers such as seminal vesicles/ejaculatory ducts, Cowper's gland, paraganglion, and verumontanum mucosal glands.[34]

Architectural Features

Architectural features are usually assessed at low- to medium-power magnification, with emphasis on spacing, size, and shape of acini (Fig. 3-2). The arrangement of the acini is diagnostically useful, providing the basis of the Gleason grade. Malignant acini usually have an irregular, haphazard arrangement and are found randomly scattered in the stroma as clusters or isolates. The spacing between malignant acini varies widely. Variation in acinar size is a useful criterion for cancer, particularly when small, irregular, abortive acini with primitive lumina

are seen at the periphery of a focus of well-differentiated carcinoma.

The acini in suspicious foci are usually small or medium-sized with irregular contours that contrast with the typically smooth and round to elongated contours of benign and hyperplastic acini. Comparison with the adjacent benign prostatic acini is always of value in the diagnosis of cancer. Well-differentiated carcinoma and the large acinar variant of Gleason grade 3 carcinoma are particularly difficult to separate from benign acini in needle biopsies because of the uniform size and spacing of acini. In such cases, greater emphasis is placed on cytologic features, immunohistochemical findings, and the presence of smaller diagnostic acini at the edge of the focus.

Although an intact basal cell layer is present along the periphery of benign acini, it is absent in prostate cancer (Fig. 3-3). This important diagnostic feature is not always easy to evaluate in routine hematoxylin-and-eosin–stained (H&E) tissue sections owing to false-negative findings with atrophy and other conditions that can mimic the appearance of cancer. Compressed stromal fibroblasts may mimic basal cells but are usually seen only focally at the periphery of acini. Small foci of adenocarcinoma sometimes cluster around or infiltrate larger benign acini that have an intact basal cell layer, further compounding diagnostic difficulties.

Cytologic Features

The cytologic features of adenocarcinoma include nuclear and nucleolar enlargement, which occurs in most malignant cells.

"Prominent" nucleoli are the cytologic hallmark of prostatic adenocarcinoma (Fig. 3-4A). Every cell has a nucleolus, so prominent nucleoli (at least 1.50 μm in diameter or larger) are sought. Pathologists do not routinely measure nucleoli

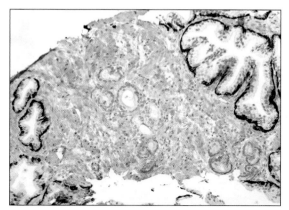

Figure 3-3. The lack of basal cell layer is the hallmark of prostate cancer, which is best highlighted by immunostaining with high-molecular-weight cytokeratin 34βE12.

for diagnosis; this determination is based on comparison with benign epithelial cells elsewhere in the specimen.

Artifacts can and often do obscure the nuclei and nucleoli. Overstaining of nuclei by hematoxylin creates one of the most common difficulties in the interpretation of suspicious cells. Differences in the preparation of biopsy specimens influence nuclear size and chromasia, so comparison with normal cells from the same specimen is useful as an internal control. Many pathologists prefer pale-staining with eosin, but this approach fails to accentuate nucleoli, which are often enlarged. In specimens with nuclear hyperchromasia and pale eosinophilic staining, pathologists often increase the light intensity and magnification to examine suggestive foci for hidden enlarged nucleoli.

Luminal Findings

Crystalloids are sharp, needle-like eosinophilic structures that are often present in the lumina

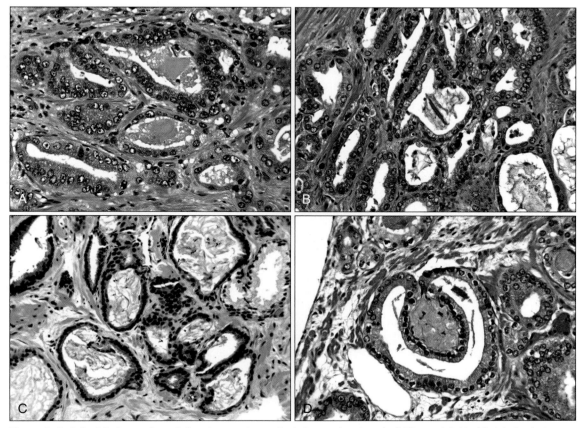

Figure 3-4. Salient features of prostatic adenocarcinoma include prominent nucleoli (**A**), crystalloids (**B**), intraluminal mucins (**C**), and collagenous nodules (**D**).

of well- and moderately differentiated carcinoma[35] (Fig. 3-4B) They are not specific for carcinoma and can be found in other conditions. The presence of crystalloids in metastatic adenocarcinoma of unknown site of origin is strong presumptive evidence of prostatic origin, although it is an uncommon finding and not conclusive.[36] Special stains highlight crystalloids, which otherwise cannot be seen by light microscopy.[36] Crystalloids stain red with a trichrome stain, blue with a toluidine blue stain and violet with the Mallory's staining and appear argyrophilic with silver stain methods. Crystalloids do not stain with periodic acid-Schiff (PAS), Alcian blue, Prussian blue, Congo red, or with immunohistochemical stains for PSA and prostatic acid phosphatase (PAP). The mechanism of crystalloid formation remains unknown, but crystalloids probably result from abnormal protein and mineral metabolism within benign and malignant acini.

Ultrastructurally, crystalloids are composed of electron-dense material that lacks the periodicity of crystals. Radiographic microanalysis reveals abundant portions of sulfur, calcium, and phosphorus, and a small amount of sodium.[35] Hard proteinaceous secretions are almost always present in adjacent acini and are probably the source of the crystalloids.

Luminal acidic sulfated and nonsulfated mucin is often seen in acini of adenocarcinoma, appearing as amorphous or delicate, threadlike, faintly basophilic secretions in routine sections (Fig. 3-4C). This mucin stains with Alcian blue and is best displayed at pH 2.5, whereas normal prostatic epithelium contains periodic acid-Schiff–reactive mucin that is neutral. Acidic mucin is not specific for carcinoma; it may be found in prostatic intraepithelial neoplasia (PIN), in atypical adenomatous hyperplasia, in sclerosing adenosis, and, rarely, in nodular hyperplasia.[37]

Occasionally, prostatic adenocarcinoma may possess intraluminal corpora amylacea. These are much more often seen in normal ducts and acini, in atypical adenomatous hyperplasia, and in verumontanum mucosal gland hyperplasia.

Stromal Findings

The stroma in cancer frequently contains young collagen, which appears lightly eosinophilic, although desmoplasia may be prominent. Muscle fibers in the stroma are sometimes split or distorted. However, this is a difficult feature to appreciate and cannot be relied on because of the resemblance to the stroma associated with benign acini.

Collagenous micronodules (or mucinous fibroplasia) (see Fig. 3-4D) are a specific but uncommon and incidental finding in prostatic adenocarcinoma—present in 0.6% of needle biopsies and 12.7% of prostatectomies. These micronodules consist of microscopic nodular masses of paucicellular eosinophilic fibrillar stroma that impinge on acinar lumina.[38] They are usually present in mucin-producing adenocarcinomas as a result of extravasation of acidic mucin into the stroma. Collagenous micronodules are not observed in benign epithelium, in nodular hyperplasia, or in PIN. Their presence may be particularly valuable in challenging needle biopsy specimens.[38]

Immunohistochemical Findings

The most important immunohistochemical markers in prostate pathology are PSA, PAP, high-molecular-weight keratin (34βE12), p63, and α-methylacyl coenzyme A racemase (AMACR). Promising new markers include prostate-specific membrane antigen (PSMA) and human glandular kallikrein 2 (hK2).[39] A useful panel of immunohistochemical stains to demonstrate a urothelial origin for a poorly differentiated carcinoma in the prostate consists of the combination of cytokeratin 7, cytokeratin 20, and thrombomodulin.

Immunohistochemical expression of PSA is useful for differentiating high-grade prostate cancer from urothelial carcinoma, colonic carcinoma, granulomatous prostatitis, and lymphoma. PSA also facilitates the identification of the site of tumor origin in metastatic adenocarcinoma. This marker can be detected in frozen sections, paraffin-embedded tissue, cellular smears, and cytologic preparations of normal and neoplastic prostatic epithelium. Staining is invariably heterogeneous. Microwave antigen retrieval is usually not necessary, even in tissues that have been immersed in formalin for years. Formalin fixation is optimal for localization of PSA, and variation in staining intensity is only partially the result of fixation and embedding effects. Immunoreactivity is preserved in decalcified specimens and may even be enhanced.

Immunohistochemical expression of PAP may also be of use in establishing a prostatic origin for a primary or metastatic adenocarcinoma.

In diagnostically difficult cases, use of monoclonal antibodies directed against high-molecular-weight cytokeratin (e.g., clone 34βE12) may be useful for the detection of retention or loss of the basal cell layer in small suspicious foci of atypical glands. This tactic is used infrequently (in less than 5% of cases), however, and only as an adjunct to the light microscopic findings. The immunohistochemical staining results should not, by themselves, be the basis for a diagnosis of malignancy, particularly in small suggestive foci. Its value lies in the ability to confirm the benign nature of a suggestive focus by showing an immunoreactive basal cell layer. Anti–keratin 34βE12 stains nearly all of the normal basal cells of the prostate; no staining occurs in the secretory and stromal cells.

A uniform absence of a basal cell layer in prostatic acinar proliferations is one of the most important diagnostic features of invasive carcinoma. Because basal cells may be unapparent by H&E stain, basal cell–specific immunostains may help to distinguish invasive prostatic adenocarcinoma from atypical, benign small acini, which can mimic cancer. Unlike prostatic carcinoma, these mimickers, such as glandular atrophy, post-atrophic hyperplasia, atypical adenomatous hyperplasia, sclerosing adenosis (atypical adenomatous hyperplasia), and radiation-induced atypia, all retain their basal cell layer.[34,40,41] Because the basal cell layer may be interrupted or not demonstrable in small numbers of benign glands, the complete absence of a basal cell layer in a small focus of acini cannot be used alone as a definitive criterion for malignancy. Rather, the absence of a basal cell layer is supportive of invasive carcinoma only in acinar proliferations that exhibit suspicious cytologic and/or architectural features on H&E staining.[40] Conversely, some early invasive prostatic carcinomas, such as microinvasive carcinomas arising in association with or independent of high-grade PIN, may have residual basal cells.[42] Intraductal spread of invasive carcinoma and entrapped benign glands are other proposed explanations for residual basal cells. Rare cases of prostatic adenocarcinoma contain sparse neoplastic glandular cells, which are immunoreactive for 34βE12, yet are not in a basal cell distribution.[43] The use of antibodies for 34βE12 is especially helpful for the diagnosis of deceptively benign-appearing variants of prostate cancer. Immunohistochemistry for cytokeratins 7 and 20 have a limited diagnostic use in prostate pathology with the exception that negative staining for both markers, which can occur in prostate adenocarcinoma, would be unusual for transitional cell (urothelial) carcinoma.[44]

A nuclear protein, p63, encoded by a gene on chromosome 3q27–29 with homology to p53 (a tumor suppressor gene), has been shown to regulate growth and development in epithelium of the skin, cervix, breast, and urogenital tract. Specific isotypes are expressed in basal cells of stratified and pseudostratified epithelia (prostate, bronchial), reserve cells of simple columnar epithelia (endocervical, pancreatic ductal), myoepithelial cells (breast, salivary glands, cutaneous apocrine/eccrine glands), urothelium, and squamous epithelium.[45] A monoclonal antibody is effective for immunohistochemistry when testing paraffin-embedded tissue following antigen retrieval. p63 has applications similar to those of high-molecular-weight cytokeratins in the diagnosis of prostatic adenocarcinoma, but with advantages such as:

- p63 stains a subset of 34βE12-negative basal cells.
- p63 is less susceptible to the staining variability of 34βE12 (particularly in TURP specimens with cautery artifact).
- p63 is easier to interpret because of its strong nuclear staining and low background intensity.

The same interpretative limitations seen with immunostaining for high-molecular weight cytokeratin (34βE12) in small atypical foci also apply to the interpretation of p63 immunohistochemistry. A correlation with morphology, both architectural and cytologic, is required.[43] Prostatic adenocarcinomas have occasional p63-immunoreactive cells, most representing entrapped benign glands or intraductal spread of carcinoma with residual basal cells.[45]

α-Methylacyl CoA Racemase (AMACR)

mRNA was recently identified as being overexpressed in prostatic adenocarcinoma by cDNA library subtraction using high-throughput RNA microarray analysis.[46] This mRNA was found to encode a racemase protein, for which polyclonal and monoclonal antibodies have been produced. These antibodies are suitable for immunohistochemical analysis because they are reactive in formalin-fixed, paraffin-embedded tissue.[47-50] Immunohistochemical studies on biopsy material with an antibody directed against AMACR (P504S) demonstrate reactivity with over 80% of prostatic adenocarcinomas.[51] Certain subtypes of prostate cancer, such as foamy gland carcinoma, atrophic carcinoma, pseudohyperplastic, and treated carcinoma show lower AMACR expression.[50,52] However, AMACR expression is not specific for prostate cancer and may be present in nodular hyperplasia (12%), atrophic glands (36%), HGPIN (over 90%),[49] and atypical adenomatous hyperplasia (17.5%).[53] AMACR immunostaining may be used as a confirmatory stain for prostatic adenocarcinoma in conjunction with H&E morphology and a basal cell–specific marker.[49] AMACR is expressed in other non-prostatic neoplasms, including urothelial and colon cancer.

An immunohistochemical cocktail containing monoclonal antibodies to cytokeratin 34βE12 and p63 is an effective basal cell stain. A combination containing antibodies against 34βE12, p63, and AMACR is also used in clinical practice (Fig. 3-5).

In 5% to 10% of prostatic carcinomas, there are zones with a large number of single or clustered neuroendocrine cells detected by chromogranin A immunostaining.[54-61] A subset of these neuroendocrine cells may also be serotonin-positive. Immunostaining for neuron-specific enolase (NSE), synaptophysin, bombesin/

gastrin-releasing peptide, and a variety of other neuroendocrine peptides may also occur in individual neoplastic neuroendocrine cells. In addition, a diffuse pattern[62] of receptors for serotonin[63] and neuroendocrine peptides[64,65] may be present. The prognostic significance of focal neuroendocrine differentiation in primary, untreated prostatic carcinoma is controversial. In advanced prostate cancer, especially androgen-independent cancer, focal neuroendocrine differentiation portends a poor prognosis[66-69] and may be a therapeutic target.[70-72]

Gleason Grading of Prostate Cancer

The Gleason grading system for prostate cancer, named after Donald F. Gleason, is the predominant grading system used around the world.[73-76] The Gleason grading system is based on glandular architecture, which can be divided into five patterns of growth (also known as grades) with different levels of differentiation. The primary and secondary pattern or grade, that is, the most prevalent and the second most prevalent pattern or grade, are added to obtain a Gleason score or sum that is to be reported.[73,77] Nuclear atypia or cytoplasmic features are not evaluated. It is important that the initial grading of prostate carcinoma be performed at low magnification. Then, one may proceed with high-power objectives to look for rare fused glands or a few individual cells. Gleason grading of prostate cancer has changed over the years in an effort to incorporate new understandings of some features of prostate cancer and to adapt to the widespread use of needle biopsies, which were unavailable at the time that Gleason originally proposed his system.

Gleason Patterns (Fig. 3-6)

- Gleason pattern 1 (Fig. 3-6A)—very well-circumscribed nodule of separate, closely packed glands that do not infiltrate into adjacent benign prostatic tissue. The glands are of intermediate size and approximately equal in size and shape. The nucleus is typically small and cytoplasm frequently is abundant and pale-staining. Nuclear and cytoplasm appearance is not taken into account in diagnosis. This pattern is exceedingly rare and usually seen in transition zone cancers.
- Gleason pattern 2 (Fig. 3-6B)—round-to-oval glands with smooth ends. The glands are more

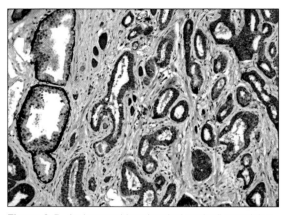

Figure 3-5. An immunohistochemical cocktail containing antibodies against high–molecular-weight cytokeratin 34βE12, p63, and α-methylacyl CoA racemase (AMACR) is useful in the diagnosis of prostate cancer.

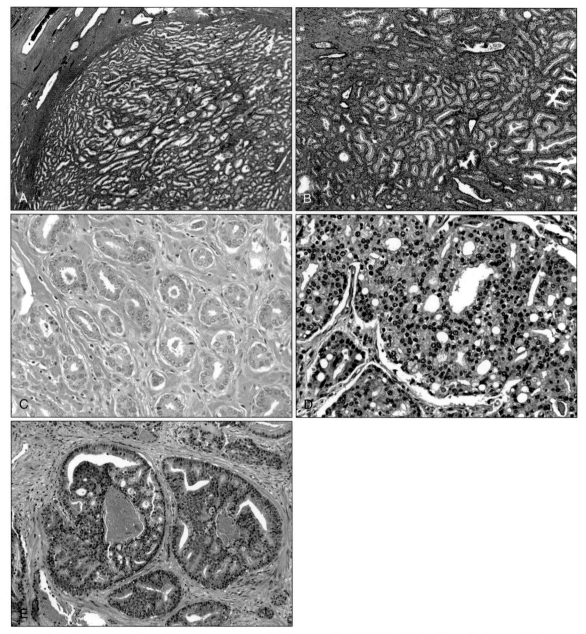

Figure 3-6. Gleason grading of prostate cancer.   A, Gleason pattern 1 is characterized by well-circumscribed nodule composed of uniformly sized glands. **B,** The malignant glands in Gleason pattern 2 show more variation in size and shape. **C,** Malignant glands in Gleason pattern 3 are infiltrative, variable in size and shape, and often angular. **D,** Malignant glands in Gleason pattern 4 are often fused, cribriform. **E,** Comedonecrosis is present in Gleason pattern 5 glands.

loosely arranged and not as uniform in size and shape as those of Gleason pattern 1. There may be minimal invasion by neoplastic glands into the surrounding non-neoplastic prostatic tissue. The glands are of intermediate size and larger than those in Gleason pattern 1. The variation in glandular size and separation between glands is less than that seen in pattern 3. Although not evaluated in Gleason grading, the cytoplasm of Gleason pattern 2 cancers is abundant and pale-staining. Gleason pattern 2 is usually seen in transition zone cancers but may occasionally be found in the peripheral zone.

■ Gleason pattern 3 (Fig. 3-6C)—the most common pattern, but morphologically heterogeneous. The glands are infiltrative and the distance between them is more variable than in patterns 1 and 2. Malignant glands often infiltrate between adjacent non-neoplastic glands. The glands of pattern 3 vary in size and shape and are often angular. Small glands are typical for pattern 3, but there may also be large and irregular. Each gland has an open lumen and is circumscribed by stroma. Cribriform pattern 3 is rare and difficult to distinguish morphologically from cribriform HGPIN, which shows the presence of basal cells. These cells are lacking in cribriform pattern 3 prostate cancer. This heterogeneous expression of Gleason grade 3 raised an initial subdivision in patterns A, B, and C, respectively.

■ Gleason pattern 4 (Fig. 3-6D)—fused, cribriform, or poorly defined and small-appearing glands. Fused glands are composed of a group of glands that are no longer completely separated by stroma. The edge of a group of fused glands is scalloped, and there are occasional thin strands of connective tissue within this group. The hypernephroid pattern described by Gleason is a rare variant of fused glands with clear or very pale-staining cytoplasm. Cribriform pattern 4 glands are large, or they may be irregular with jagged edges. In contrast to fused glands, there are no strands of stroma within a cribriform gland. Most cribriform invasive cancers should be assigned a pattern 4 rather than pattern 3. Poorly defined glands do not have a lumen that is completely encircled by epithelium.

■ Gleason pattern 5 (Fig. 3-6E)—almost complete loss of glandular lumina, which are only occasionally present. The epithelium forms solid sheets, solid strands, or single cells invading the stroma; comedonecrosis may be present. Care must be applied when assigning a Gleason pattern 4 or 5 to limited cancer on needle biopsy to exclude an artifact of tangential sectioning of lower-grade cancer.

Gleason Scores in Prostate Needle Biopsies

Gleason Score 2–4. The diagnosis of Gleason score 2–4 on needle biopsies should be made "rarely, if ever," and the reasons are compelling[78]: (1) Gleason score 2–4 cancer is extraordinarily rare in needle biopsies compared with transurethral resection specimens; (2) there is poor reproducibility, as found among experts[79–81]; (3) the correlation with the prostatectomy score is poor; and (4) a low score of Gleason 2–4 may misguide clinician into believing that there is an indolent tumor.[82] A recent consensus stated that a Gleason score of $1 + 1 = 2$ is a grade that should not be diagnosed, regardless of the type of specimen, with extremely rare exceptions. It is believed that most of these cases diagnosed in the era of Gleason would today be referred to as adenosis (atypical adenomatous hyperplasia) because of improved techniques for the recognition of basal cells.[78,83,84] Cribriform morphology is not allowed within Gleason pattern 2.[85]

Gleason Pattern 3. Gleason pattern 3 tumors consist of variably sized individual glands. Although most cribriform-pattern tumors should be diagnosed as Gleason pattern 4, rare cribriform lesions may be classified as pattern 3.[75,85,86] These rare cribriform pattern 3 tumors consist of round, well-circumscribed glands of the same size as normal glands. "Individual cells" would not be allowed within Gleason pattern 3.

Gleason Pattern 4 in Gleason Score 7 Tumors. Gleason pattern 4 tumors consist of fused glandular masses and most cribriform lesions. The importance of determining the percentage of Gleason 4 pattern in Gleason score 7 tumors is rapidly becoming apparent.[78,86,87] In recently generated nomograms, patients with Gleason score $4 + 3$ versus $3 + 4$ are stratified differently.[88] Whether or not the percentage of pattern 4 tumors should be included in the report remains optional at the present time. Small, ill-defined glands with poorly formed glandular lumina also warrant the diagnosis of Gleason pattern 4, as stated by a recent consensus.[78]

Gleason Pattern 5. Comedonecrosis, when seen in solid nests or cribriform masses, should be regarded as Gleason pattern 5. However, the definition of comedonecrosis requires intraluminal necrotic cells and/or nuclear debris (karyorrhexis).[78]

Tertiary Pattern. Another important change recently incorporated in current practice is the recognition and reporting of the tertiary pattern in needle biopsies. This includes tumors with patterns 3, 4, and 5 in various proportions on a biopsy. Tertiary patterns are uncommon, but when the worst Gleason grade is the tertiary pattern, it should influence the final Gleason score. Therefore, the primary pattern and the highest grade should be recorded following the rule of "the most and the worst."[78] For example, a case with primary Gleason pattern 3, secondary pattern 4, and tertiary pattern 5 should be assigned a Gleason score of 8. These tumors should be classified overall as high grade (Gleason score 8–10).[89,90]

Needle Biopsy with Different Cores Showing Different Grades. This phenomenon occurs when one or more of the cores show pure high-grade cancer (i.e., Gleason score 4 + 4 = 8) and the other cores show pattern 3 (3 + 3, 3 + 4 or 4 + 3) cancer. If one reports the grades of each core separately, the highest-grade tumor (Gleason score 8) would typically be the one selected by the clinician as the grade of the entire case. Others give instead an overall score for the entire case. For example, in a case with Gleason score 4 + 4 = 8 on one core and pattern 3 (3 + 3 = 6, 3 + 4 = 7, 4 + 3 = 7) on other cores, the overall score for the entire case would be Gleason score 4 + 3 = 7 or 3 + 4 = 7, depending on whether pattern 4 or 3 predominated. It has been demonstrated that when one core is Gleason score 4 + 4 = 8 with other cores having pattern 3, the pathologic stage at radical prostatectomy is comparable to cases with all needle cores having Gleason score 4 + 4 = 8.[2,76,78,86,91,92] Thus, the use of the highest core grade in cases where there are multiple cores of different grades is advocated; this provides additional support for the practice of giving cores a separate grade rather than an overall score for the entire case.[78,93] A recent survey concluded that 81% of urologists used the highest Gleason score on a positive biopsy to determine treatment, regardless of the overall percentage of involvement.[94] Consequently, it has been recommended to assign individual Gleason scores to separate cores as long as the cores are submitted in separate containers, or in the same container but specified by the urologist as to their location (i.e., by different colors of ink). In addition, one has the option to also give an overall score at the end of the case.[87,95]

When a container contains multiple pieces of tissue and it cannot be determined whether the core is intact, it is recommended to only give an overall score for that container.[78]

Gleason Scores in Radical Prostatectomy Specimens

In specimens from tumors in radical prostatectomy, one should assign the Gleason score based on the primary and secondary patterns with a comment on the tertiary pattern, if present.[2,78,86]

Gleason Scores 2–4. Gleason scores 2–4 are rarely seen as the grade of the main tumor in radical prostatectomies performed for stages T1c or T2 disease. These tumors are typically seen as incidental foci of tumor in patients with multifocal adenocarcinomas of the prostate and within the transition zone in TURP specimens.[78,83,86] The situation in which Gleason scores 2–4 tumor represents the major tumor at radical prostatectomy, performed after incidentally finding carcinoma upon TURP (stages T1a and T1b), is uncommon. In one study, Gleason score 2–4 was the grade of the main tumor in 2% of radical prostatectomy specimens; this represents a disproportionate number of T1a and T1b tumors compared with what is seen in today's practice. All men with Gleason scores 2–4 tumor at radical prostatectomy are considered surgically cured.[78,86]

Gleason Scores 5–6. It is important to recognize that most tumors with Gleason scores 5–6 are cured after radical prostatectomy.[78,96]

Gleason Score 7. Patients whose tumors have a Gleason score of 7 have a significantly worse prognosis than those with a Gleason score of 6. Given the adverse prognosis associated with Gleason pattern 4, one would expect that whether a tumor is Gleason score 3 + 4 or 4 + 3 would influence prognosis.[96] Several studies addressing Gleason score 3 + 4 were compared with Gleason score 4 + 3 at radical prostatectomy with somewhat conflicting results.[3,88,97,98] Most investigations have shown that Gleason score 4 + 3 presents a worse prognosis.

Gleason Scores 8–10. Gleason scores 8–10 may account for only 7% of the grades seen at radical prostatectomy, but patients with these Gleason scores have highly aggressive tumors at such an advanced stage that they are not amenable to surgical therapy alone. Overall, patients with Gleason scores 8–10 at radical prostatectomy have a 15% chance of having no evidence of disease at 15 years after surgery.[95,96]

Percent Gleason Pattern 4/5. The percentage of high-grade tumor (i.e., the combined percentage of Gleason pattern 4/5) has been proposed as the preferred method for grading prostate cancer because this value is predictive of disease progression.[99] It has recently been demonstrated that classifying tumors based on the combined percent of pattern 4/5 is more predictive than stratifying patients into Gleason score alone. Therefore, it is recommended that this percentage be included in the surgical pathology report.[9,14]

Tertiary Gleason Pattern. In contrast to needle biopsies, a higher percentage of radical prostatectomies contain more than two grades, and over 50% of them contain at least three grades.[30] The progression rates of Gleason scores 5–6 tumors with a tertiary component of Gleason pattern 4 are almost the same as those of pure Gleason score 7 tumors. Patients with Gleason score 7 tumors with a tertiary pattern 5 experience progression rates after radical prostatectomy approximating those with pure Gleason 8 tumors.[89] On the other hand, there appears to be no such significance to a tertiary pattern 5 in cases of Gleason 4 + 4 = 8 tumors. Because Gleason score 8 tumors are already aggressive, the existence of pattern 5 elements adds no additional adverse properties. Prostate cancers in radical prostatectomy specimens should be graded routinely (primary and secondary patterns) with a comment in the report noting the presence of a tertiary element.[9,14,30,98] In the setting of high-grade cancer (score 8–10), one should ignore lower-grade patterns if they occupy less than 5% of the area of the tumor.[87,100]

Tumors with One Predominant Pattern and a Small Percentage of Higher-Grade Tumor. Some controversy still exists regarding how to grade tumors in which a single low-grade pattern constitutes more than 95% of the tumor, with only a very small percentage of higher-grade tumor. For example, for a tumor composed of more than 95% Gleason pattern 3 and less than 5% pattern 4, some experts would assign a

Gleason score 3 + 3 = 6, since it has been proposed that over 5% of a pattern should be present for it to be incorporated within the Gleason score. Others might grade the tumor as Gleason score 3 + 4 = 7. A high-grade component, even if it constitutes less than 5% of the whole tumor, seems to have a significant adverse influence.[78,82]

Radical Prostatectomy Specimens with Separate Tumor Nodules. It has been recommended that radical prostatectomy specimens be processed in an organized fashion whereby assessment can be made as to whether one is dealing with a dominant nodule or separate tumor nodules.[87] Some suggest that a separate grade be assigned to each dominant tumor nodule(s). Most often, the dominant nodule is the largest tumor, which is also the tumor associated with the highest stage and the highest grade.[30]

Correlation between Needle Biopsy and Radical Prostatectomy Gleason Scores. Several studies address the correlation between Gleason scores in needle biopsies and the corresponding radical prostatectomy specimens.[77,93] Although earlier studies used thicker (14-gauge) needle biopsies,[101,102] more recent series are based on thin-core (18-gauge) needles used in conjunction with biopsy guns attached to transrectal ultrasound. Sextant or other modes of systematic sampling are typically performed in more current series. In a recent compilation of data from 3789 patients from 18 studies, exact correlation of Gleason scores was found in 43% of cases and correlation plus or minus 1 Gleason core unit was seen in 77% of cases.[103] Undergrading of carcinoma in needle biopsy is the most common problem, occurring in 42% of all reviewed cases. Overgrading of carcinoma in needle biopsies may also occur, but this was only found in 15% of cases. In general, adverse findings on needle biopsy accurately predict adverse findings in the radical prostatectomy specimen. By contrast, favorable findings on the needle biopsy do not necessarily predict favorable findings in the radical prostatectomy specimens, largely because of sampling error.

Sampling error is due to the small amount of tissue that is removed by thin-core needle biopsies. The average 20-mm, 18-gauge core samples approximately 0.04% of the average gland volume (40 mL). The most common type of sampling error occurs when a high-grade component is within the radical prostatectomy specimen that is not sampled on needle biopsy.[90] This typically occurs when the tumor in a needle biopsy is graded as Gleason score 3 + 3 = 6, and the corresponding radical prostatectomy contains a Gleason pattern 4 component, which was not sampled on the biopsy.

Overgrading can result from sampling error in cases in which the high-grade pattern may represent only a very minor element in the radical prostatectomy specimen but is selectively represented in needle biopsy. However, undergrading is more commonly encountered. Gleason scores of minimal adenocarcinoma in needle biopsies show a reasonably strong correlation with radical prostatectomy scores, but the Gleason scores do not have the same power to predict extraprostatic extension and positive margin status as they do in nonminimal carcinomas.

Variants and Unusual Subtypes of Prostate Cancer

Most prostate cancers are acinar adenocarcinomas. Unusual histologic variants or types of prostatic carcinoma account for about 5% to 10% of carcinomas that originate in the prostate gland.[3,15,18]

Ductal Adenocarcinoma

The ductal subtype of adenocarcinoma (Fig. 3-7A) is composed of larger glands that are lined by tall pseudostratified columnar cells. *Endometrial carcinoma* originally described this entity because of its morphologic similarity to endometrium. In pure form, ductal adenocarcinoma accounts for 0.2% to 0.8% of prostate cancers.[104-106] More commonly, it is seen with an acinar component. Most studies have demonstrated that ductal adenocarcinoma is aggressive. Some studies reported that 25% to 40% of cases had metastases at the time of diagnosis with a poor 5-year survival rate that ranged from 15% to 43%.[105,107,108] Limited ductal adenocarcinoma on biopsy warrants definitive therapy. Although these cancers are less hormonally responsive than acinar adenocarcinoma, androgen deprivation therapy may provide palliative relief.

Serum PSA levels in patients with ductal adenocarcinoma may be normal, especially in patients with only centrally located tumors. In most cases, transurethral resections performed for diagnosis or relief of urinary obstruction provide sufficient diagnostic tissue. Transrectal needle core biopsies may also obtain diagnostic tissue when the tumor is more peripherally located.[109] In addition, areas of ductal adenocarcinoma may be incidentally identified in prostatectomy specimens.

Ductal adenocarcinoma may be located centrally around the prostatic urethra or—more frequently—peripherally and admixed with typical acinar adenocarcinoma. A centrally located ductal adenocarcinoma may also be associated with a peripherally situated acinar adenocarcinoma. Centrally occurring tumors appear as exophytic, polypoid, or papillary masses protruding into the urethra around the verumontanum. Peripherally occurring tumors typically show a white-gray firm appearance similar to that of acinar adenocarcinoma. Periurethral or centrally located ductal adenocarcinoma may cause hematuria, urinary urgency, and eventually urinary retention. In these cases, there may be no abnormalities on rectal examination. Tumors arising peripherally may lead to enlargement or induration of the prostate.

Ductal adenocarcinoma is characterized by tall columnar cells with abundant—usually amphophilic—cytoplasm, which forms a single or pseudostratified epithelial layer reminiscent of endometrial carcinoma. Although the cytoplasm of ductal adenocarcinoma is often amphophilic, it may occasionally appear clear. In some cases, there are numerous mitoses and marked cytologic atypia. In others, the cytologic atypia is minimal, which makes diagnosis difficult particularly on needle biopsy. Peripherally located tumors are often admixed with cribriform, glandular, or solid patterns, as seen in acinar adenocarcinoma.

Ductal adenocarcinoma should be graded as Gleason score 4 + 4 = 8, while retaining the diagnostic term of ductal adenocarcinoma to denote the unique clinical and pathologic features of this variant. In some cases, comedonecrosis is present, in which case they could be considered equivalent to Gleason pattern 5. Ductal adenocarcinoma displays a variety of architectural patterns that are often intermingled,[110] including papillary, cribriform, individual gland, and solid patterns.

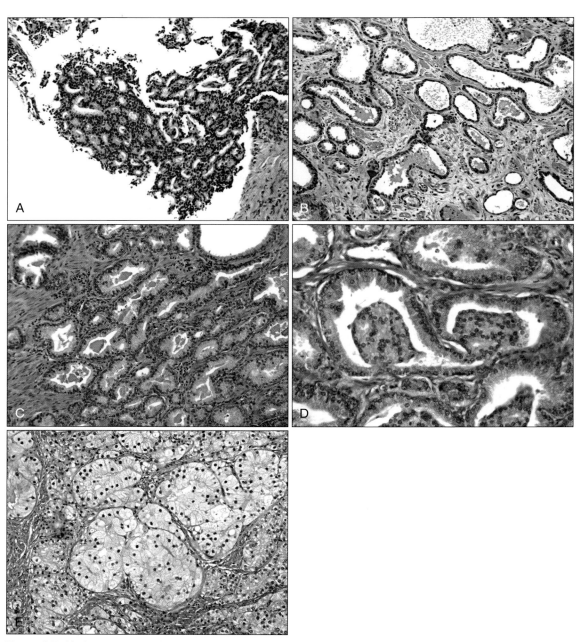

Figure 3-7. Variants of prostatic adenocarcinoma. A, Ductal adenocarcinoma. **B,** Atrophic adenocarcinoma.
C, Pseudohyperplastic adenocarcinoma. **D,** Adenocarcinoma with glomeruloid feature. **E,** Foamy gland adenocarcinoma.

Immunohistochemically, ductal adenocarcinoma is strongly positive for PSA and PAP. Tumor cells are typically negative for basal cell–specific high-molecular-weight cytokeratin (detected by 34βE12); however, preexisting ducts may be positive for this marker.

Ductal adenocarcinomas usually spread along the urethra or into the prostatic ducts, with or without stromal invasion. Other patterns of spread are similar to that of acinar prostatic adenocarcinoma with invasion to extraprostatic tissues and metastasis to pelvic lymph nodes or distal organs. Ductal adenocarcinomas appear to have a tendency to metastasize to the lungs and penis.

Ductal adenocarcinoma must be distinguished from urothelial carcinoma, ectopic prostatic tissue, benign prostatic polyps, and proliferative papillary urethritis. Also, one of the more difficult lesions to distinguish from ductal adenocarcinoma is cribriform-pattern high-grade prostatic intraepithelial neoplasia (HGPIN). Some patterns of ductal adenocarcinoma may represent ductal carcinoma in situ.

Atrophic Adenocarcinoma

Most prostate cancers have abundant cytoplasm. An unusual variant of prostate cancer resembles benign atrophy owing to its scant cytoplasm (see Fig. 3-7B). Although ordinary prostate cancers may develop atrophic cytoplasm as a result of treatment (see Morphology of Prostate Cancer after Therapy), atrophic prostate cancers are usually not associated with a treatment history.[111,112]

The diagnosis of carcinoma in atrophic adenocarcinoma may be based on several features. First, atrophic prostate cancer may demonstrate a truly infiltrative pattern of growth with individual small atrophic glands situated between larger benign glands. In contrast, benign atrophy has a lobular configuration. A characteristic finding in some benign cases of atrophy is the presence of a centrally dilated atrophic gland surrounded by clustered smaller glands, a pattern that has been termed "post-atrophic hyperplasia."[113] Although the glands of benign atrophy may appear to be infiltrative on needle biopsy, they are not truly infiltrative, because individual benign atrophic glands do not infiltrate between the larger benign glands. Although some forms of atrophy are associated with fibrosis, atrophic prostate cancers lack such a desmoplastic stromal response. Atrophic prostate cancer may also be differentiated from benign atrophy by the presence of marked cytologic atypia. Atrophy may show enlarged nuclei and prominent nucleoli, although not the huge eosinophilic nucleoli seen in some atrophic prostate cancers. Finally, the presence of a component of conventional acinar carcinoma can help in recognizing the malignant nature of the adjacent atrophic cancer glands. Immunostaining for high-molecular-weight cytokeratin is extremely helpful in difficult cases.

Pseudohyperplastic Adenocarcinoma

Pseudohyperplastic prostate cancer resembles benign prostate glands in that the neoplastic glands are large with branching and papillary infoldings[114,115] (see Fig. 3-7C). The recognition of cancer with this pattern is based on the architectural pattern of numerous closely packed glands as well as nuclear features more typical of carcinoma. Some pseudohyperplastic adenocarcinomas consist of numerous large glands that are almost back to back with straight even luminal borders and abundant cytoplasm. Comparably sized benign glands either have papillary infoldings or are atrophic. The presence of cytologic atypia in some of these glands further distinguishes them from benign glands. It is almost always helpful to verify pseudohyperplastic cancer with the use of immunohistochemistry to verify the absence of basal cells.

Pseudohyperplastic cancer, despite its benign appearance, may be associated with typical intermediate-grade cancer and can exhibit aggressive behavior (i.e., extraprostatic extension).

Adenocarcinoma with Glomeruloid Features

Prostatic adenocarcinoma with glomeruloid features is characterized by intraluminal ball-like clusters of cancer cells, reminiscent of renal glomeruli (see Fig. 3-7D). Glomeruloid structures in the prostate represent an uncommon but distinctive pattern of growth that is specific for malignancy. Glomeruloid features can be a useful diagnostic clue for malignancy, particularly in some challenging needle biopsy specimens. This pattern of growth is usually seen in high-grade adenocarcinoma, often with extraprostatic extension. Glomeruloid features have not been observed in any benign or premalignant lesions, including hyperplasia and intraepithelial neoplasia.[116]

Foamy Gland Adenocarcinoma

Foamy gland cancer is a variant of acinar adenocarcinoma of the prostate and is characterized by abundant foamy-appearing cytoplasm with a very low nuclear-to-cytoplasmic ratio. Although the cytoplasm has a xanthomatous appearance, it does not contain lipid, but rather empty vacuoles.[117] More typical cytologic features of adenocarcinoma, such as nuclear enlargement and prominent nucleoli, are frequently absent, making this lesion difficult to recognize as carcinoma, especially on biopsy material. Characteristically, the nuclei in foamy gland carcinoma are small and densely hyperchromatic. These nuclei are typically round, even more so than those of benign prostatic secretory cells. This variant is recognized as carcinoma by its architectural pattern of crowded and/or infiltrative glands, and dense, pink, acellular secretions are frequently seen in association with these tumors.[118] In most cases, foamy gland cancer is seen in association with ordinary adenocarcinoma of the prostate.

Despite foamy gland cancer's benign cytology, almost all such cases are associated with a high-grade component of ordinary adenocarcinoma. Consequently, foamy gland carcinoma appears best classified as an intermediate-grade carcinoma.

Oncocytic Adenocarcinoma

Oncocytic prostatic adenocarcinomas are composed of large cells with granular, eosinophilic cytoplasm. Tumor cells have round to ovoid hyperchromatic nuclei and are strongly immunoreactive for PSA. Numerous mitochondria are seen on ultrastructural examination. High Gleason grade,[119,120] elevated serum PSA,[120] and metastasis of similar morphology[119] have been reported with this variant.

Lymphoepithelioma-Like Carcinoma

Lymphoepithelioma-like carcinoma is an undifferentiated carcinoma characterized by malignant cells arranged in a syncytial pattern with an associated heavy lymphocytic infiltrate. Malignant cells are PSA-positive. An associated acinar adenocarcinoma has been noted.[121,122] In situ hybridization has been negative for Epstein-Barr virus.[121] The clinical significance of this entity remains uncertain.

Mucinous and Signet Ring Cell Adenocarcinoma

The diagnosis of mucinous adenocarcinoma of the prostate gland should be made when at least 25% of the tumor resected contains lakes of extracellular mucin (Fig. 3-8A). Mucinous (colloid) adenocarcinoma of the prostate gland is one of the least common morphologic variants of prostatic carcinoma.[123–125] In contrast to bladder adenocarcinomas, mucinous adenocarcinomas of the prostate rarely contain mucin-positive signet ring cells.

Mucinous prostate adenocarcinomas behave aggressively.[123–125] In the largest reported series,

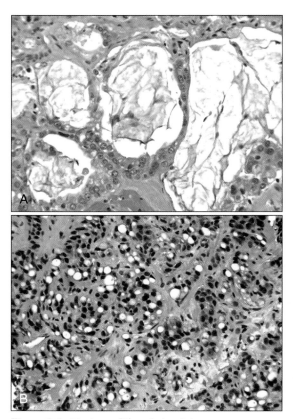

Figure 3-8. Mucinous **(A)** and signet ring adenocarcinoma **(B)**.

7 of 12 patients died of tumor (mean 5 years) and 5 were alive with disease (mean 3 years). Although these tumors are not as hormonally responsive as their nonmucinous counterparts, some tumors respond to androgen withdrawal. Mucinous prostate adenocarcinomas have a propensity to lead to bone metastases, and patients have increased serum PSA levels with advanced disease. There is no consensus on how mucinous (colloid) carcinoma should be scored.[78] Some authors suggest that a Gleason score of 8 is to be assigned, whereas others recommend ignoring mucin and grading the tumor based on the underlying architectural pattern.

Some carcinomas of the prostate have a signet ring cell appearance; yet the vacuoles do not contain intracytoplasmic mucin[126] (Fig. 3-8B) These vacuolated cells may be present in single glands, in sheets of cells, or as singly invasive cells. Only a few cases of prostate cancer have been reported with mucin-positive signet ring cells.[127,128]

When confronted with a mucinous prostatic tumor, one should exclude other mucinous tumors of nonprostatic origin by using morphologic assessment, immunohistochemistry, and clinical information.

Squamous Cell Carcinoma

Squamous cell carcinomas may originate either in the periurethral glands or in the prostatic glandular acini and probably arise from the lining basal cells via a divergent differentiation pathway.[129,130] Approximately 50% of adenosquamous carcinomas arise in prostate cancer patients subsequent to endocrine therapy or radiation therapy.[131] The incidence of squamous cell carcinoma of the prostate is less than 0.6% of all prostate cancers.[132,133] Even more infrequent is the incidence of adenosquamous carcinoma of the prostate. Both squamous cell carcinomas and adenosquamous carcinomas tend to metastasize rapidly with a predilection for the bones.[133,134]

Most, if not all, pure squamous cell carcinomas are manifested clinically by local symptoms such as urinary outflow obstruction and occasionally with associated bone pain and hematuria. Adenosquamous carcinomas may be detected by increased serum PSA but more typically are detected on transurethral resections performed to relieve obstruction of urinary outflow.[131] A proportion of cases shows an initial response to hormone therapy.[135,136]

By definition, pure squamous cell carcinomas do not contain glandular features and are identical with squamous cell carcinomas of other organs. Primary prostatic squamous cell carcinomas must be distinguished on clinical grounds from secondary involvement of the gland by squamous carcinomas of the urinary bladder or urethra. Histologically, squamous cell carcinoma must be distinguished from squamous metaplasia, which is sometimes seen with infarction or after hormonal therapy.

Adenosquamous carcinomas are defined by the presence of both glandular (acinar) and squamous carcinoma components. The glandular tumor component generally expresses PSA and PAP, whereas the squamous component displays positivity for high-molecular-weight cytokeratins on immunohistochemistry.[131]

Transitional Cell (Urothelial) Carcinoma

The incidence of primary urothelial carcinoma is less than 1% of prostatic tumors in adults[137] (Fig. 3-9A). Patients with invasive bladder carcinoma show involvement of the prostate gland in up to 45% of cases.[138-140] Primary urothelial carcinoma is usually located within the proximal prostatic ducts. Many cases are locally advanced at diagnosis and replace the prostate gland. Primary urothelial carcinoma presents in a similar fashion to that of other prostatic masses with urinary obstruction and hematuria. Digital rectal examination is abnormal in most but is infrequently the presenting sign.[141] There are limited data on PSA levels in patients with urothelial carcinoma of the prostate. For patients with either primary or secondary urothelial carcinoma of the prostate, the single most important prognostic parameter is the presence of prostatic stromal invasion. With stromal invasion or extension beyond the confines of the prostate, the prognosis is poor.[142-145]

Most cases of urothelial carcinoma are diagnosed by transurethral resection or, less often, by needle biopsy.[141] In all suspected cases, the possibility of secondary involvement of the prostate by a primary bladder cancer must be excluded; the bladder tumor can be occult and random biopsies may be necessary to exclude this possibility.[146]

In situ carcinoma can spread along ducts and involve acini, or, similar to bladder carcinoma in situ, the tumor can spread along ejaculatory ducts and into seminal vesicles. Initial spread of urothelial carcinomas of the prostate is by invasion of prostatic stroma. Local spread beyond the confines of the prostate may occur. Metastases are to regional lymph nodes and bone.[147] Bone metastases are osteolytic. These tumors are staged as urethral tumors.[148] For tumors involving the prostatic ducts, there is a T1 category for invasion of subepithelial connective tissue that is distinct from invasion of prostatic stroma (T2). The prognostic importance of these categories has been confirmed in clinical studies.[142] The full range of histologic types and grades of urothelial neoplasia can be seen in primary and secondary urothelial neoplasms of the prostate.[142]

Small Cell Carcinoma

Small cell carcinomas of the prostate are histologically identical with small cell carcinomas of the lung[149,150] (see Fig. 3-9B). In approximately 50% of the cases, the tumors are mixed small cell carcinoma and adenocarcinoma of the prostate. Neurosecretory granules have been

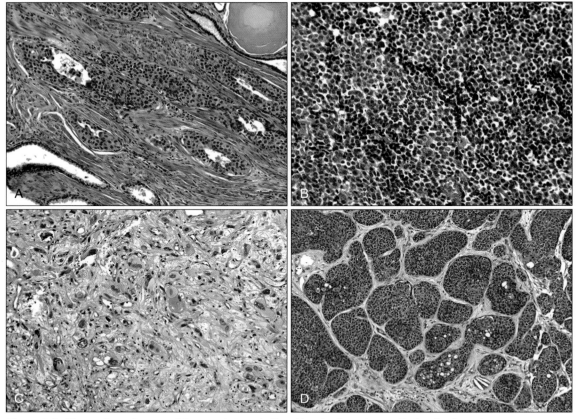

Figure 3-9. Unusual carcinoma of the prostate.   **A,** Transitional cell carcinoma. **B,** Small cell carcinoma.
C, Sarcomatoid carcinoma. **D,** Basal cell carcinoma.

demonstrated within several prostatic small cell carcinomas. Using immunohistochemical techniques, small cell components are negative for PSA and PAP. There are conflicting studies as to whether small cell carcinomas of the prostate are positive for thyroid transcription factor-1 (TTF-1).

The average survival of patients with small cell carcinoma of the prostate is less than 1 year. There is no difference in prognosis between patients with pure small cell carcinomas and those with mixed glandular and small cell carcinomas. The appearance of a small cell component within the course of prostatic adenocarcinoma usually indicates an aggressive terminal phase of the disease.

Sarcomatoid (Carcinosarcoma) Carcinoma

Considerable controversy exists in the literature regarding the nomenclature and histogenesis of sarcomatoid carcinomas (see Fig. 3-7C). In some series, carcinosarcoma and sarcomatoid carcinoma are considered as separate entities based on the presence of specific mesenchymal elements in the former. However, given their otherwise similar clinicopathologic features and identically poor prognosis, these two lesions are best considered as one entity. Sarcomatoid carcinoma of the prostate is a rare neoplasm composed of both malignant epithelial and malignant spindle cell and/or mesenchymal elements.[151-155] Sarcomatoid carcinoma may be present in the initial pathologic material (synchronous presentation), or the patient may have a history of adenocarcinoma treated by radiation and/or hormonal therapy.[156] Serum PSA is within normal limits in most cases. Nodal and distant organ metastases at diagnosis are common.[152,156,157] The five-year survival rate is less than 40%.[152]

The gross appearance of this malignancy often resembles sarcomas. Microscopically, sarcomatoid carcinoma is composed of a glandular component showing variable Gleason score.[152,157] The sarcomatoid component often consists of a nonspecific malignant spindle cell proliferation. Among the specific mesenchymal elements that may be seen in these neoplasms are osteosarcoma, chondrosarcoma, rhabdomyosarcoma, leiomyosarcoma, liposarcoma, angiosarcoma, and multiple types of heterologous differentiation.[152,156] Sarcomatoid carcinoma should be differentiated from the rare carcinoma with metaplastic, benign-appearing bone or cartilage in the stroma.

By immunohistochemistry, epithelial elements react with antibodies against PSA and/or pancytokeratins, whereas spindle cell elements react with markers of soft tissue tumors and variably express cytokeratins.

Basal Cell Carcinoma

Basal cell carcinomas are rare (see Fig. 3-9D). Basal cell carcinoma of the prostate includes malignant basaloid proliferations (basaloid carcinomas) and also neoplasms that resemble, to a certain degree, adenoid cystic carcinomas of the salivary glands.[158–161] A large number of terms have been used for these neoplasms and related growths, such as adenoid basal cell tumor, adenoid cystic tumor, adenoid cystlike tumor, basal cell carcinoma, and adenoid basal proliferation of uncertain significance. Some of these cases most likely represent adenoid cystlike hyperplasia. The difficulty in classification of these proliferations resides in the fact that they are rare, there is no agreement on histologic criteria, and follow-up is available for only a few cases. Histologic grading of basal cell carcinoma is generally not performed. Limited data on patient outcomes have revealed a few cancer-specific deaths, indicating that basal cell carcinoma of the prostate is a potentially aggressive neoplasm.

Grossly, the tumors were white and solid, sometimes with microcysts. Microscopically, several growth arrangements may be evident, including large basaloid nests with peripheral palisading and necrosis, a florid basal cell hyperplasia–like pattern, or an adenoid basal cell hyperplasia–like pattern (adenoid cystic carcinoma pattern). Infiltrative permeation, extraprostatic extension, perineural invasion, necrosis, and stromal desmoplasia are characteristics of basal cell carcinoma that can help in differentiating it from basal cell hyperplasia. The differential diagnosis of basal cell carcinoma also includes poorly differentiated prostatic adenocarcinoma and urothelial carcinoma. Poorly differentiated adenocarcinoma may grow in solid nests as does basal cell carcinoma. Lack of immunoreactivity for p63 and 34βE12, however, is helpful in recognizing conventional adenocarcinoma, although it has been reported that this tumor occasionally expresses p63. As with basal cell carcinoma, urothelial carcinoma may exhibit a solid growth pattern with peripheral palisading and central necrosis and may express high level of p63. However, urothelial carcinoma expresses CK20 and CK7. Basal cell carcinoma is positive for CK7 and negative for CK20.

Morphology of Prostate Cancer after Therapy

Radiation Therapy

Radiation therapy can be given as an external-beam radiation, interstitial seed implants, or as a combination of the two. The histologic effects of these treatments on the cancer are identical (Fig. 3-10A). After radiation therapy, the prostate gland is usually small and hard. Radiation therapy affects prostate cancer variably, with some glands showing marked radiation effect and others showing no evidence of radiation damage.[41,162,163] Architecturally, carcinoma showing radiation treatment effect typically loses the glandular pattern, resulting in clustered cells or individual cells. Cytologically, the cytoplasm of the tumor cells is pale, increased in volume, and often vacuolated. There is often a greater variation of nuclear size than in nonirradiated prostate cancer, and the nuclei may be pyknotic or large with clumped chromatin. Nucleoli are often lost.[164–170] Paradoxically, the nuclear atypia in prostate carcinoma showing radiation effect is less than that seen in radiation atypia of benign glands. The stroma is often sclerosed, particularly after radioactive seed implantation. In the latter, the stromal hyalinization is often sharply delineated. Biopsy findings may predict prognosis; positive biopsies without treatment effect have a worse outcome than negative biopsies, and cancer with treatment effect has an intermediate prognosis.[171] Immunohistochemistry with antibodies against high-molecular-weight cytokeratin (34βE12) or

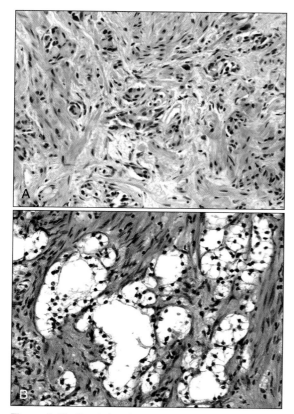

Figure 3-10. Prostatic adenocarcinoma after radiation therapy **(A)** and hormonal therapy **(B)**.

p63 is useful to distinguish cancer from benign glands with effects due to radiation therapy.

After radiation therapy, prostatic biopsy results should be categorized as no evidence of cancer, cancer showing no or minimal radiation effect, cancer showing significant radiation effect, or a combination of these. Although various systems exist to grade radiation effects, these are not recommended for routine clinical practice.

Hormonal Therapy

Hormonal therapy results in a significant overall reduction in the volume of prostate cancer compared with untreated disease in radical prostatectomy specimens from patients with clinically confined disease. In general, histologic response seems to correlate with the tumor patterns and the Gleason grades observed before the androgen ablation therapy is initiated. Moreover, the morphologic changes following total androgen ablation are more pronounced than those seen

after hormonal monotherapy (i.e., luteinizing hormone-releasing hormone analogue or antiandrogen). Residual prostate cancer invading the prostatic capsule, peri-prostatic soft tissue, seminal vesicles, or metastasizing to pelvic lymph nodes shows therapy-induced changes similar to those of adenocarcinomas confined within the prostate gland.[172–180]

Treated tumors show neoplastic acini that appear shrunken (see Fig. 3-10B). Areas of individual infiltrating tumor cells separated by abundant connective tissue and a decreased frequency of intraluminal crystalloids are seen. The epithelial tumor cells show cytoplasmic clearing due to the coalescence of vacuoles and to overall cellular enlargement resulting from the altered permeability of ruptured cell membranes. The nuclear chromatin shows various changes, which range from a mild condensation that barely allows distinction between coarse chromatin granules (corresponding to heterochromatin) and finely dispersed chromatin (corresponding to euchromatin) to a tightly condensed state similar to that observed in apoptosis.[181] As in treated PIN, apoptotic bodies are easily identifiable in all epithelial cell layers. Intraluminal macrophages and sloughed epithelial cells are also seen. The hallmark of untreated adenocarcinoma is the presence of tumor nuclei that are frequently multinucleolated, with the nucleoli being prominent (mean diameter 1.47 μm), marginated, and surrounded by perinuclear halos. In treated cases, the nucleoli become inconspicuous without margination and have a decreased mean diameter of 1.09 μm. The nucleolar diameter is below 1.0 μm in 20% of hormonally treated tumors.[172] The treated tumors with pretherapy cribriform and solid/trabecular patterns (primary Gleason grades 4 and 5) show nuclear and cytoplasmic changes that are less pronounced than in the lower-grade acinar patterns.

The post-therapy stroma displays reduced capillary vascularity, variable degrees of fibrosis, and variable densities of lymphocytic infiltrates, which are often intermingled with mast cells, plasma cells, and eosinophils. Infiltrates of foamy histiocytes, difficult to distinguish from prostate cancer cells with clear cytoplasm, are sometimes present.[182]

Periprostatic fibrosis, obscuring the normal cleavage plane and making surgical treatment more difficult, has been reported after hormonal therapy.[183] The longer patients receive hormonal therapy before surgery, the more fibrosis is observed around the prostate. Currently, there are no detailed qualitative and quantitative histologic studies on the degree of fibrosis and its specific location after hormone therapy. Based on a preliminary morphologic evaluation, it appears that there is an increased thickness of the fibrous connective tissue septa that usually traverse the adipose tissue surrounding the capsule. Foci in which the fatty tissue is totally obliterated by fibrous connective tissue are sometimes present laterally, posteriorly, and around the seminal vesicles. The possibility that this feature represents tumor-induced stroma in which cancer cells have regressed secondary to hormonal therapy cannot be excluded.

Because of therapy-induced morphologic changes, grading of residual prostate cancer based on standard Gleason criteria is not accurate and is therefore discouraged.[177] Conflicting evidence exists regarding pathologic downstaging, with some studies suggesting benefit and others asserting no benefit of androgen manipulation before radical prostatectomy.

Prognosis of Prostate Cancer

Prognostic factor assessment in a given cancer allows selection of an appropriate treatment plan. It allows for prediction of outcome in individual patients and also prediction of general outcomes after a therapeutic intervention. Prognostic factors are also important for education of patients and of caregivers.

In addition to providing important prognostic information, the surgical pathology report of a prostate needle biopsy with carcinoma has become critical in providing information that guides the subsequent management of the cancer. The surgical pathology report should thus be comprehensive, but succinct, and should provide relevant information in a consistent fashion to urologists, radiation oncologists, oncologists and—ultimately—to the patient.[184,185]

Surgical pathology reports for radical prostatectomy specimens should likewise include clinically relevant information derived from the macroscopic and microscopic examination of the radical prostatectomy and pelvic lymph node specimens. Separately, some other extensively studied biologic and clinical factors, whose importance remains to be validated in statistically robust studies, may be recorded.

TNM Staging

Current recommended protocols for the pathologic examination of prostatectomy specimens advocate TNM Staging System of the American Joint Committee on Cancer (AJCC) and the International Union Against Cancer (UICC) for carcinoma of the prostate.[148] Clinical staging (cTNM) is usually accomplished by the referring physician prior to treatment during the initial evaluation of the patient or when pathologic classification is not possible. The prefix symbol "p" refers to the pathologic TNM stage (pTNM), as opposed to the clinical stage "c." Pathologic staging is based on the gross and microscopic examination of the prostate specimen. By AJCC/UICC convention, the designation "T" of the TNM classification refers exclusively to the first resection of a primary tumor. Therefore, pT is based either on a resection of the primary tumor or on a biopsy that is adequate to evaluate the highest pT category (e.g., a biopsy of the seminal vesicle or of periprostatic adipose tissue). The pN stage requires removal of lymph node tissue adequate to validate the presence or absence of a lymph node metastasis. The pM stage requires histologic documentation of metastatic prostate cancer at distant sites.

Residual tumor within a resection specimen after previous (neoadjuvant) treatment of any type (radiation therapy alone, chemotherapy alone, or any combined-modality treatment) is codified by the TNM system using a prescript "y" to indicate the post-treatment status of the tumor (e.g., ypT1). The pathologic staging of residual disease may be a predictor of postoperative outcome. In addition, the ypTNM system provides a standardized framework for the collection of data needed to accurately evaluate new neoadjuvant therapies. Tumor that is locally recurrent after a documented disease-free interval following surgical resection is staged according to the TNM categories but modified with the prefix "r" (e.g., rpT1).

The TNM staging system for prostate cancer was initially adopted for worldwide use in 1992, with subsequent revisions published in 1997 and 2002. The 1997 revision merged palpable tumors occupying less than half a lobe with larger tumors in a single lobe (formerly 1992 T2a and T2b) into a single category (T2a) and changed the T2b category to designate palpable tumors involving both lobes (formerly 1992 T2c). In 2002, the sixth edition of the AJCC staging system refuted the two-tiered classification and reverted back to the three-tiered system for T2 cancers.[148] In a series of 369 totally embedded, serially sectioned, whole-mount radical prostatectomies, unilateral tumors histologically occupying more than half a single lobe (pT2b) were not identified.[186] Thus, a true pT2b prostate cancer (based on the 2002 TNM staging criteria) probably does not exist.

Important staging parameters that can be easily assessed on examination of radical prostatectomy specimens include extraprostatic extension (pT3a) (Fig. 3-11A). and seminal vesicle involvement (pT3b) (Fig. 3-11B). Histologically, the prostatic capsule is not well defined.[187] In areas, there may appear to be a fibrous or fibromuscular band at the edge of the prostate; however, in other areas, normal prostatic glands extend out to the edge of the prostate without any appearance of a capsule. Because the prostate lacks a discrete capsule, the term "extraprostatic extension" (EPE) has replaced "capsular penetration" to describe tumor that has extended out of the prostate into periprostatic soft tissue.[188,189] Tumor abutting or admixed with fat constitutes extraprostatic extension. Extraprostatic extension may also be reported when tumor involves perineural spaces in the neurovascular bundles, even in the absence of periprostatic fat involvement.

Difficulty in diagnosing extraprostatic extension arises when tumor extends out of the prostatic gland and induces a dense desmoplastic response in the periprostatic adipose tissue.[11,13,187,190,191] This is most commonly seen in prostatectomy specimens obtained after endocrine neoadjuvant therapy. Because of the desmoplastic response, it can be difficult to judge whether the tumor has extended out of the gland or is within the fibrous tissue of the prostate. The best way of assessing whether extraprostatic extension has occurred is to look at the adjacent edge of the prostate (where there is no tumor) on scanning magnification and to follow the edge of the gland to the area in question to see whether the normal rounded contour of the gland has been retained or has been altered by a protuberance representing extension of tumor into the periprostatic tissue. A similar approach may be applied when assessing extraprostatic extension in locations with little fat, such as the anterior prostate and bladder neck regions. In these locations, extraprostatic extension is diagnosed when the tumor extends beyond the confines of the normal glandular prostate. At the apex, tumor admixed with skeletal muscle elements does not constitute extraprostatic extension.[192]

The degree of extraprostatic extension varies from only a few glands outside the prostate to more extensive extraprostatic spread. The amount of extraprostatic extension carries prognostic importance. In a recent study, Sung et al.[191] found that the radial distance of extraprostatic tumor measured by ocular micrometer is an independent prognostic factor for pT3 prostate cancer. Two-year and 4-year PSA recurrence-free survival rates were 62% and 35%, respectively, for patients with radial distance of more than 0.75 mm, compared with 35% and 18%, respectively, for those with radial distance

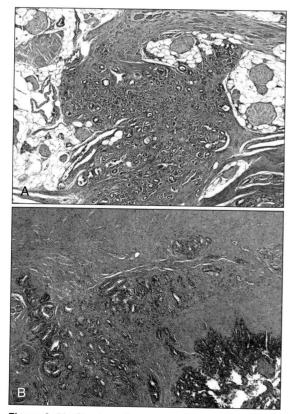

Figure 3–11. Staging of prostate cancer.
A, Extraprostatic extension. **B,** Seminal vesicle invasion.

of 0.75 mm. The added independent predictive knowledge regarding risk of PSA recurrence makes radial distance a potentially useful incorporation for future TNM staging systems to substage pT3a.[191]

Seminal vesicle invasion (SVI) is defined as cancer invading into the muscular coat of the seminal vesicle.[193,194] Seminal vesicle invasion has been shown in numerous studies to be a significant prognostic indicator.[195-198] Three mechanisms by which prostate cancer invades the seminal vesicles were described by Ohori et al.[194] as follows: (1) extension up the ejaculatory duct complex; (2) spread across the base of the prostate without other evidence of extraprostatic extension or involvement from tumor invading the seminal vesicles from the periprostatic and periseminal vesicle adipose tissue; and (3) an isolated tumor deposit without continuity with the primary prostate cancer tumor focus.

In most cases, seminal vesicle invasion occurs in prostate cancers with extraprostatic extension; however, in a minority of cases, it cannot be documented. Of these patients with seminal vesicle invasion and without extraprostatic extension, many had only minimal involvement of the seminal vesicles by their cancer or had involvement of only the portion of the seminal vesicles that is at least partially intraprostatic. Patients in this category have been reported to have a favorable prognosis, similar to patients without seminal vesicle invasion.[193]

Routine biopsy sampling may occasionally contain extraprostatic fat or seminal vesicle tissue. If cancer is noted to involve these structures, the finding indicates pT3 disease. The presence of seminal vesicle invasion or extraprostatic fat involvement in the needle biopsy is highly correlative with similar findings at radical prostatectomy. Extraprostatic fat invasion on needle biopsy is highly predictive of recurrence (79% recurrence rate, compared with a 43% failure rate in cases with extraprostatic extension not detected by needle biopsy). Fat is not present within the normal prostate.[190] Hence, tumor in adipose tissue in a needle biopsy specimen can be safely interpreted as extraprostatic extension.[190] Ganglion cells and skeletal muscle involvement by tumor are not equivalent to extraprostatic extension, since both may frequently be found within the prostate.

In seminal vesicle or extraprostatic fat–targeted biopsies, it is important not only to diagnose cancer, but also to determine whether or not the targeted tissue is represented. In a biopsy that is positive for carcinoma, if the intended tissue is not present and its absence is not specified in the report, then the likelihood of misinterpretation of cancer stage by the treating clinician is high. Distinction between the seminal vesicle epithelium and the ejaculatory duct epithelium may be impossible in limited biopsy specimens, although occasionally the seminal vesicle can be distinguished if its smooth muscle wall is present. In contrast, ejaculatory duct epithelium has a rim of fibrous tissue that is rich in thin blood vessels. If the distinction between seminal vesicle/ejaculatory duct tissue is not feasible, diagnostic terminology such as "adenocarcinoma of the prostate with invasion of seminal vesicle/ejaculatory duct tissue" may be used. Seminal vesicle invasion in radical prostatectomy should demonstrate tumor within the muscular wall.

Cancer Grade

Gleason grading, both in needle biopsy and radical prostatectomy specimens, remains as one of the most significant factors in the clinical decision-making process. The choice of radiation therapy, radical prostatectomy, or other therapies is initially based on the Gleason score in the needle biopsy. In addition to helping guide treatment, the Gleason grade predicts pathologic stage, margin status, biochemical failure, local recurrences, lymph node metastases, disease progression, and distant metastasis after prostatectomy.[2,7,9,91,98,163,199,200] In practice, Gleason scores of 7–10 are associated with worse prognoses, whereas Gleason scores of 5–6 are associated with lower progression rates after therapy.[82,83,201] In recent years, Gleason scores have been included in clinical nomograms, which are being used with increasing frequency to predict disease progression.[3,88,202,203] A recent consensus conference organized by the members of the International Society of Urological Pathology (ISUP) has dealt with the current application of the Gleason system.[78] The Gleason grading system is recommended as the international standard for grading prostate cancer.[204]

Histologic Type

Since acinar adenocarcinoma makes up an overwhelming majority of the histologic types of cancer that may be found in prostate needle biopsy specimens, it is not necessary to specify such cancers as acinar or conventional type in pathology reports. Carcinomas of the prostate with architectural or cytologic variations, such as atrophic, pseudohyperplastic, and so on, are descriptive terms to describe variations in prostate cancer to help pathologists recognize diagnostic pitfalls that have no known prognostic significance. They may be commented on in a microscopic description but do not deserve specific mention in the final diagnosis.

In recent years, many unusual histologic forms have been identified, including ductal adenocarcinoma, mucinous adenocarcinoma, signet ring cell adenocarcinoma, adenosquamous carcinoma, small cell carcinoma, and sarcomatoid carcinoma. The biologic behavior of many of these variants may differ from typical adenocarcinoma, and proper clinical management depends on the accurate diagnosis of these neoplasms and their separation from tumors arising from extraprostatic sites. The former three diagnoses can be made only on examination of radical prostatectomy or transurethral resection specimens. If seen in needle biopsy specimens, the diagnostic terminology must be adenocarcinoma of prostate with ductal features; adenocarcinoma of prostate with signet ring cell features; and adenocarcinoma of prostate with mucinous differentiation. Small cell carcinoma, sarcomatoid carcinoma, and adenosquamous carcinoma may be diagnosed on needle biopsies. No formal studies have demonstrated that these histologic variants, if found in needle biopsies, are of prognostic or predictive importance; however, the often-aggressive outcome associated with such tumors suggests the value of this exercise.

Volume of Cancer

Prostate Biopsy

The amount of tumor in prostate needle cores from biopsies is an important pathologic parameter that must be reported.[205] The extent of involvement of needle cores by prostatic adenocarcinoma has been shown to correlate with Gleason score, with tumor volume, with surgical margin status, and with the pathologic stage in radical prostatectomy specimens[96,206] The extent of needle core involvement, including bilateral involvement, has also been shown to predict recurrence, postprostatectomy progression, and unresponsiveness to radiation therapy in univariate and often in multivariate analysis.[96,206–208] It is a parameter included in some recent nomograms that were created to predict both radiation therapy failure and pathologic stage and seminal vesicle invasion after radical prostatectomy.[206,207,209,210]

The amount of cancer in a biopsy specimen depends on many factors, including prostate volume, cancer volume, cancer distribution, technical procedure, number of biopsy cores obtained, and the cohort of patients being evaluated. There is a lack of consensus in the literature as to the best method of reporting the extent of tumor involvement. The report should provide the number of involved cores and, if possible, should include the overall percentage of involvement in individual cores. In addition, one or both of the following more detailed methods of determining tumor extent should be performed: reporting the linear length of cancer in millimeters (e.g., total tumor length in all biopsies; longest single length of tumor)[211] or providing a percentage estimate of involvement of each of the cores derived by visual estimation (e.g., overall percentage of cancer in all biopsies; percentage of each core involved; reporting the percentage of cancer involvement in increments of 5% or 10% is appropriate).[212] A problem with these otherwise straightforward methods occurs with extreme fragmentation of the needle biopsy specimen, making assessment of the number of cores and the percentage of cancer within each core difficult. Highly fragmented tissue may be overcome by providing a composite (global) percentage of involvement of cancer in all needle biopsy tissue, and this may be a slightly more accurate indicator of the amount of cancer in the prostate gland itself. Although a direct correlation exists between high tumor burden in needle biopsies and the likelihood of an adverse outcome, low tumor burden in needle biopsies is not necessarily an indicator of low-volume and low-stage cancer in the prostatectomy specimen.[213]

Bilateral cancer, which may indicate multifocality, is indirectly suggestive of greater tumor volume. This parameter is easily assessed since needle biopsies of each side are typically submitted as separate specimens. In patients not subsequently treated by radical prostatectomy, this is a critical factor in assigning pathologic stage.

Radical Prostatectomy

A critical and controversial topic concerns whether tumor volume is an independent prognostic parameter after controlling for other routinely assessed variables, such as Gleason grade and tumor stage. There is one situation in which it is important to give some estimate of tumor volume at radical prostatectomy. As a consequence of screening for prostate cancer, we have seen an increase in the resection of prostates harboring so-called "clinically insignificant cancers." The pathologist needs to specify in the pathology report that these tumors are "small" or "minute" (i.e., less than 0.5 mL) so that patients may understand that they are cured of their disease.[214,215]

A consensus for a standard method of volume determination has not yet been achieved. Volume is most precisely determined by stereologic methods, using either planimetry or point counting based on overlaid grids.[216,217] However, the time and labor involved in these approaches will probably not lead to wide acceptance. In a recent study, maximum tumor diameter is a significant predictor of biochemical recurrence and correlates with preoperative PSA, tumor volume measured by the grid method, Gleason score, and pathologic stage, and it predicts biochemical recurrence independent of these parameters.[218] Inclusion of maximum tumor diameter in surgical pathology reports for radical prostatectomies may be considered. It has been recommended that, at the very least, the proportion (percentage) of prostatic tissue involved by tumor be included for all specimens,[7] although its role as an independent predictor of patient outcome has been questioned.[219,220]

More recently, Marks et al.[221] found that the ratio of tumor positive tissue blocks to the total number of blocks submitted (positive-block ratio) can be used as an independent prognostic indicator for PSA recurrence. Using a multivariate Cox regression model, controlling for pathologic stage, Gleason score, lymph node metastasis, and surgical margin status, positive-block ratio was an independent predictor of PSA recurrence. This simple method of tumor measurement appears to be promising for quantifying tumor volume and could be used with ease in all pathology practices.[221]

Positive Surgical Margins in Radical Prostatectomy

Patients with positive surgical margins have a significantly increased risk of progression compared with those with negative margins.[11,13,222] Surgical margins are inked during the gross dissection of the radical prostatectomy specimen to facilitate the microscopic assessment of these margins. Surgical margins should be designated as "negative" if tumor is not present at the inked margin or as "positive" if tumor cells touch the ink at the margin[11,13] (Fig. 3-12A). Positive surgical margins should not be interpreted as extraprostatic extension.[11,13,219,223] If the surgical margin is positive, the pathologist should state this explicitly, although this finding is not relied on for pathologic staging. The examining pathologist should be aware of false-positive margins due to the penetration of ink into cracks that may be present on the external surface. The main causes for difficulty in assessing margins include situations in which cancer is very close to, but not clearly touching, the inked margins.

The specific locations of positive margins should be documented, and there should be some indication (e.g., number of positive blocks, linear extent in millimeters) of the extent of margin positivity, although a recent study did not find the significance of linear extent of margin positivity.[224] The apex should be closely examined because of its unusual susceptibility to positive margins.

Although margin positivity does not directly impact the TNM staging system, there are situations in which this variable does influence the pathologic stage as determined by the pathologist. For example, there is no full consensus on the definition of the "T" category in situations in which the prostate base/bladder neck is involved and the margin is positive. This problem is linked to the fact that the basal prostatic stroma blends imperceptibly into the bladder neck musculature and therefore is linked to the difficulty in defining the exact transition point from prostate base to bladder neck, even though the latter is composed of distinct large bundles of smooth muscle fibers. Microscopic involvement of bladder neck muscle fibers in radical prostatectomy specimens should be defined as

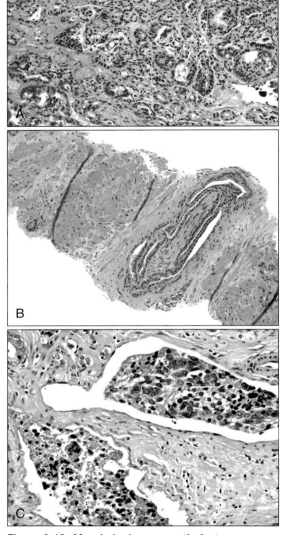

Figure 3-12. Morphologic prognostic factors.
A, Positive surgical margins. **B,** Perineural invasion.
C, Lymphovascular invasion.

pT4.[225] Other researchers[226] believe that gross involvement of the bladder neck must be present to warrant a pT4 stage and that microscopic involvement of bladder neck muscle fibers, by itself, should not be equated with a pT4 designation. Poulos et al.[227] found that bladder neck involvement is an independent predictor of patient outcome.

Tumor remaining in a patient after therapy with curative intent (e.g., surgical resection) is categorized by a system known as "R" classification. This classification may be used by the surgeon to indicate the known or assumed status of the completeness of the surgical resection. For the pathologist, the R classification is relevant only to the margins of surgical resection specimens; patients with tumor involving the resection margins on pathologic examination may be assumed to have residual tumor. Such patients may be classified according to whether the involvement is macroscopic or microscopic.

The pathology report may also indicate the presence of normal prostate tissue at the surgical resection margin. This might help the urologist explain why the serum PSA in patients with such a feature remains detectable after radical prostatectomy. Thus, a detectable postoperative serum PSA value (especially when values are very low) is not always linked to tumor recurrence and persistence but to incomplete resection of the prostate gland. The most common location of benign prostatic glandular tissue at the surgical margin was the apex.[228] It was uncommon in the anterior or posterior prostate. In that study, the presence of benign prostatic epithelial tissue at the inked surgical margins was not associated with postoperative PSA recurrence.[228]

Perineural Invasion

Prostate Biopsy

Perineural invasion is one of the major mechanisms by which prostate cancer spreads out of the gland. Perineural, circumferential, or intraneural invasion is defined as the presence of prostate cancer juxtaposed intimately along, around, or within a nerve (see Fig. 3-12B). Other descriptors of perineural invasion that may strengthen the prognostic significance of this parameter include extensive (multifocal) perineural invasion and perineural invasion involving a greater nerve diameter.[229] Involvement of nerves within adipose tissue (extraprostatic nerves) by cancer indicates extraprostatic extension and deserves notation in the pathology report when present.

Although perineural invasion in needle biopsy specimens is not an independent predictor of prognosis when the Gleason score, serum PSA, and extent of cancer are considered, most studies indicate that its presence correlates with extraprostatic extension (38–93%).[230-232] Recent data suggest that this finding may independently predict lymph node metastasis and postsurgical progression.[231,233] The presence or absence of perineural invasion on needle biopsy may also be important in planning nerve-sparing surgery.[234] Some of the data from the radiation oncology literature suggest that perineural invasion is an independent risk factor for predicting adverse outcome after external-beam radiation therapy. Therefore, in patients with high Gleason score and perineural invasion, adjuvant hormonal therapy or dose escalation has been advocated.[231,235]

Radical Prostatectomy

Perineural invasion is almost ubiquitously present in radical prostatectomy specimens,[236] and pathologists may not document it within radical prostatectomy pathology reports. As with all other parameters, the key question is whether the presence of perineural (intraprostatic) invasion in the prostatectomy specimen is an independent predictor of outcome. At this time, it is not entirely clear whether there are differences in prognosis between patients with intraprostatic and extraprostatic perineural invasion.[7]

Vascular/Lymphatic Invasion

Microvascular invasion consists of tumor cells within endothelial-lined spaces (see Fig. 3-12C). A cellular reaction in the adjacent stroma is not required for diagnosis. Also, pathologists do not differentiate between vascular and lymphatic channels because of the difficulty and lack of reproducibility of such a distinction by routine light microscopic examination.[237] Microvascular invasion may be confused with fixation-associated retraction artifact of acini. Immunohistochemical stains directed against endothelial cells such as factor VIII-related antigen, *Ulex europaeus*, CD31, or CD34 may aid in the detection of lymphovascular invasion.[237]

Since lymphovascular invasion, as studied in radical prostatectomy specimens, correlates with lymph node metastasis, biochemical recurrence, distant metastasis, and cancer death,[10] its presence in the needle biopsy is likely to have similar correlations. However, this feature is very rarely seen in needle biopsy specimens and should be mentioned in the report only if identified.[238,239]

By AJCC/UICC criteria, vessel invasion (lymphatic or venous) does not affect the T category (indicating local extent of tumor) in prostate cancer staging, unlike the staging of tumors from some other organs. Lymphatic and venous invasion by tumor are coded separately. The TNM system uses the categories "L" and "V" to indicate the presence of lymphatic or venous invasion. Most of the time when vascular invasion is noted, it is present in tumors with fairly advanced pathology.

Pelvic Lymph Node Assessment

The adverse prognosis associated with metastatic disease in the pelvic lymph nodes is universally accepted. The incidence of pelvic lymph node metastases at the time of radical prostatectomy has decreased over the last couple of decades.[192] As a consequence of this declining incidence, concerns have been raised as to whether pelvic lymphadenectomy is necessary in all patients, especially those with a low risk of having positive lymph nodes as determined by preoperative clinicopathologic findings. The major factor contributing to this decreased incidence of regional lymph node metastasis is the widespread use of serum PSA testing, which, in turn, leads to both better patient selection as to who is a good candidate for surgery and to the earlier detection of prostate cancer.

The handling of lymphadenectomy specimens at the time of surgery is controversial and depends on the philosophy of the urologist. Some urologists abort the radical prostatectomy in patients with positive lymph nodes identified by frozen section at the time of surgery since surgery will not be curative. Other urologists proceed with radical prostatectomy when positive lymph nodes are found intraoperatively, as long as patients are projected to have a long survival and might benefit in terms of local control. The pathologist should try to optimize the identification of metastatic disease at the time of frozen section. It is not practical to freeze all the pelvic lymph nodes, especially given the low likelihood of finding metastatic disease even on permanent sections. A more reasonable approach would be to identify clinical parameters preoperatively that are associated with such a low risk of lymph node metastases that frozen sections need not be performed.

In many incidences, the only lymph node metastasis that is present is located within a small lymph node that is not grossly recognized. All the adipose tissue from the pelvic lymphadenectomy specimens should be carefully searched. The detection of pelvic lymph node metastases may be enhanced through special techniques. In particular, micrometastases can be immunohistochemically detected using a cocktail of antibodies to keratin.

The metastatic tumor volume in lymph nodes is an important prognostic factor and should be documented by the pathologist.[200,240,241] Several parameters should be mentioned in the pathology reports including the number of positive nodes, the number of lymph nodes sampled, the largest dimension of tumor metastasis, and extranodal extension.

Atypical Small Acinar Proliferation, Suspicious for But Not Diagnostic of Malignancy

Terminology, such as "atypical small acinar proliferation [ASAP] suspicious for but not diagnostic of malignancy," also referred to as atypical focus suspicious for but not diagnostic of malignancy, is used to render a descriptive diagnosis for a needle biopsy containing a small group of glands that are suspicious for adenocarcinoma, but which lack sufficient cytologic and/or architectural atypia to establish a definitive diagnosis.[2,6,201,242–245] Thus, this is descriptive terminology meant to convey diagnostic uncertainty. It is a broad diagnostic "umbrella" or category that encompasses benign lesions mimicking malignant glandular proliferations and undersampled, small foci of carcinoma that harbor some of the features needed for a definitive diagnosis of malignancy.[2] This term does not represent a specific diagnostic entity and should not be interpreted as a condition synonymous with high-grade prostatic intraepithelial neoplasia (HGPIN).

Incidence and Clinical Features

Approximately 5% of needle biopsies are diagnosed as atypical focus suspicious for but not diagnostic of malignancy (range 0.7% to 23.4%).[242,246–248] No clinical features are contributory to or predictive of atypical small acinar proliferations suspicious for malignancy.[242,244–247,249–251] Ages range from 40 to 95, with a mean patient age in the seventh decade. These men are typically biopsied to rule out prostate cancer after either an elevated serum PSA or after an abnormal digital rectal examination. The median PSA level is usually only modestly elevated, ranging from 6 to 8 ng/mL, but very high PSA levels (greater than 50 ng/mL) have been seen. Only few transrectal ultrasound results have been reported.[246]

Diagnosis

This noncommittal category encompasses a variety of lesions including benign mimickers of cancer and small foci of adenocarcinoma, which, for a variety of reasons, cannot be accurately diagnosed[252] (Fig. 3-13). These lesions may be composed of acini of small size, that is, smaller than normal ducts and acini, but may also include glands with a diameter similar to that of normal ducts and acini.[2]

Benign lesions that are considered to be problematic and that may mimic malignant glandular proliferations have changed over the years. In the past, seminal vesicle tissue was considered one of the common mimickers of adenocarcinoma of the prostate.[253] Adenosis and complete atrophy have also been found to be common problems in previous years.[254] Currently, partial atrophy is one of the most common benign mimickers of cancer.[255] In part, the atypical diagnoses that may result from the evaluation of

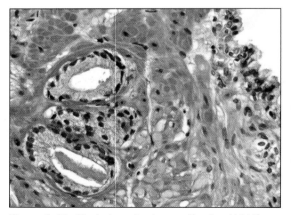

Figure 3-13. Atypical small acinar proliferation (ASAP), suggestive of but not diagnostic of malignancy.

partial atrophy are related to negative immuno-staining for high-molecular-weight cytokeratin and for p63 and to positive immunostaining for AMACR (see section that follows).

Other factors that may prevent a definitive diagnosis of carcinoma on needle biopsy include marginal or imperfect sampling of the tumor. This results in a biopsy with an atypical or sus-picious focus that is very small and that con-tains only a small number of acini. In some cases, the atypical focus is present only at the edge of the core or at its tip, where infiltration between benign acini cannot be appreciated. In these cases, if the glands do not show promi-nent cytologic and architectural atypia, a defi-nite diagnosis of cancer may not be possible. Mechanical distortion from the needle biopsy can result in crush artifact of a few atypical glands and obscure cytologic detail. Problems with fixation and processing, especially with sections that are too thick or overstained, can also prevent definitive diagnosis because of poor histologic detail. Prominent atrophy in or near a small focus of cancer confounds this diagnos-tic difficulty.

Another factor that may hamper accurate interpretation is the fact that not all cancers display the classic features of malignancy. The absence of convincing cytologic features of malignancy and/or a clustered growth pattern can prevent a definite diagnosis in some cases. Prominent inflammatory changes are common and can obscure the cytologic features of a small focus of carcinoma. In addition, it can be difficult to differentiate malignant features from the reactive changes and distortion that may occur in benign glands as a result of inflammation.[252]

The combination of HGPIN and atypical small acinar proliferation suspicious for malig-nancy is found in 16% to 31% of cases.[242,245,256] This combination may be seen in two distinct patterns.[243] There may be discrete and discon-tinuous foci of HGPIN and atypical foci suspi-cious for but not diagnostic of malignancy. Alternatively, the two lesions may coexist when there is definite HGPIN but when one cannot distinguish small outpouchings or tangential sec-tions of the HGPIN from carcinoma associated with the HGPIN.[257] In addition to these two scenarios, HGPIN may involve small acini and thus may be difficult to distinguish from invasive cancer.[258]

Immunohistochemical Findings

Basal Cell Immunostains. Immunohisto-chemical stains, such as p63 (nuclear stain)[259] and high-molecular-weight cytokeratin that is detected by the antibody 34βE12 (cytoplasmic stain)[260] can aid in the investigation of atypical glandular proliferations by staining basal cells. Cancer lacks a basal cell layer, so the presence of basal cells in an atypical focus effectively excludes cancer from consideration. Conversely, the absence of a basal cell layer in a small focus that is highly suspicious for cancer supports the diagnosis of cancer. However, negative staining for basal cell markers is, by itself, not diagnostic of cancer. False-negative staining can arise from technical problems, including tissue changes induced by the surgical procedure (e.g., cautery artifact with transurethral resection of the pros-tate), imperfect specimen fixation, and varia-tions in processing and antigen retrieval.[261] Negative staining should be interpreted only when there is confirmatory positive staining in adjacent benign glands. Staining variability with negative staining of benign glands, including glands displaying atrophy and inflammation-associated changes, has also been reported.[43] Some benign lesions may have negative or dis-continuous staining with basal cell markers.[262] In particular, fully developed atrophy typically stains fairly uniformly and intensely with basal cell markers, whereas partial atrophy often has negative or discontinuous staining with these markers.[255] The combination of two specific basal cell stains (34βE12 and p63) increases the sensitivity of basal cell detection compared with using either marker alone.[263,264] However, even with the combination of these markers, certain benign conditions and mimickers of cancer have cells that fail to react with these immunohisto-chemical stains.

α-Methylacyl CoA Racemase. Racemase (AMACR) immunoreactivity converted diagno-ses of atypical foci to diagnoses of cancer in approximately 10% of cases.[265] The addition of anti-racemase antibodies to those of anti-keratin 34βE12 may allow a cancer diagnosis to be rendered in approximately 30% of cases that might previously have been called atypical focus or HGPIN.[252] Use of a p63/racemase cocktail resolved 87% of cases with more diagnosed as cancer than as benign.[245,266,267]

Clinical Significance

Predictive Value for Subsequent Cancer.
The incidences of detecting carcinoma on repeat needle biopsy after a diagnosis of isolated atypical foci in the initial biopsy ranged from 17% to 60%, with the mean value approximately 41%.[242,244,245,247–251,267–273] A decrease in the predictive value for a subsequent cancer diagnosis has been claimed in some recent series.[245,269] For instance, Schlesinger et al.[245] found that isolated atypical foci have a predictive value of 37% for cancer; this is only a slight decrease from the 45% predictive value observed between 1989 and 1996. Various explanations have been offered to explain such an observation, such as the use of extended biopsy techniques, advances in immunostaining, and previous PSA testing; moreover, multiple biopsies from the same patient have been reported.[245,269]

Attempts have been made to place atypical small acinar proliferations into three tiers, such as "favor benign," "uncertain" (or equivocal), and "favor carcinoma" (highly suspicious).[244,249,250] Such stratification has not been shown to significantly influence the risk of subsequent detection of carcinoma on repeat biopsy. Even when a benign diagnosis is favored, up to 44% of patients (range 20–44%) were diagnosed with carcinoma on repeat biopsy.[244,249,250,274,275] This three-tier stratification offers low reproducibility with 63% interobserver agreement in one study.[250,276]

Associated clinical parameters in patients with diagnoses of atypical small acinar proliferations have limited value in predicting the presence of cancer on repeat biopsy.[277] Initial mean PSA concentrations were higher in those with malignant cells present in subsequent biopsies than in those whose repeat biopsies were negative for malignancy. Park et al.[251] reported that digital rectal examination and patient age were independent predictors of cancer in 45 patients with "atypia" on needle biopsy; however, other studies have found that serum PSA and digital rectal examination findings are not predictive of cancer on subsequent biopsy.[245,267,278]

The mean cancer detection rate on repeat biopsy in patients who have both an atypical focus and HGPIN is 53%, which is significantly higher than that seen with patients having only an isolated atypical focus.[103] Leite et al.[278] observed a high percentage of prostate cancer (72.5%) in men with initial biopsies demonstrating HGPIN associated with an atypical focus. Scattoni et al.[267] observed adenocarcinoma in 58% of repeat biopsies from patients with both lesions on initial biopsy, whereas cancer was present in only 35% of repeat biopsies from patients with isolated atypical foci in the initial biopsy. These figures are similar to those reported by Kronz et al.,[257] who found that HGPIN with adjacent small atypical glands on prostate biopsy had a 46% follow-up cancer detection rate. By contrast, Schlesinger et al.[245] reported that atypical small acinar proliferations associated with HGPIN predicted cancer in 33% of the cases, slightly lower than the reported predictive value for atypical small acinar proliferations alone (37%). Of particular interest is the unique observation by Brausi et al.,[273] who found cancer in 100% of 25 patients with isolated atypical small acinar proliferations suspicious for malignancy who underwent prostatectomy. This led these authors to suggest that immediate surgery was the treatment of choice for young patients with atypical small acinar proliferations suggestive of malignancy.

Adenocarcinomas that are found on repeat biopsy are mainly of intermediate grade, with Gleason scores of 5 and 6; however, 30% are high grade with Gleason scores of 7 to 10.[249,250]

Re-Biopsy Strategy

Given the documented high risk of cancer in patients with atypical foci suspicious for but not diagnostic of malignancy, it is reasonable to consider re-biopsy within 3 to 4 months after an initial biopsy observation of atypical glands. Most carcinomas on repeat biopsy are found within 6 months.[249,250]

It seems logical that focusing on sites with documented atypical foci will provide a greater diagnostic yield for malignancy on repeat biopsy. However, the best re-biopsy strategy is controversial. Some authors recommend a sextant biopsy technique and additional biopsies directed to the site of the atypical glands or to the ipsilateral site.[249] Allen et al.[279] found that 85% of all cancers detected on repeat biopsy exist either in the same sextant, adjacent ipsilateral, or adjacent contralateral sextant biopsies as the initial atypical focus. Thus, they suggest a re-biopsying strategy to include not just the initial atypical site but also adjacent ipsilateral and contralateral sites. The researchers recommend obtaining several cores from the atypical location, two cores each from adjacent locations, and one each from other sextant locations. Park et al.[251] calculated significantly increased odds of finding cancer at the same site of the initial atypical prostate biopsy: 65% probability, which increases to 88% when including adjacent sites. On a multisite scheme study, Scattoni et al.[267] found precise spatial concordance between atypical small acinar proliferations and cancer in only 33% of the cases, similar to the likelihood of finding cancer in an adjacent site or in a nonadjacent site.

A second diagnosis of an atypical focus on repeat biopsy is seen in about 6% of cases. These patients probably should undergo a second re-biopsy. Consideration for additional re-biopsy sessions should also be based on clinical findings (serum PSA and digital rectal examination results) and clinical judgment.[244,247,249,280]

High-Grade Prostatic Intraepithelial Neoplasia

Prostatic intraepithelial neoplasia (PIN) is a neoplastic transformation of the secretory epithelial lining of prostatic ducts and acini. This process is confined within the epithelium and is thus "intraepithelial." Initially, PIN was divided into three grades.[281] Subsequently, it has been recommended that the classification should be simplified into a two-tier system: low grade (previous grade I) and high grade (previous grades II and III).[282] The prevalence of this neoplastic process increases with age. HGPIN shows a strong association with cancer in terms of coexistence within the same gland and in the same spatial distribution.[283] Reported incidence of HGPIN in needle biopsies of the prostate was 4% to 6%.[5] The Japanese and European literatures report a slightly lower frequency. Sixteen percent to 31% of cases of HGPIN are associated with atypical foci of glands suspicious for malignancy.[243,268] HGPIN is relatively uncommon in transurethral resection of the prostate (TURP) specimens with two studies reporting an incidence of 2.3% and 2.8%, respectively.[284,285]

The prevalence of HGPIN in radical prostatectomy specimens removed for prostate cancer is remarkably high (85–100%), reflecting the strong association between this lesion and prostate cancer.[5] HGPIN was present in 82% of step-sectioned autopsy prostates with cancer, but only in 43% of benign prostates from patients of similar age.[281] Qian et al.[286] found that 86% of whole-mount radical prostatectomy specimens with cancer contained HGPIN, usually within 2 mm of the cancer. The extent of HGPIN in prostates with cancer is also increased compared with those without cancer. HGPIN is more extensive in small cancers than in larger cancers, presumably because of "overgrowth" or obliteration of HGPIN by larger cancers.

The predominant location of HGPIN is the peripheral zone of the prostate, which is also the location in which most cancers arise. The majority of HGPIN foci are exclusively in the peripheral zone (or nontransition zone; in one study, 63% of the cases) or simultaneously in the peripheral and transition zones (36%); only rare cases (1%) are exclusively in the transition zone.[287] Other authors have reported a higher percentage of HGPIN in the transition zone, with a range of 2% to 37% of cases.[285] Kovi et al.[288] reported the highest frequency of involvement of the transition zone (37%) in prostatectomies with cancer, whereas they found a significantly lower percentage in studies of TURP specimens. HGPIN and cancer are usually multicentric.[286] HGPIN is multicentric in 72% of radical prostatectomies with cancer, including 63% of those involving the nontransition zone and 7% of those involving the transition zone. Two percent of cases have separate foci of HGPIN in all zones.

Treatment is currently not indicated after a needle biopsy diagnosis of HGPIN. In particular, prophylactic radical prostatectomy or radiation is not acceptable for patients who have HGPIN only.[5] Patients with isolated HGPIN in needle biopsy may be considered for enrollment into clinical trials with a chemoprevention agent.[5]

Diagnosis

The classification of PIN into low-grade and high-grade categories is based on the cytologic characteristics of the secretory cells. The nuclei of cells composing low-grade PIN (LGPIN) are enlarged, vary in size, have normal or slightly increased chromatin content, and possess small or inconspicuous nucleoli. High-grade PIN (HGPIN), by contrast, is characterized by cells with large nuclei of relatively uniform size, having increased chromatin content (which may be irregularly distributed) and prominent nucleoli that are similar to those of carcinoma cells. Similar to adenocarcinoma, the cytoplasm in most cases of HGPIN is immunoreactive with an antibody directed against α-methylacyl-CoA racemase. The basal cell layer, as best demonstrated with immunohistochemical techniques (antibodies directed against the nuclear p63 protein and against the cytoplasmic high-molecular-weight cytokeratin 34βE12), is intact or rarely interrupted in LGPIN, but may have frequent disruptions in HGPIN.

There is an inversion of the normal orientation of epithelial proliferation in HGPIN lesions. Proliferation (evaluated immunohistochemically with the Ki-67 antibody) occurs in the basal cell compartment in benign epithelium; however, in HGPIN, epithelial proliferation predominantly occurs on the luminal side of the ducts and acini.[287,289]

Early stromal invasion, which represents the earliest evidence of carcinoma, occurs in HGPIN at sites of acinar outpouching and basal cell disruption. This is present in about 2% of HGPIN lesions and is seen just as frequently in all architectural patterns[287,289] (see text that follows). Foci of HGPIN in association with small cancers are lined by a crowded and pseudostratified epithelium, in contrast to the simple columnar or cuboidal lining of the malignant acini. In some cases, a small tubular malignant acinus appears to originate abruptly from a dysplastic duct wall.[287,289]

Architectural Patterns and Variants

Although the cytologic features of low-grade and high-grade PIN are fairly constant, the architecture is variable with a spectrum ranging from a flattened epithelium to a florid cribriform proliferation. There are four main patterns of HGPIN: tufting, micropapillary, cribriform, and flat[290] (Fig. 3-14). Although most cases have multiple patterns, the tufting pattern is the most

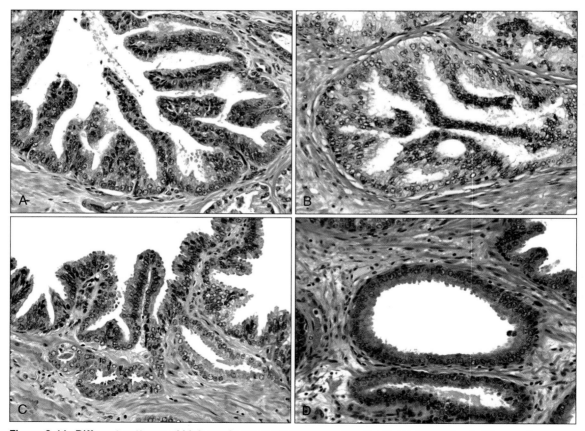

Figure 3-14. Different patterns of high-grade prostatic intraepithelial neoplasia (HGPIN).   A, Micropapillary pattern. **B,** Cribriform pattern. **C,** Tufting. **D,** Flat.

common, being present in 97% of cases. No known clinically significant differences have been found among the architectural patterns of HGPIN. Their recognition appears to be only of interest diagnostically.

Other less common variants of HGPIN include lesions with signet ring cells, small cell neuroendocrine differentiation, mucinous features, foamy cytoplasm, inverted pattern, and/or squamous differentiation. The presence of HGPIN with various histologic patterns provides additional support for the close relationship between HGPIN and the multiple variants of invasive prostate carcinoma.

Differential Diagnosis

The differential diagnosis of HGPIN includes several benign and malignant lesions. The former include atypia induced by inflammation, infarction, radiation, transitional cell metaplasia, basal cell hyperplasia with or without atypia, clear cell cribriform hyperplasia, and normal ejaculatory duct and seminal vesicle epithelium. Malignant lesions to be distinguished from HGPIN include transitional cell carcinoma involving prostatic ducts and acini and cribriform acinar and cribriform ductal carcinomas. Transitional cell carcinomas involving ducts and acini are usually high-grade tumors with significant cellular pleomorphism, numerous mitoses, and occasional foci of comedonecrosis. Immunoreactivity for PSA and prostatic acid phosphatase is not observed.

HGPIN Morphology after Treatment

Androgen Deprivation Therapy

There is a marked decrease in the prevalence and extent of PIN in patients after androgen deprivation therapy compared with untreated patients. The cellular changes in HGPIN that result from this therapy are similar to those seen in adenocarcinomas following endocrine therapy. The loss of epithelial cells with androgen deprivation is due to acceleration of apoptosis.[287,291] Blockade of 5α-reductase with drugs such as finasteride appears to induce little morphologic changes on HGPIN, unlike with other forms of androgen deprivation therapy. The incidence of PIN was unchanged in one study after 1 year of treatment with finasteride.[292]

Radiation Therapy

After radiation therapy, PIN retains the features characteristic of untreated HGPIN and is readily recognized in tissue specimens.[162] The most common patterns of PIN seen after radiation therapy are tufting and micropapillary patterns, similar to those most commonly seen in untreated patients. The prevalence and extent of HGPIN are decreased with radiation therapy.

Isolated HGPIN in Prostate Needle Biopsy

HGPIN does not result in any abnormalities on digital rectal examination. HGPIN may be indistinguishable from cancer on transrectal ultrasound examination, in which it appears as a hypoechoic lesion.[5] HGPIN by itself does not appear to elevate serum pPSA levels.

On repeat biopsy, the cancer detection rate is about 20% after an initial diagnosis of benign prostatic tissue and 16% after an initial diagnosis of LGPIN.[274] In the past, the mean incidence of carcinoma detection on re-biopsy after a diagnosis of HGPIN in needle biopsy tissue was about 36%.[245,270,293] In recent years, a significant decline in the predictive value of cancer after an initial diagnosis of HGPIN has been observed.[243,245] According to Epstein and Herawi,[243] the median risk of cancer on a subsequent biopsy after a diagnosis of HGPIN is 24.1%, which is not much higher than the risk reported in the literature for repeat biopsy following a benign diagnosis. A slightly lower (weighted average) value (21%) was observed by Schlesinger et al.[245] This recent trend toward lower cancer detection rates after a diagnosis of HGPIN may be attributable to stage migration, to lower cancer volumes in highly screened populations, to more extensive tissue sampling, and to the use of new biopsy strategies with the addition of more lateral biopsies.[5] These findings may have implications in designing follow-up regimens for patients with an isolated diagnosis of HGPIN. Other factors, such as patient age, family history of prostate cancer, serum PSA levels, and digital rectal examination findings should be considered in clinical management.

There are two situations in which isolated HGPIN can still show a high predictive value for carcinoma in repeat biopsy. A combination of HGPIN and adjacent atypical glands confers a higher risk for subsequent diagnosis of carcinoma compared with HGPIN alone, averaging a 53% detection rate on repeat biopsy.[243,245,268,294] Also, when there is plurifocality of HGPIN,[295–297] the cancer detection rate on repeat biopsy has been shown in some studies to be significantly greater than in patients with monofocal HGPIN. By contrast, Naya et al.[295] demonstrated that the number of biopsy specimens positive for HGPIN on initial biopsy was not associated with an increased likelihood of prostate cancer on repeat biopsy.[295]

Re-Biopsy Strategy

Current standards of care recommend that patients with isolated HGPIN be re-biopsied at 0- to 6-month intervals for 2 years, regardless of the serum PSA level and digital rectal examination findings, and thereafter at 12-month intervals for life. However, this recommendation may change with emerging data indicating a lower risk of prostate carcinoma following a needle biopsy showing HGPIN.[5] It is not clear whether serum PSA and digital rectal examination findings provide additional information regarding the likelihood of finding carcinoma on re-biopsy in patients with HGPIN.[5] Data are inconsistent as to whether the extent of HGPIN and/or its architectural pattern predicts risk of subsequent carcinoma. Genetic abnormalities and/or immunophenotypes of HGPIN are not currently used to assess risk for subsequent detection of carcinoma.

The re-biopsy technique should entail at least systematic sextant re-biopsy of the entire gland,[298] since HGPIN is a general risk factor for carcinoma throughout the gland. Thirty-five percent of carcinomas would have been missed if only the side with the initially detected HGPIN had been re-biopsied. The majority (80–90%) of cases of carcinomas are detected on the first re-biopsy after a HGPIN diagnosis. Re-biopsy may also detect persistent HGPIN in 5% to 43% of cases.[298] When HGPIN is associated with atypical small acinar proliferations, it is reasonable to consider re-biopsy within 3 to 4 months after the initial biopsy. It is assumed that a greater diagnostic yield for malignancy will be achieved by focusing on sites with documented atypical foci.

A few studies have found that HGPIN on TURP specimens places an individual at higher risk for the subsequent detection of cancer.[284,285] Among 14 patients with HGPIN and benign prostatic hyperplasia followed up for up to 7 years (mean 5.9 years), 3 (21.4%) developed prostatic cancer.[285] Mean serum PSA concentration was higher in those who developed cancer compared with those who did not (8.1 versus 4.6 ng/mL, respectively). All subsequent cancers apparently arose in the peripheral zone and were detected by needle biopsy. By contrast, a long-term study from Norway demonstrated no association between the presence of HGPIN on TURP and the incidence of subsequent cancer.[299] In a younger man with HGPIN on TURP, it may be recommended that needle biopsies be performed to rule out a peripheral zone cancer. In an older man without elevated serum PSA levels, clinical follow-up is probably sufficient. When HGPIN is found on TURP, some pathologists recommend sectioning deeper into the corresponding block, and most pathologists recommend processing the entire specimen to identify any small foci of carcinoma that may be present in the tissue.

Other Proposed Preneoplastic Lesions and Conditions

There are other possible findings in the prostate that may be premalignant (LGPIN, atrophy, malignancy-associated foci, atypical adenomatous hyperplasia, more recently, proliferative inflammatory atrophy),[300–302] but the data for these are less compelling than the data for HGPIN.

References

1. Bostwick DG: Evaluating prostate needle biopsy: therapeutic and prognostic importance. Ca Cancer J Clin 47:297–319, 1997.
2. Amin M, Boccon-Gibod L, Egevad L, et al: Prognostic and predictive factors and reporting of prostate carcinoma in prostate needle biopsy specimens. Scand J Urol Nephrol Suppl:20–33, 2005.
3. Srigley JR, Amin M, Boccon-Gibod L, et al: Prognostic and predictive factors in prostate cancer: historical perspectives and recent international consensus initiatives. Scand J Urol Nephrol 216(Suppl:8–19): 2005.
4. Bostwick DG, Montironi R: Prostatic intraepithelial neoplasia and the origins of prostatic carcinoma. Pathol Res Pract 191:828–832, 1995.
5. Cheng L, Paterson RF, Beck SD, et al: Prostatic intraepithelial neoplasia: an update. Clin Prostate Cancer 3:26–30, 2004.
6. Bostwick DG, Meiers I: Atypical small acinar proliferation in the prostate: clinical significance in 2006. Arch Pathol Lab Med 130:952–957, 2006.
7. Bostwick DG, Grignon DJ, Hammond EH, et al: Prognostic factors in prostate cancer. College of American Pathologists consensus statement 1999. Arch Pathol Lab Med 124:995–1000, 2000.

8. Bostwick DG, Qian J, Schlesinger C: Contemporary pathology of prostate cancer. Urol Clin N Am 30:181–207, 2003.

9. Cheng L, Koch MO, Juliar BE, et al: The combined percentage of Gleason patterns 4 and 5 is the best predictor of cancer progression after radical prostatectomy. J Clin Oncol 23:2911–2917, 2005.

10. Cheng L, Jones TD, Lin H, et al: Lymphovascular invasion is an independent prognostic factor in prostatic adenocarcinoma. J Urol 174:2181–2185, 2005.

11. Cheng L, Darson MF, Bergstralh EJ, et al: Correlation of margin status and extraprostatic extension with progression of prostate carcinoma. Cancer 86:1775–1782, 1999.

12. Cheng L, Slezak J, Bergstralh EJ, et al: Dedifferentiation in the metastatic progression of prostate carcinoma. Cancer 86:657–663, 1999.

13. Cheng L, Slezak J, Bergstralh EJ, et al: Preoperative prediction of surgical margin status in prostate cancer patients treated by radical prostatectomy. J Clin Oncol 18:2862–2868, 2000.

14. Cheng L, Davidson DD, Lin H, et al: Gleason percent pattern 4/5 predicts survival after radical prostatectomy. Cancer 110:1967–1972, 2007.

15. Nelson WG, De Marzo AM, Isaacs WB: Prostate cancer. N Engl J Med 349:366–381, 2003.

16. Nelson WG, De Marzo AM, DeWeese TL: The molecular pathogenesis of prostate cancer: implications for prostate cancer prevention. Urology 57:39–45, 2001.

17. Visakorpi T: The molecular genetics of prostate cancer. Urology 62:3–10, 2003.

18. Crawford ED: Epidemiology of prostate cancer. Urology 62:3–12, 2003.

19. Bostwick DG, Burke HB, Djakiew D, et al: Human prostate cancer risk factors. Cancer 101:2371–2490, 2004.

20. Cheng L, Lloyd RV, Weaver AL, et al: The cell cycle inhibitors p21WAF1 and p27KIP1 are associated with survival in patients treated by salvage prostatectomy after radiation therapy. Clin Cancer Res 6:1896–1899, 2000.

21. Cheng L, Pan C, Zhang JT, et al: Loss of 14-3-3σ in prostate cancer and its precursors. Clin Cancer Res 10:3064–3068, 2004.

22. Cheng L, Sebo TJ, Cheville JC, et al: P53 protein overexpression is associated with increased cell proliferation in patients with locally recurrent prostate carcinoma after radiation therapy. Cancer 85:1293–1299, 1999.

23. Cheng L, Leibovich BC, Bergstralh EJ, et al: p53 alteration in regional lymph node metastases from prostate carcinoma: a marker for progression? Cancer 85:2455–2459, 1999.

24. Cheng L, Bostwick DG, Li G, et al: Allelic imbalance in the clonal evolution of prostate carcinoma. Cancer 85:2017–2022, 1999.

25. Cheng L, Song SY, Pretlow TG, et al: Evidence of independent origin of multiple tumors from patients with prostate cancer. J Natl Cancer Inst 90:233–237, 1998.

26. Katona TM, Neubauer BL, Iversen PW, et al: Elevated expression of angiogenin in prostate cancer and its precursors. Clin Cancer Res 11:8358–8363, 2005.

27. Byar DP, Mostofi FK: Carcinoma of the prostate: prognostic evaluation of certain pathologic features in 208 radical prostatectomies. Cancer 30:5–13, 1972.

28. McNeal JE: Origin and development of carcinoma in the prostate. Cancer 23:24–34, 1969.

29. Epstein JI, Walsh PC, Carmichael M, et al: Pathologic and clinical findings to predict tumor extent of nonpalpable (stage T1c) prostate cancer. JAMA 271:368–374, 1994.

30. Arora R, Koch MO, Eble JN, et al: Heterogeneity of Gleason grade in multifocal adenocarcinoma of the prostate. Cancer 100:2362–2366, 2004.

31. Greene DR, Egawa S, Neerhut G, et al: The distribution of residual cancer in radical prostatectomy specimens in stage A prostate cancer. J Urol 146:1069–1076, 1991.

32. Greene DR, Wheeler TM, Egawa S, et al: Relationship between clinical stage and histological zone of origin in early prostate cancer: morphometric analysis. Br J Urol 68:499–509, 1991.

33. Greene DR, Wheeler TM, Egawa S, et al: A comparison of the morphological features of cancer arising in the transition zone and in the peripheral zone of the prostate. J Urol 146:1069–1076, 1991.

34. Srigley JR: Benign mimickers of prostatic adenocarcinoma. Mod Pathol 17:328–348, 2004.

35. Del Rosario AD, Bui HX, Abdulla M, et al: Sulfur-rich prostatic intraluminal crystalloids: a surgical pathologic and electron probe x-ray microanalytic study. Hum Pathol 24:1159–1167, 1993.

36. Molberg KH, Mikhail A, Vuitch F: Crystalloids in metastatic prostatic adenocarcinoma. Am J Clin Pathol 101:266–268, 1994.

37. Goldstein NS, Qian J, Bostwick DG: Mucin expression in atypical adenomatous hyperplasia of the prostate. Hum Pathol 26:887–891, 1995.

38. Bostwick DG, Wollan P, Adlakha K: Collagenous micronodules in prostate cancer. A specific but infrequent diagnostic finding. Arch Pathol Lab Med 119:444–447, 1995.

39. Darson MF, Pacelli A, Roche P, et al: Human glandular kallikrein 2 (hK2) expression in prostatic intraepithelial neoplasia and adenocarcinoma: a novel prostate cancer marker. Urology 49:857–862, 1997.

40. Hendrick L, Epstein JI: Use of keratin 903 as an adjunct in the diagnosis of prostate carcinoma. Am J Surg Path 13:389–396, 1989.

41. Cheng L, Cheville JC, Bostwick DG: Diagnosis of prostate cancer in needle biopsies after radiation therapy. Am J Surg Pathol 23:1173–1183, 1999.

42. Oliai BR, Kahane H, Epstein JI: Can basal cells be seen in adenocarcinoma of the prostate?: an immunohistochemical study using high molecular weight cytokeratin (clone 34betaE12) antibody. Am J Surg Pathol 26:1151–1160, 2002.

43. Shah RB, Zhou M, LeBlanc M, et al: Comparison of the basal cell-specific markers, 34betaE12 and p63, in the diagnosis of prostate cancer. Am J Surg Pathol 26:1161–1168, 2002.

44. Genega EM, Hutchinson B, Reuter VE, et al: Immunophenotype of high-grade prostatic adenocarcinoma and urothelial carcinoma. Mod Pathol 13:1186–1191, 2000.

45. Kaufmann O, Fietze E, Mengs J, et al: Value of p63 and cytokeratin 5/6 as immunohistochemical markers for the differential diagnosis of poorly differentiated and undifferentiated carcinomas. Am J Clin Pathol 116:823–830, 2001.

46. Xu J, Stolk JA, Zhang X, et al: Identification of differentially expressed genes in human prostate cancer using subtraction and microarray. Cancer Res 60:1677–1682, 2000.

47. Beach R, Gown AM, De Peralta-Venturina MN, et al: P504S immunohistochemical detection in 405 prostatic specimens including 376 18-gauge needle biopsies. Am J Surg Pathol 26:1588–1596, 2002.

48. Jiang Z, Woda BA, Rock KL, et al: P504S: a new molecular marker for the detection of prostate carcinoma. Am J Surg Pathol 25:1397–1404, 2001.

49. Zhou M, Chinnaiyan AM, Kleer CG, et al: Alpha-methylacyl-CoA racemase: a novel tumor marker over-expressed in several human cancers and their precursor lesions. Am J Surg Pathol 26:926–931, 2002.

50. Sung MT, Jiang Z, Montironi R, et al: Alpha-methylacyl-CoA racemase (P504S)/34betaE12/p63 triple cocktail stain in prostatic adenocarcinoma after hormonal therapy. Hum Pathol 38:332–341, 2007.

51. Jiang Z, Wu CL, Woda BA, et al: P504S/alpha-methylacyl-CoA racemase: a useful marker for diagnosis of small foci of prostatic carcinoma on needle biopsy. Am J Surg Pathol 26:1169–1174, 2002.

52. Jiang Z, Woda BA, Wu CL, et al: Discovery and clinical application of a novel prostate cancer marker: alpha-methylacyl CoA racemase (P504S). Am J Clin Pathol 122:275–289, 2004.

53. Yang XJ, Wu CL, Woda BA, et al: Expression of alpha-Methylacyl-CoA racemase (P504S) in atypical adenomatous hyperplasia of the prostate. Am J Surg Pathol 26:921–925, 2002.

54. Abrahamsson PA: Neuroendocrine differentiation in prostatic carcinoma. Prostate 39:135–148, 1999.

55. Abrahamsson PA, Wadstrom LB, Alumets J, et al: Peptide-hormone- and serotonin-immunoreactive tumour cells in carcinoma of the prostate. Pathol Res Pract 182:298–307, 1987.

56. Bonkhoff H: Neuroendocrine differentiation in human prostate cancer. Morphogenesis, proliferation and androgen receptor status. Ann Oncol 12 (Suppl 2):S141–S144, 2001.

57. di Sant'Agnese PA: Neuroendocrine differentiation in carcinoma of the prostate. Diagnostic, prognostic, and therapeutic implications. Cancer 70:254–268, 1992.

58. di Sant'Agnese PA: Neuroendocrine differentiation in human prostatic carcinoma. Hum Pathol 23:287–296, 1992.

59. Hansson J, Abrahamsson PA: Neuroendocrine pathogenesis in adenocarcinoma of the prostate. Ann Oncol 12(Suppl 2): S145–S152, 2001.
60. Helpap B, Kloppel G: Neuroendocrine carcinomas of the prostate and urinary bladder: a diagnostic and therapeutic challenge. Virchows Arch 440:241–248, 2002.
61. Helpap B, Kollermann J: Immunohistochemical analysis of the proliferative activity of neuroendocrine tumors from various organs. Are there indications for a neuroendocrine tumor-carcinoma sequence? Virchows Arch 438:86–91, 2001.
62. Ishimaru H, Kageyama Y, Hayashi T, et al: Expression of matrix metalloproteinase-9 and bombesin/gastrin-releasing peptide in human prostate cancers and their lymph node metastases. Acta Oncol 41:289–296, 2002.
63. Abdul M, Anezinis PE, Logothetis CJ, et al: Growth inhibition of human prostatic carcinoma cell lines by serotonin antagonists. Anticancer Res 14:1215–1220, 1994.
64. Hansson J, Bjartell A, Gadaleanu V, et al: Expression of somatostatin receptor subtypes 2 and 4 in human benign prostatic hyperplasia and prostatic cancer. Prostate 53:50–59, 2002.
65. Sun B, Halmos G, Schally AV, et al: Presence of receptors for bombesin/gastrin-releasing peptide and mRNA for three receptor subtypes in human prostate cancers. Prostate 42:295–303, 2000.
66. Cheville JC, Tindall D, Boelter C, et al: Metastatic prostate carcinoma to bone: clinical and pathologic features associated with cancer-specific survival. Cancer 95:1028–1036, 2002.
67. Jiborn T, Bjartell A, Abrahamsson PA: Neuroendocrine differentiation in prostatic carcinoma during hormonal treatment. Urology 51:585–589, 1998.
68. Krijnen JL, Bogdanowicz JF, Seldenrijk CA, et al: The prognostic value of neuroendocrine differentiation in adenocarcinoma of the prostate in relation to progression of disease after endocrine therapy. J Urol 158:171–174, 1997.
69. Tarle M, Ahel MZ, Kovacic K: Acquired neuroendocrine-positivity during maximal androgen blockade in prostate cancer patients. Anticancer Res 22:2525–2529, 2002.
70. Berruti A, Dogliotti L, Mosca A, et al: Effects of the somatostatin analog lanreotide on the circulating levels of chromogranin-A, prostate-specific antigen, and insulin-like growth factor-1 in advanced prostate cancer patients. Prostate 47:205–211, 2001.
71. Schally AV, Comaru-Schally AM, Plonowski A, et al: Peptide analogs in the therapy of prostate cancer. Prostate 45:158–166, 2000.
72. Zaky Ahel M, Kovacic K, Kraljic I, et al: Oral estramustine therapy in serum chromogranin A-positive stage D3 prostate cancer patients. Anticancer Res 21:1475–1479, 2001.
73. Gleason DF: Classification of prostatic carcinomas. Cancer Chemother Rep 50:125–128, 1966.
74. Gleason DF, Mellinger GT: Prediction of prognosis for prostatic adenocarcinoma by combined histological grading and clinical staging. Veterans administration cooperative urologic research group. J Urol 111:58–64, 1974.
75. Gleason DF: Histologic grading of prostate cancer: a perspective. Hum Pathol 23:273–279, 1992.
76. Bailar JC, 3rd, Mellinger GT, Gleason DF: Survival rates of patients with prostatic cancer, tumor stage, and differentiation–preliminary report. Cancer Chemother Rep 50:129–136, 1966.
77. Bostwick DG: Gleason grading of prostatic needle biopsies: correlation with grade 316 matched prostatectomies. Am J Surg Pathol 18:796–803, 1994.
78. Epstein JI, Allsbrook WC, Jr, Amin MB, et al: The 2005 International Society of Urological Pathology (ISUP) Consensus Conference on Gleason Grading of Prostatic Carcinoma. Am J Surg Pathol 29:1228–1242, 2005.
79. Egevad L, Allsbrook WC, Jr, Epstein JI: Current practice of Gleason grading among genitourinary pathologists. Hum Pathol 36:5–9, 2005.
80. Allsbrook WC, Jr, Mangold KA, Johnson MH, et al: Interobserver reproducibility of Gleason grading of prostatic carcinoma: urologic pathologists. Hum Pathol 32:74–80, 2001.
81. Allsbrook WC, Jr, Mangold KA, Johnson MH, et al: Interobserver reproducibility of Gleason grading of prostatic carcinoma: general pathologist. Hum Pathol 32:81–88, 2001.
82. Epstein JI, Partin AW, Sauvageot J, et al: Prediction of progression following radical prostatectomy: a multivariate analysis of 721 men with long-term follow-up. Am J Surg Pathol 20:286–292, 1996.
83. Epstein JI: Gleason score 2–4 adenocarcinoma of the prostate on needle biopsy: a diagnosis that should not be made [Letter]. Am J Surg Pathol 24:477–478, 2000.
84. Lopez-Beltran A, Qian J, Montironi R, et al: Atypical adenomatous hyperplasia (adenosis) of the prostate: DNA ploidy analysis and immunophenotype. Int J Surg Pathol 13:167–173, 2005.
85. Amin MB, Schultz DS, Zarbo RJ: Analysis of cribriform morphology in prostatic neoplasia using antibody to high-molecular-weight cytokeratins. Arch Pathol Lab Med 118:260–264, 1994.
86. Epstein JI, Amin M, Boccon-Gibod L, et al: Prognostic factors and reporting of prostate carcinoma in radical prostatectomy and pelvic lymphadenectomy specimens. Scand J Urol Nephrol Suppl:34–63, 2005.
87. Montironi R, Mazzucchelli R, Scarpelli M, et al: Gleason grading of prostate cancer in needle biopsies or radical prostatectomy specimens: contemporary approach, current clinical significance and sources of pathology discrepancies. BJU Int 95:1146–1152, 2005.
88. Makarov DV, Sanderson H, Partin AW, et al: Gleason score 7 prostate cancer on needle biopsy: is the prognostic difference in Gleason scores 4 + 3 and 3 + 4 independent of the number of involved cores? J Urol 167:2440–2442, 2002.
89. Pan C, Potter SR, Partin AW, et al: The prognostic significance of tertiary Gleason patterns of higher grade in radical prostatectomy specimens: a proposal to modify the Gleason grading system. Am J Surg Pathol 24:563–569, 2000.
90. Rubin MA, Dunn R, Kambham N, et al: Should a Gleason score be assigned to a minute focus of carcinoma on prostate biopsy? Am J Surg Pathol 24:1634–1640, 2000.
91. Augustin H, Eggert T, Wenske S, et al: Comparison of accuracy between the Partin tables of 1997 and 2001 to predict final pathological stage in clinically localized prostate cancer. J Urol 171:177–181, 2004.
92. Babaian RJ, Troncoso P, Bhadkamkar VA, et al: Analysis of clinicopathologic factors predicting outcome after radical prostatectomy. Cancer 91:1414–1422, 2001.
93. Poulos CK, Daggy JK, Cheng L: Preoperative prediction of Gleason grade in radical prostatectomy specimens: the influence of different Gleason grades from multiple positive biopsy sites. Mod Pathol 18:228–234, 2005.
94. Rubin MA, Bismar TA, Curtis S, et al: Prostate needle biopsy reporting: how are the surgical members of the Society of Urologic Oncology using pathology reports to guide treatment of prostate cancer patients? Am J Surg Pathol 28:946–952, 2004.
95. Mian BM, Troncoso P, Okihara K, et al: Outcome of patients with Gleason score 8 or higher prostate cancer following radical prostatectomy alone. J Urol 167:1675–1680, 2002.
96. Kattan MW, Eastham JA, Wheeler TM, et al: Counseling men with prostate cancer: a nomogram for predicting the presence of small, moderately differentiated, confined tumors. J Urol 170:1792–1797, 2003.
97. Sakr WA, Tefilli MV, Grignon DJ, et al: Gleason score 7 prostate cancer: a heterogeneous entity? Correlation with pathologic parameters and disease-free survival. Urology 56:730–734, 2000.
98. Hattab EM, Koch MO, Eble JN, et al: Tertiary Gleason pattern 5 is a powerful predictor of biochemical relapse in patients with Gleason score 7 prostatic adenocarcinoma. J Urol 175:1695–1699, 2006.
99. Stamey T, McNeal J, Yemoto C, et al: Biological determinants of cancer progression in men with prostate cancer. JAMA 281:1395–1400, 1999.
100. Montironi R, Scarpelli M, Lopez-Beltran A: Carcinoma of the prostate: inherited susceptibility, somatic gene defects and androgen receptors. Virchows Arch 444:503–508, 2004.
101. Garnett JE, Oyasu R, Grayhack JT: The accuracy of diagnostic biopsy specimens in predicting tumor grades by Gleason's classification of radical prostatectomy specimens. J Urol 131:690–693, 1984.
102. Mills SE, Fowler JE, Jr: Gleason histologic grading of prostatic carcinoma. Correlations between biopsy and prostatectomy specimens. Cancer 57:346–349, 1986.
103. Humphrey P: Prostate Pathology. Chicago: ASCP Press, 2003.
104. Bostwick DG, Kindrachuk RW, Rouse RV: Prostatic adenocarcinoma with endometrioid features. Clinical, pathologic, and ultrastructural findings. Am J Surg Pathol 9:595–609, 1985.

105. Epstein JI, Woodruff JM: Adenocarcinoma of the prostate with endometrioid features. A light microscopic and immunohistochemical study of ten cases. Cancer 57:111–119, 1986.

106. Green LF, Farrow GM, Ravits JM: Prostatic adenocarcinoma. J Urol Pathol 2:319–325, 1979.

107. Christensen WN, Steinberg G, Walsh PC, et al: Prostatic duct adenocarcinoma. Findings at radical prostatectomy. Cancer 67:2118–2124, 1991.

108. Ro JY, Ayala AG, Wishnow KI, et al: Prostatic duct adenocarcinoma with endometrioid features: immunohistochemical and electron microscopic study. Semin Diagn Pathol 5:301–311, 1988.

109. Brinker DA, Potter SR, Epstein JI: Ductal adenocarcinoma of the prostate diagnosed on needle biopsy: correlation with clinical and radical prostatectomy findings and progression. Am J Surg Pathol 23:1471–1479, 1999.

110. Bostwick DG: Neoplasms of the Prostate. St. Louis: Mosby, 1997.

111. Cina SJ, Epstein JI: Adenocarcinoma of the prostate with atrophic features. Am J Surg Pathol 21:289–295, 1997.

112. Egan AJ, Lopez-Beltran A, Bostwick DG: Prostatic adenocarcinoma with atrophic features: malignancy mimicking a benign process. Am J Surg Pathol 21:931–935, 1997.

113. Amin MB, Tamboli P, Varma M, et al: Postatrophic hyperplasia of the prostate gland. Am J Surg Pathol 23:925–931, 1999.

114. Humphrey PA, Kaleem Z, Swanson PE, et al: Pseudohyperplastic prostatic adenocarcinoma. Am J Surg Pathol 22:1239–1246, 1998.

115. Levi AW, Epstein JI: Pseudohyperplastic prostatic adenocarcinoma on needle biopsy and simple prostatectomy. Am J Surg Pathol 24:1039–1046, 2000.

116. Pacelli A, Lopez-Beltran A, Egan AJ, et al: Prostatic adenocarcinoma with glomeruloid features. Hum Pathol 29:543–546, 1998.

117. Tran TT, Sengupta E, Yang XJ: Prostatic foamy gland carcinoma with aggressive behavior: clinicopathologic, immunohistochemical, and ultrastructural analysis. Am J Surg Pathol 25:618–623, 2001.

118. Nelson RS, Epstein JI: Prostatic carcinoma with abundant xanthomatous cytoplasm. Foamy gland carcinoma. Am J Surg Pathol 20:419–426, 1996.

119. Ordonez NG, Ro JY, Ayala AG: Metastatic prostatic carcinoma presenting as an oncocytic tumor. Am J Surg Pathol 16:1007–1012, 1992.

120. Pinto JA, Gonzalez JE, Granadillo MA: Primary carcinoma of the prostate with diffuse oncocytic changes. Histopathology 25:286–288, 1994.

121. Adlakha K, Bostwick D: Lymphoepithelioma-like carcinoma of prostate. J Urol 2:319–325, 1994.

122. Randolph TL, Amin MB, Ro JY, et al: Histologic variants of adenocarcinoma and other carcinomas of prostate: pathologic criteria and clinical significance. Mod Pathol 10:612–629, 1997.

123. Epstein JI, Lieberman PH: Mucinous adenocarcinoma of the prostate gland. Am J Surg Pathol 9:299–308, 1985.

124. Ro JY, Grignon DJ, Ayala AG, et al: Mucinous adenocarcinoma of the prostate: histochemical and immunohistochemical studies. Hum Pathol 21:593–600, 1990.

125. Saito S, Iwaki H: Mucin-producing carcinoma of the prostate: review of 88 cases. Urology 54:141–144, 1999.

126. Ro JY, el-Naggar A, Ayala AG, et al: Signet-ring-cell carcinoma of the prostate. Electron-microscopic and immunohistochemical studies of eight cases. Am J Surg Pathol 12:453–460, 1988.

127. Hejka AG, England DM: Signet ring cell carcinoma of prostate. Immunohistochemical and ultrastructural study of a case. Urology 34:155–158, 1989.

128. Uchijima Y, Ito H, Takahashi M, et al: Prostate mucinous adenocarcinoma with signet ring cell. Urology 36:267–268, 1990.

129. Dhom G: Histopathology of prostate carcinoma. Diagnosis and differential diagnosis. Pathol Res Pract 179:277–303, 1985.

130. Gray GF, Jr, Marshall VF: Squamous carcinoma of the prostate. J Urol 113:736–738, 1975.

131. Bassler TJ, Jr., Orozco R, Bassler IC, et al: Adenosquamous carcinoma of the prostate: case report with DNA analysis, immunohistochemistry, and literature review. Urology 53:832–834, 1999.

132. Mott LJ: Squamous cell carcinoma of the prostate: report of 2 cases and review of the literature. J Urol 121:833–835, 1979.

133. Nabi G, Ansari MS, Singh I, et al: Primary squamous cell carcinoma of the prostate: a rare clinicopathological entity. Report of 2 cases and review of literature. Urol Int 66:216–219, 2001.

134. Gattuso P, Carson HJ, Candel A, et al: Adenosquamous carcinoma of the prostate. Hum Pathol 26:123–126, 1995.

135. Accetta PA, Gardner WA, Jr.: Adenosquamous carcinoma of prostate. Urology 22:73–75, 1983.

136. Ishigooka M, Yaguchi H, Tomaru M, et al: Mixed prostatic carcinoma containing malignant squamous element. Reports of two cases. Scand J Urol Nephrol 28:425–427, 1994.

137. Greene LF, Mulcahy JJ, Warren MM, et al: Primary transitional cell carcinoma of the prostate. J Urol 110:235–237, 1973.

138. Mahadevia PS, Koss LG, Tar IJ: Prostatic involvement in bladder cancer. Prostate mapping in 20 cystoprostatectomy specimens. Cancer 58:2096–2102, 1986.

139. Nixon RG, Chang SS, Lafleur BJ, et al: Carcinoma in situ and tumor multifocality predict the risk of prostatic urethral involvement at radical cystectomy in men with transitional cell carcinoma of the bladder. J Urol 167:502–505, 2002.

140. Wood DP, Jr, Montie JE, Pontes JE, et al: Transitional cell carcinoma of the prostate in cystoprostatectomy specimens removed for bladder cancer. J Urol 141:346–349, 1989.

141. Oliai BR, Kahane H, Epstein JI: A clinicopathologic analysis of urothelial carcinomas diagnosed on prostate needle biopsy. Am J Surg Pathol 25:794–801, 2001.

142. Cheville JC, Dundore PA, Bostwick DG, et al: Transitional cell carcinoma of the prostate: clinicopathologic study of 50 cases. Cancer 82:703–707, 1998.

143. Bodner DR, Cohen JK, Resnick MI: Primary transitional cell carcinoma of the prostate. J Urol (Paris) 92:121–122, 1986.

144. Laplante M, Brice M, 2nd: The upper limits of hopeful application of radical cystectomy for vesical carcinoma: does nodal metastasis always indicate incurability? J Urol 109:261–264, 1973.

145. Shen SS, Lerner SP, Muezzinoglu B, et al: Prostatic involvement by transitional cell carcinoma in patients with bladder cancer and its prognostic significance. Hum Pathol 37:726–734, 2006.

146. Sawczuk I, Tannenbaum M, Olsson CA, et al: Primary transitional cell carcinoma of prostatic periurethral ducts. Urology 25:339–343, 1985.

147. Takashi M, Sakata T, Nagai T, et al: Primary transitional cell carcinoma of prostate: case with lymph node metastasis eradicated by neoadjuvant methotrexate, vinblastine, doxorubicin, and cisplatin (M-VAC) therapy. Urology 36:96–98, 1990.

148. Greene FL, Page DL, Fleming ID, et al: American Joint Committee on Cancer Staging Manual, 6th ed . New York: Springer, 2002.

149. Ro JY, Tetu B, Ayala AG, et al: Small cell carcinoma of the prostate. II. Immunohistochemical and electron microscopic studies of 18 cases. Cancer 59:977–982, 1987.

150. Tetu B, Ro JY, Ayala AG, et al: Small cell carcinoma of the prostate. Part I. A clinicopathologic study of 20 cases. Cancer 59:1803–1809, 1987.

151. Delahunt B, Eble JN, Nacey JN, et al: Sarcomatoid carcinoma of the prostate: progression from adenocarcinoma is associated with p53 over-expression. Anticancer Res 19:4279–4283, 1999.

152. Dundore PA, Cheville JC, Nascimento AG, et al: Carcinosarcoma of the prostate. Report of 21 cases. Cancer 76:1035–1042, 1995.

153. Lopez-Beltran A, Pacelli A, Rothenberg HJ, et al: Carcinosarcoma and sarcomatoid carcinoma of the bladder: clinicopathological study of 41 cases. J Urol 159:1497–1503, 1998.

154. Reuter VE: Sarcomatoid lesions of the urogenital tract. Semin Diagn Pathol 10:188–201, 1993.

155. Shannon RL, Ro JY, Grignon DJ, et al: Sarcomatoid carcinoma of the prostate. A clinicopathologic study of 12 patients. Cancer 69:2676–2682, 1992.

156. Luque Barona RJ, Gonzalez Campora CR, Vicioso Recio L, et al: Synchronous prostatic carcinosarcoma: report of 2 cases and review of the literature. Actas Urol Esp 24:173–178, 2000.

157. Poblet E, Gomez-Tierno A, Alfaro L: Prostatic carcinosarcoma: a case originating in a previous ductal adenocarcinoma of the prostate. Pathol Res Pract 196:569–572, 2000.

158. Devaraj LT, Bostwick DG: Atypical basal cell hyperplasia of the prostate. Immunophenotypic profile and proposed classifi-

cation of basal cell proliferations. Am J Surg Pathol 17:645–659, 1993.

159. Iczkowski KA, Montironi R: Adenoid cystic/basal cell carcinoma of the prostate strongly expresses HER-2/neu. J Clin Pathol 59:1327–1330, 2006.

160. Iczkowski KA, Ferguson KL, Grier DD, et al: Adenoid cystic/basal cell carcinoma of the prostate: clinicopathologic findings in 19 cases. Am J Surg Pathol 27:1523–1529, 2003.

161. Ali TZ, Epstein JI: Basal cell carcinoma of the prostate: a clinicopathologic study of 29 cases. Am J Surg Pathol 31:697–705, 2007.

162. Cheng L, Cheville JC, Pisansky TM, et al: Prevalence and distribution of prostatic intraepithelial neoplasia in salvage radical prostatectomy specimens after radiation therapy. Am J Surg Pathol 23:803–808, 1999.

163. Cheng L, Sebo TJ, Slezak J, et al: Predictors of survival in prostate cancer patients treated with salvage prostatectomy after radiation therapy. Cancer 83:2164–1671, 1998.

164. Dhom G, Degro S: Therapy of prostatic cancer and histopathologic follow-up. Prostate 3:531–542, 1982.

165. Gaudin PB: Histopathologic effects of radiation and hormonal therapies on benign and malignant prostate tissue. J Urol Pathol 8:55–67, 1998.

166. Helpap B: Treated prostatic carcinoma. Histological, immunohistochemical and cell kinetic studies. Appl Pathol 3:230–241, 1985.

167. Helpap B: Fundamentals on the pathology of prostatic carcinoma after brachytherapy. World J Urol 20:207–212, 2002.

168. Helpap B, Koch V: Histological and immunohistochemical findings of prostatic carcinoma after external or interstitial radiotherapy. J Cancer Res Clin Oncol 117:608–614, 1991.

169. Herr HW, Whitmore WF, Jr: Significance of prostatic biopsies after radiation therapy for carcinoma of the prostate. Prostate 3:339–350, 1982.

170. Lytton B, Collins JT, Weiss RM, et al: Results of biopsy after early stage prostatic cancer treatment by implantation of 125I seeds. J Urol 121:306–309, 1979.

171. Crook J, Malone S, Perry G, et al: Postradiotherapy prostate biopsies: what do they really mean? Results for 498 patients. Int J Radiat Oncol Biol Phys 48:355–367, 2000.

172. Vailancourt L, Ttu B, Fradet Y, et al: Effect of neoadjuvant endocrine therapy (combined androgen blockade) on normal prostate and prostatic carcinoma. A randomized study. Am J Surg Path 20:86–93, 1996.

173. Montironi R, Magi-Galluzzi C, Muzzonigro G, et al: Effects of combination endocrine treatment on normal prostate, prostatic intraepithelial neoplasia, and prostatic adenocarcinoma. J Clin Pathol 47:906–913, 1994.

174. Armas OA, Aprikian AG, Melamed J, et al: Clinical and pathobiological effects of neoadjuvant total androgen ablation therapy on clinically localized prostatic adenocarcinoma. Am J Surg Pathol 18:979–991, 1994.

175. Magi-Galluzzi C, Montironi R, Giannulis I, et al: Prostatic invasive adenocarcinoma. Effect of combination endocrine therapy (LHRH agonist and flutamide) on the expression and location of proliferating cell nuclear antigen (PCNA). Pathol Res Pract 189:1154–1160, 1993.

176. Murphy WM, Soloway MS, Barrows GH: Pathologic changes associated with androgen deprivation therapy for prostate cancer. Cancer 68:821–828, 1991.

177. Reuter VE: Pathological changes in benign and malignant prostatic tissue following androgen deprivation therapy. Urology 49:16–22, 1997.

178. Smith DM, Murphy WM: Histologic changes in prostate carcinomas treated with leuprolide (luteinizing hormone-releasing hormone effect). Distinction from poor tumor differentiation. Cancer 73:1472–1477, 1994.

179. Tetu B, Srigley JR, Boivin JC, et al: Effect of combination endocrine therapy (LHRH agonist and flutamide) on normal prostate and prostatic adenocarcinoma. A histopathologic and immunohistochemical study. Am J Surg Pathol 15:111–120, 1991.

180. Van de Voorde WM, Van Poppel HP, Verbeken EK, et al: Morphologic and neuroendocrine features of adenocarcinoma arising in the transition zone and in the peripheral zone of the prostate. Mod Pathol 8:591–598, 1995.

181. Akakura K, Bruchovsky N, Goldenberg SL, et al: Effects of intermittent androgen suppression on androgen-dependent tumors. Apoptosis and serum prostate-specific antigen. Cancer 71:2782–2790, 1993.

182. Van de Voorde WM, Elgamal AA, Van Poppel HP, et al: Morphologic and immunohistochemical changes in prostate cancer after preoperative hormonal therapy. A comparative study of radical prostatectomies. Cancer 74:3164–1675, 1994.

183. Schulman CC, Wildschutz T, Zlotta AR: Neoadjuvant hormonal treatment prior to radical prostatectomy: facts and open questions. Eur Urol 32:41–47, 1997.

184. Bostwick DG, Adolfsson J, Burke HB, et al: Epidemiology and statistical methods in prediction of patient outcome. Scand J Urol Nephrol Suppl:94–110, 2005.

185. Montironi R, Mazzucchelli R, Scarpelli M, et al: Prostate carcinoma II: prognostic factors in prostate needle biopsies. BJU Int 97:492–497, 2006.

186. Eichelberger LE, Cheng L: Does pT2b prostate carcinoma exist? Critical appraisal of the 2002 TNM classification of prostate carcinoma. Cancer 100:2573–2576, 2004.

187. Hong H, Koch MO, Foster RS, et al: Anatomic distribution of periprostatic adipose tissue: a mapping study of 100 radical prostatectomy specimens. Cancer 97:1639–1643, 2003.

188. Mazzucchelli R, Santinelli A, Lopez-Beltran A, et al: Evaluation of prognostic factors in radical prostatectomy specimens with cancer. Urol Int 68:209–215, 2002.

189. Grignon DJ, Sakr WA: Pathologic staging of prostate carcinoma: what are the issues? Cancer 78:337–340, 1996.

190. Sung MT, Eble JN, Cheng L: Invasion of fat justifies assignment of stage pT3a in prostatic adenocarcinoma. Pathology 38:309–311, 2006.

191. Sung MT, Lin H, Koch MO, et al: Radial distance of extraprostatic extension measured by ocular micrometer is an independent predictor of prostate-specific antigen recurrence: a new proposal for the substaging of pT3a prostate cancer. Am J Surg Pathol 31:311–318, 2007.

192. Bostwick DG, Montironi R: Evaluating radical prostatectomy specimens: therapeutic and prognostic importance. Virchows Arch 430:1–16, 1997.

193. Epstein JI, Partin AW, Potter SR, et al: Adenocarcinoma of the prostate invading the seminal vesicle: prognostic stratification based on pathologic parameters. Urology 56:283–288, 2000.

194. Ohori M, Scardino PT, Lapin SL, et al: The mechanisms and prognostic significance of seminal vesicle involvement by prostate cancer. Am J Pathol 17:1252–1261, 1993.

195. Catalona WJ, Smith DS: Cancer recurrence and survival rates after anatomic radical retropubic prostatectomy for prostate cancer: intermediate-term results. J Urol 160:2428–2434, 1998.

196. D'Amico AV, Whittington R, Malkowicz SB, et al: A multivariate analysis of clinical and pathological factors that predict for prostate specific antigen failure after radical prostatectomy for prostate cancer. J Urol 154:131–138, 1995.

197. Debras B, Guillonneau B, Bougaran J, et al: Prognostic significance of seminal vesicle invasion on the radical prostatectomy specimen. Rationale for seminal vesicle biopsies. Eur Urol 33:271–277, 1998.

198. Tefilli MV, Gheiler EL, Tiguert R, et al: Prognostic indicators in patients with seminal vesicle involvement following radical prostatectomy for clinically localized prostate cancer. J Urol 160:802–806, 1998.

199. Cheng L, Slezak J, Bergstralh EJ, et al: Dedifferentiation in the metastatic progression of prostate cancer. Cancer 86:657–663, 1999.

200. Cheng L, Zincke H, Blute ML, et al: Risk of prostate carcinoma death in patients with lymph node metastasis. Cancer 91:66–73, 2001.

201. Boccon-Gibod L, van der Kwast TH, Montironi R, et al: Handling and pathology reporting of prostate biopsies. Eur Urol 46:177–181, 2004.

202. Kattan MW, Stapleton AMF, Wheeler TM, et al: Evaluation of a nomogram used to predict the pathologic stage of clinically localized prostate carcinoma. Cancer 79:528–537, 1997.

203. Partin AW, Kattan MW, Subong EN, et al: Combination of prostate-specific antigen, clinical stage, and Gleason score to predict pathological stage of localized prostate cancer. JAMA 277:1445–1451, 1997.

204. Eble JN, Epstein JI, Sauter G, et al: WHO Classification of Tumours : Pathology and Genetics. Tumours of the Urinary

and Male Reproductive System. Lyon, France: IARC Press, 2004.

205. Poulos CK, Daggy JK, Cheng L: Prostate needle biopsies: multiple variables are predictive of final tumor volume in radical prostatectomy specimens. Cancer 101:527–532, 2004.

206. Freedland SJ, Aronson WJ, Terris MK, et al: Percent of prostate needle biopsy cores with cancer is a significant independent predictor of prostate specific antigen recurrence following radical prostatectomy: results from the search database. J Urol 169:2136–2141, 2003.

207. Freedland SJ, Csathy GS, Dorey F, et al: Percent prostate needle biopsy tissue with cancer is more predictive of biochemical failure or adverse pathology after radical prostatectomy than prostate specific antigen or Gleason score. J Urol 167:516–520, 2002.

208. Gancarczyk KJ, Wu H, McLeod DG, et al: Using the percentage of biopsy cores positive for cancer, pretreatment PSA, and highest biopsy Gleason sum to predict pathologic stage after radical prostatectomy: the Center for Prostate Disease Research nomograms. Urology 61:589–595, 2003.

209. Kronz JD, Allan CH, Shaikh AA, et al: Predicting cancer following a diagnosis of high-grade prostatic intraepithelial neoplasia on needle biopsy: data on men with more than one follow-up biopsy. Am J Surg Pathol 25:1079–1085, 2001.

210. Kestin LL, Goldstein NS, Vicini FA, et al: Percentage of positive biopsy cores as predictor of clinical outcome in prostate cancer treated with radiotherapy. J Urol 168:1994–1999, 2002.

211. Lewis JS, Vollmer RT, Humphrey PA: Carcinoma extent in prostate needle biopsy tissue in the prediction of whole gland tumor volume in a screening population. Am J Clin Pathol 118:442–450, 2002.

212. Epstein JI: Diagnosis and reporting of limited adenocarcinoma of the prostate on needle biopsy. Mod Pathol 17:307–315, 2004.

213. Thorson P, Vollmer RT, Arcangeli C, et al: Minimal carcinoma in prostate needle biopsy specimens: diagnostic features and radical prostatectomy follow-up. Mod Pathol 11:543–551, 1998.

214. Cheng L, Poulos CK, Pan CK, et al: Preoperative prediction of small volume cancer (<0.5 ml) in radical prostatectomy specimens. J Urol 174:898–902, 2005.

215. Cheng L, Jones TD, Pan CX, et al: Anatomic distribution and pathologic characterization of small-volume prostate cancer (<0.5 ml) in whole-mount prostatectomy specimens. Mod Pathol 18:1022–1026, 2005.

216. Humphrey PA, Vollmer RT: Intraglandular tumor extent and prognosis in prostatic carcinoma: application of a grid method to prostatectomy specimens. Hum Pathol 21:799–804, 1990.

217. Eichelberger LE, Koch MO, Daggy JK, et al: Predicting tumor volume in radical prostatectomy specimens from patients with prostate cancer. Am J Clin Pathol 120:386–391, 2003.

218. Eichelberger LE, Koch MO, Eble JN, et al: Maximum tumor diameter is an independent predictor of prostate specific antigen recurrence in prostate cancer. Mod Pathol 18:886–890, 2005.

219. Emerson RE, Koch MO, Jones TD, et al: The influence of extent of surgical margin positivity on prostate specific antigen recurrence. Am J Clin Pathol 58:1028–1032, 2005.

220. Jones TD, Koch MO, Lin H, et al: Visual estimation of tumour extent is not an independent predictor of prostate specific antigen recurrence. BJU Int 96:1253–1257, 2005.

221. Marks RA, Lin H, Koch MO, et al: Positive-block ratio in radical prostatectomy specimens is an independent predictor of prostate-specific antigen recurrence. Am J Surg Pathol 31:877–881, 2007.

222. Wieder JA, Soloway MS: Incidence, etiology, location, prevention and treatment of positive surgical margins after radical prostatectomy for prostate cancer. J Urol 160:299–315, 1998.

223. Emerson RE, Koch MO, Daggy JK, et al: Closest distance between tumor and resection margin in radical prostatectomy specimens: lack of prognostic significance. Am J Surg Pathol 29:225–229, 2005.

224. Marks RA, Koch MO, Lopez-Beltran A, et al: Relationship between the extent of surgical margin positivity and prostate-specific antigen recurrence in radical prostatectomy specimens. Hum Pathol 38:1207–1211, 2007.

225. Hoedemaeker RF, Vis AN, Van der Kwast TH: Staging prostate cancer. Microsc Res Tech 51:423–429, 2000.

226. True LD: Surgical pathology examination of the prostate gland. Practice survey by American Society of Clinical Pathologists. Am J Clin Pathol 102:572–579, 1994.

227. Poulos CK, Koch MO, Eble JN, et al: Bladder neck invasion is an independent predictor of prostate-specific antigen recurrence. Cancer 101:1563–1568, 2004.

228. Kernek KM, Koch MO, Daggy JK, et al: The presence of benign prostatic glandular tissue at surgical margins does not predict PSA recurrence. J Clin Pathol 58:725–728, 2005.

229. Maru N, Ohori M, Kattan MW, et al: Prognostic significance of the diameter of perineural invasion in radical prostatectomy specimens. Hum Pathol 32:828–833, 2001.

230. Anderson PR, Hanlon AL, Patchefsky A, et al: Perineural invasion and Gleason 7–10 tumors predict increased failure in prostate cancer patients with pretreatment PSA <10 ng/ml treated with conformal external beam radiation therapy. Int J Radiat Oncol Biol Phys 41:1087–1092, 1998.

231. Quinn DI, Henshall SM, Brenner PC, et al: Prognostic significance of preoperative factors in localized prostate carcinoma treated with radical prostatectomy: importance of percentage of biopsies that contain tumor and the presence of biopsy perineural invasion. Cancer 97:1884–1893, 2003.

232. Vargas SO, Jiroutek M, Welch WR, et al: Perineural invasion in prostate needle biopsy specimens. Correlation with extraprostatic extension at resection. Am J Clin Pathol 111:223–228, 1999.

233. Sebo TJ, Cheville JC, Riehle DL, et al: Predicting prostate carcinoma volume and stage at radical prostatectomy by assessing needle biopsy specimens for percent surface area and cores positive for carcinoma, perineural invasion, Gleason score, DNA ploidy and proliferation, and preoperative serum prostate specific antigen. Cancer 91:2196–2204, 2001.

234. Holmes GF, Walsh PC, Pound CR, et al: Excision of the neurovascular bundle at radical prostatectomy in cases with perineural invasion on needle biopsy. Urology 53:752–756, 1999.

235. Beard CJ, Chen MH, Cote K, et al: Perineural invasion is associated with increased relapse after external beam radiotherapy for men with low-risk prostate cancer and may be a marker for occult, high-grade cancer. Int J Radiat Oncol Biol Phys 58:19–24, 2004.

236. Ng JC, Koch MO, Daggy JK, et al: Perineural invasion in radical prostatectomy specimens: lack of prognostic significance. J Urol 172:2249–2251, 2004.

237. Salomao DR, Graham SD, Bostwick DG: Microvascular invasion in prostate cancer correlates with pathologic stage. Arch Pathol Lab Med 119:1050–1054, 1995.

238. Ito K, Nakashima J, Mukai M, et al: Prognostic implication of microvascular invasion in biochemical failure in patients treated with radical prostatectomy. Urol Int 70:297–302, 2003.

239. Shariat SF, Khoddami SM, Saboorian H, et al: Lymphovascular invasion is a pathological feature of biologically aggressive disease in patients treated with radical prostatectomy. J Urol 171:1122–1127, 2004.

240. Cheng L, Bergstralh EJ, Cheville JC, et al: Cancer volume of lymph node metastasis predicts progression in prostate cancer. Am J Surg Pathol 22:1491–1500, 1998.

241. Cheng L, Pisansky TM, Ramnani DM, et al: Extranodal extension in lymph node-positive prostate cancer. Mod Pathol 13:113–118, 2000.

242. Cheville JC, Reznicek MJ, Bostwick DG: The focus of "atypical glands, suspicious for malignancy" in prostatic needle biopsy specimens: incidence, histologic features, and clinical follow-up of cases diagnosed in a community practice [see comments]. Am J Clin Pathol 108:633–640, 1997.

243. Epstein JI, Herawi M: Prostate needle biopsies containing prostatic intraepithelial neoplasia or atypical foci suspicious for carcinoma: implications for patient care. J Urol 175:820–834, 2006.

244. Iczkowski KA, MacLennan GT, Bostwick DG: Atypical small acinar proliferation suspicious for malignancy in prostate needle biopsies: clinical significance in 33 cases. Am J Surg Pathol 21:1489–1495, 1997.

245. Schlesinger C, Bostwick DG, Iczkowski KA: High-grade prostatic intraepithelial neoplasia and atypical small acinar proliferation: predictive value for cancer in current practice. Am J Surg Pathol 29:1201–1207, 2005.

246. Bostwick DG, Qian J, Frankel K: The incidence of high grade prostatic intraepithelial neoplasia in needle biopsies. J Urol 154:1791–1794, 1995.
247. Kahane H, Sharp JW, Shuman GB, et al: Utilization of high molecular weight cytokeratin on prostate needle biopsies in an independent laboratory. Urology 45:981–986, 1995.
248. Borboroglu PG, Sur RL, Roberts JL, et al: Repeat biopsy strategy in patients with atypical small acinar proliferation or high grade prostatic intraepithelial neoplasia on initial prostate needle biopsy. J Urol 166:866–870, 2001.
249. Chan TY, Epstein JI: Follow-up of atypical prostate needle biopsies suspicious for cancer. Urology 53:351–355, 1999.
250. Iczkowski KA, Bassler TJ, Schwob VS, et al: Diagnosis of "suspicious for malignancy" in prostate biopsies: predictive value for cancer. Urology 51:749–758, 1998.
251. Park S, Shinohara K, Grossfeld GD, et al: Prostate cancer detection in men with prior high grade prostatic intraepithelial neoplasia or atypical prostate biopsy. J Urol 165:1409–1414, 2001.
252. Samaratunga H, Gardiner RA, Yaxley J, et al: Atypical prostatic glandular proliferations on needle biopsy: diagnostic implications, use of immunohistochemistry, and clinical significance. Anal Quant Cytol Histol 28:104–110, 2006.
253. Srigley JR: Small-acinar patterns in the prostate gland with emphasis on atypical adenomatous hyperplasia and small-acinar carcinoma. Semin Diagn Pathol 5:254–272, 1988.
254. Epstein JI: Diagnostic criteria of limited adenocarcinoma of the prostate on needle biopsy. Hum Pathol 26:223–229, 1995.
255. Herawi M, Parwani AV, Irie J, et al: Small glandular proliferations on needle biopsies: most common benign mimickers of prostatic adenocarcinoma sent in for expert second opinion. Am J Surg Pathol 29:874–880, 2005.
256. Iczkowski KA, Bostwick DG: Criteria for biopsy diagnosis of minimal volume prostatic adenocarcinoma: analytic comparison with nondiagnostic but suspicious atypical small acinar proliferation. Arch Pathol Lab Med 124:98–107, 2000.
257. Kronz JD, Shaikh AA, Epstein JI: High-grade prostatic intraepithelial neoplasia with adjacent small atypical glands on prostate biopsy. Hum Pathol 32:389–395, 2001.
258. Mai KT, Yazdi HM, Belanger E, et al: High grade prostatic intraepithelial neoplasia involving small ducts and acini. Histopathology 46:475–477, 2005.
259. Signoretti S, Waltregny D, Dilks J, et al: p63 is a prostate basal cell marker and is required for prostate development. Am J Pathol 157:1769–1775, 2000.
260. Ramnani DM, Bostwick DG: Basal cell-specific anti-keratin antibody 34betaE12: optimizing its use in distinguishing benign prostate and cancer. Mod Pathol 12:443–444, 1999.
261. Montironi R, Vela-Navarrete R, Lopez-Beltran A, et al: 2005 update on pathology of prostate biopsies with cancer. Eur Urol 49:441–447, 2006.
262. Bostwick DG, Srigley J, Grignon D, et al: Atypical adenomatous hyperplasia of the prostate: morphologic criteria for its distinction from well-differentiated carcinoma. Hum Pathol 24:819–832, 1993.
263. Shah RB, Kunju LP, Shen R, et al: Usefulness of basal cell cocktail (34betaE12 + p63) in the diagnosis of atypical prostate glandular proliferations. Am J Clin Pathol 122:517–523, 2004.
264. Zhou M, Shah R, Shen R, et al: Basal cell cocktail (34betaE12 + p63) improves the detection of prostate basal cells. Am J Surg Pathol 27:365–371, 2003.
265. Zhou M, Aydin H, Kanane H, et al: How often does alpha-methylacyl-CoA-racemase contribute to resolving an atypical diagnosis on prostate needle biopsy beyond that provided by basal cell markers? Am J Surg Pathol 28:239–243, 2004.
266. Hameed O, Humphrey PA: Immunohistochemistry in diagnostic surgical pathology of the prostate. Semin Diagn Pathol 22:88–104, 2005.
267. Scattoni V, Roscigno M, Freschi M, et al: Predictors of prostate cancer after initial diagnosis of atypical small acinar proliferation at 10 to 12 core biopsies. Urology 66:1043–1047, 2005.
268. Moore CK, Karikehalli S, Nazeer T, et al: Prognostic significance of high grade prostatic intraepithelial neoplasia and atypical small acinar proliferation in the contemporary era. J Urol 173:70–72, 2005.
269. Postma R, Roobol M, Schroder FH, et al: Lesions predictive for prostate cancer in a screened population: first and second screening round findings. Prostate 61:260–266, 2004.
270. O'Dowd GJ, Miller MC, Orozco R, et al: Analysis of repeated biopsy results within 1 year after a noncancer diagnosis. Urology 55:553–559, 2000.
271. Hoedemaeker RF, Kranse R, Rietbergen JBW, et al: Evaluation of prostate needle biopsies in a population-based screening study. Cancer 85:145–152, 1999.
272. Fadare O, Wang S, Mariappan MR: Practice patterns of clinicians following isolated diagnoses of atypical small acinar proliferation on prostate biopsy specimens. Arch Pathol Lab Med 128:557–560, 2004.
273. Brausi M, Castagnetti G, Dotti A, et al: Immediate radical prostatectomy in patients with atypical small acinar proliferation. Over treatment? J Urol 172:906–908, 2004.
274. Girasole CR, Cookson MS, Putzi MJ, et al: Significance of atypical and suspicious small acinar proliferations, and high grade prostatic intraepithelial neoplasia on prostate biopsy: implications for cancer detection and biopsy strategy. J Urol 175:929–933, 2006.
275. Montironi R, Scattoni V, Mazzucchelli R, et al: Atypical foci suspicious but not diagnostic of malignancy in prostate needle biopsies (also referred to as "atypical small acinar proliferation suspicious for but not diagnostic of malignancy"). Eur Urol 50:666–674, 2006.
276. Keane PF, Ilesley IC, O'Donoghue PN, et al: Pathological classification and follow-up of prostatic lesions initially diagnosed as "suspicious of malignancy." Br J Urol 66:306–311, 1990.
277. Descazeaud A, Rubin MA, Allory Y, et al: What information are urologists extracting from prostate needle biopsy reports and what do they need for clinical management of prostate cancer? Eur Urol 48:911–915, 2005.
278. Leite KR, Mitteldorf CA, Camara-Lopes LH: Repeat prostate biopsies following diagnoses of prostate intraepithelial neoplasia and atypical small gland proliferation. Int Braz J Urol 31:131–136, 2005.
279. Allen EA, Kahane H, Epstein JI: Repeat biopsy strategies for men with atypical diagnoses or initial prostate needle biopsy. Urol 52:803–807, 1998.
280. Ellis WJ, Brawer MK: Repeat prostate needle biopsy: who needs it? J Urol 153:1496–1498, 1995.
281. McNeal JE, Bostwick DG: Intraductal dysplasia: a premalignant lesion of the prostate. Hum Pathol 17:64–71, 1986.
282. Bostwick DG: Prostatic intraepithelial neoplasia (PIN): current concepts. J Cell Biochem 16H (Suppl):9–10, 1992.
283. Sakr WA, Grignon DJ, Haas GP, et al: Age and racial distribution of prostatic intraepithelial neoplasia. Eur Urol 30:138–144, 1996.
284. Gaudin PB, Sesterhenn IA, Wojno KJ, et al: Incidence and clinical significance of high-grade prostatic intraepithelial neoplasia in TURP specimens. Urology 49:558–563, 1997.
285. Pacelli A, Bostwick DG: Clinical significance of high-grade prostatic intraepithelial neoplasia in transurethral resection specimens. Urology 50:355–359, 1997.
286. Qian J, Wollan P, Bostwick DG: The extent and multicentricity of high-grade prostatic intraepithelial neoplasia in clinically localized prostatic adenocarcinoma. Hum Pathol 28:143–148, 1997.
287. Montironi R, Mazzucchelli R, Algaba F, et al: Morphological identification of the patterns of prostatic intraepithelial neoplasia and their importance. J Clin Pathol 53:655–665, 2000.
288. Kovi J, Jackson MA, Heshmat MY: Ductal spread in prostatic carcinoma. Cancer 56:1566–1573, 1985.
289. Bostwick DG, Liu L, Brawer MK, et al: High-grade prostatic intraepithelial neoplasia. Rev Urol 6:171–179, 2004.
290. Bostwick DG, Amin MB, Dundore P, et al: Architectural patterns of high-grade prostatic intraepithelial neoplasia. Hum Pathol 24:298–310, 1993.
291. Scattoni V, Montironi R, Mazzucchelli R, et al: Pathological changes of high-grade prostatic intraepithelial neoplasia and prostate cancer after monotherapy with bicalutamide 150 mg. BJU Int 98:54–58, 2006.
292. Cote RJ, Skinner EC, Salem CE, et al: The effect of finasteride on the prostate gland in men with elevated serum prostate-specific antigen levels. Br J Cancer 78:413–418, 1998.
293. Epstein JI, Potter SR: The pathological interpretation and significance of prostate needle biopsy findings: implications and current controversies. J Urol 166:402–410, 2001.
294. Izawa JI, Lega I, Downey D, et al: Do all patients with high-grade prostatic intraepithelial neoplasia on initial prostatic

biopsy eventually progress to clinical prostate cancer? BJU Int 96:320–323, 2005.

295. Naya Y, Ayala AG, Tamboli P, et al: Can the number of cores with high-grade prostate intraepithelial neoplasia predict cancer in men who undergo repeat biopsy? Urology 63:503–508, 2004.

296. Herawi M, Kahane H, Cavallo C, et al: Risk of prostate cancer on first re-biopsy within 1 year following a diagnosis of high grade prostatic intraepithelial neoplasia is related to the number of cores sampled. J Urol 175:121–124, 2006.

297. Roscigno M, Scattoni V, Freschi M, et al: Monofocal and plurifocal high-grade prostatic intraepithelial neoplasia on extended prostate biopsies: factors predicting cancer detection on extended repeat biopsy. Urology 63:1105–1110, 2004.

298. Joniau S, Goeman L, Pennings J, et al: Prostatic intraepithelial neoplasia (PIN): importance and clinical management. Eur Urol 48:379–385, 2005.

299. Harvei S, Skjorten FJ, Robsahm TE, et al: Is prostatic intraepithelial neoplasia in the transition/central zone a true precursor of cancer? A long-term retrospective study in Norway. Br J Cancer 78:46–49, 1998.

300. Cheng L, Shan A, Cheville JC, et al: Atypical adenomatous hyperplasia of the prostate: a premalignant lesion? Cancer Res 58:389–391, 1998.

301. De Marzo AM, Marchi VL, Epstein JI, et al: Proliferative inflammatory atrophy of the prostate. Am J Pathol 155:1985–1992, 1999.

302. De Marzo AM, Platz EA, Sutcliffe S, et al: Inflammation in prostate carcinogenesis. Nat Rev Cancer 7:256–269, 2007.

Expectant Management

4

Danil V. Makarov, Christopher A. Warlick, and H. Ballentine Carter

KEY POINTS

- Prostate cancer represents a heterogeneous set of diseases with a wide range of outcomes.
- Many men have prostate cancer at autopsy, fewer are diagnosed with prostate cancer during their lifetimes, and fewer still die of prostate cancer.
- Initial insights into the natural history of prostate cancer came from nonrandomized, retrospective data.
- The common selection criteria for expectant management of prostate cancer include clinical stage, prostate-specific antigen (PSA), Gleason score, and other pathologic surrogates for low-volume tumors.
- Several groups have demonstrated good oncologic outcomes among men carefully selected for the conservative management of prostate cancer.
- Efforts are underway to standardize selection and intervention criteria for expectant management.
- Novel biomarkers are needed to better predict the outcomes of men considered for enrollment into expectant management protocols.

Introduction

Prostate cancer is the most commonly diagnosed nondermatologic malignancy among men in the United States.[1] Despite its widespread prevalence, it is well known that prostate cancers exhibit a diverse range of outcomes. Although autopsy series have demonstrated that 42% of men older than 50 years harbor prostate cancer, we also know that only 16% of all men will ever be diagnosed with prostate cancer (lifetime risk) and that only 3% of men ultimately die of the disease.[2–4]

From the adage, "more men die with prostate cancer than of prostate cancer" was born the concept that perhaps not all men with prostate cancer need aggressive treatment of their disease. Indeed, in an examination of trends in the treat-

ment of prostate cancer from the CaPSURE database, Harlan and associates[5] and then Cooperberg and associates[6] have demonstrated that a not insignificant proportion of men diagnosed with prostate cancer are electing conservative treatment of their disease. However, this number is probably lower than might be expected (Fig. 4-1). In this chapter, we examine the development of expectant management as an option for men with prostate cancer, we examine the landmark studies establishing the natural history of untreated prostate cancer, and we examine the design and outcomes of several institutions' efforts to study expectant management in a rigorous fashion.

Rationale for Expectant Management

Because the morbidity of treatment of prostate cancer may be severe, regardless of modality, the challenge to the clinician is to determine which prostate cancers need treatment and which do not.[7–9] Mean (SEM) time to prostate cancer-specific mortality in patients with non-palpable (T1) lesions has been demonstrated to be 17 (1.8) years and 11.7 (1.2) years for patients with clinically palpable lesions (T2 or greater)[10] (Fig. 4-2). It is evident when comparing these estimates of lengthy survival time with the expectations of life in a 65-year-old man (17.1 years) and a 75-year-old man (10.7 years) living in the United States in 2004 that not all men diagnosed with prostate cancer need to be treated for it.[3]

The annual age-adjusted prostate cancer death rate in the United States has declined steadily since the early 1990s[1] (Fig. 4-3). The annual age-adjusted prostate cancer incidence

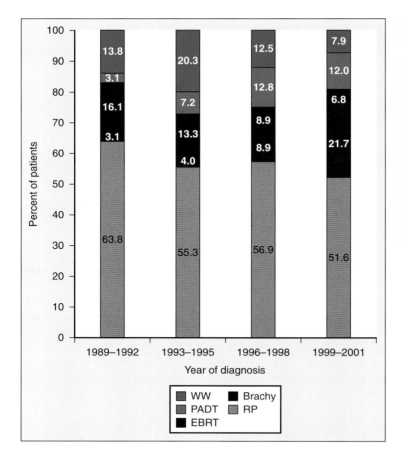

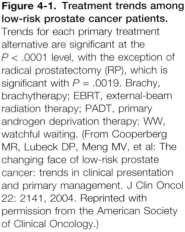

Figure 4-1. Treatment trends among low-risk prostate cancer patients. Trends for each primary treatment alternative are significant at the $P < .0001$ level, with the exception of radical prostatectomy (RP), which is significant with $P = .0019$. Brachy, brachytherapy; EBRT, external-beam radiation therapy; PADT, primary androgen deprivation therapy; WW, watchful waiting. (From Cooperberg MR, Lubeck DP, Meng MV, et al: The changing face of low-risk prostate cancer: trends in clinical presentation and primary management. J Clin Oncol 22: 2141, 2004. Reprinted with permission from the American Society of Clinical Oncology.)

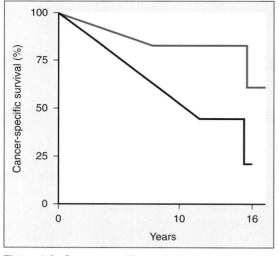

Figure 4-2. Cancer-specific survival rate curves for patients with microscopic (T1, green) and palpable (T2-3, red) tumor during 1976–1983. (From Horan AH, McGehee M: Mean time to cancer-specific death of apparently clinically localized prostate cancer: policy implications for threshold ages in prostate-specific antigen screening and ablative therapy. BJU Int 85:1063, 2000.)

rates rose steadily until their peak in 1991 and then decreased and reached a plateau in the last 8 years to a level much higher than in the pre-PSA (prostate-specific antigen) era[1] (Fig. 4-4). Moreover, 90% of newly diagnosed patients present with local or regional disease.[1] This trend (stage migration)—whether the result of earlier detection or changes in disease biology—has created a dramatic shift in the clinical stage of newly diagnosed prostate cancer patients.[11]

Despite these trends toward the detection of more, but less significant cancers, the potential to diagnose still greater numbers of men with even more favorable characteristics has been suggested by data from the control arm of the Prostate Cancer Prevention Trial. Even among a cohort of men with low PSA (less than 4.0 ng/mL) and normal digital rectal examinations (DRE), prostate cancer was found in 15.2% when they underwent a biopsy (not for a specific cause) at the end of the study; however, only 2% of cancers in this group were high grade (Table 4-1).[12] Cancer was even found in men

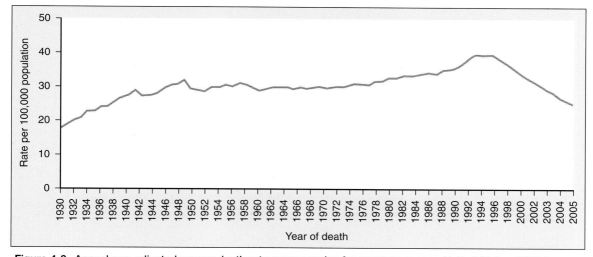

Figure 4-3. Annual age-adjusted cancer death rate among males for prostate cancer, United States, 1930 to 2005.   Rates are age-adjusted to the 2000 U.S. standard population. Note that because of changes in ICD coding, numerator information has changed over time. Rates for cancers of the lung and bronchus, colon and rectum, and liver are affected by these changes. (Adapted from Jemal A, Siegel R, Ward E, et al: Cancer statistics, 2009. CA Cancer J Clin 59:225–249, 2009, Figure 4. © 2009 American Cancer Society. Reprinted with permission of John Wiley & Sons, Inc.)

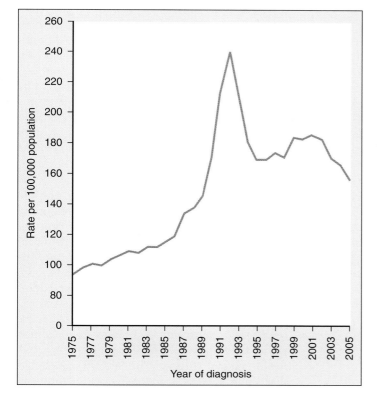

Figure 4-4. Annual age-adjusted prostate cancer incidence rates among males, United States, 1975 to 2005. Rates are age-adjusted to the 2000 U.S. standard population and adjusted for delays in reporting. (Adapted from Jemal A, Siegel R, Ward E, et al: Cancer statistics, 2009. CA Cancer J Clin 59:225–249, 2009, Figure 3. © 2009 American Cancer Society. Reprinted with permission of John Wiley & Sons, Inc.)

Table 4-1. Relationship of the Prostate-Specific Antigen (PSA) Level to the Prevalence of Prostate Cancer and High-Grade Disease

PSA Level	No. of Men (N = 2950)	Men with Prostate Cancer (N = 449) No. of Men (%)	Men with High-Grade Prostate Cancer (N = 67) No./Total No. (%)	Sensitivity	Specificity
≤0.5 ng/mL	486	32 (6.6)	4/32 (12.5)	1.0	0.0
0.6–1.0 ng/mL	791	80 (10.1)	8/80 (10.0)	0.93	0.18
1.1–2.0 ng/mL	998	170 (17.0)	20/170 (11.8)	0.75	0.47
2.1–3.0 ng/mL	482	115 (23.9)	22/115 (19.1)	0.37	0.80
3.1–4.0 ng/mL	193	52 (26.9)	13/52 (25.0)	0.12	0.94

High-grade disease was defined by a Gleason score of 7 or greater. The population was restricted to men with a PSA level of 4.0 ng/mL or less throughout the study. Therefore, the definitions of sensitivity and specificity are restricted to cutoff values of <4.0 ng/mL (the cutoff values are equal to the lower value of the ranges in the PSA column [0.0, 0.6, 1.1, 2.1, and 3.1 ng/mL]). Sensitivity was defined as the proportion of men with cancer who had a PSA value above the cutoff among all men with cancer who had a PSA value of 4.0 ng/mL or less. Specificity was defined in a like manner.

From Thompson IM, Pauler DK, Goodman PJ, et al.: Prevalence of prostate cancer among men with a prostate-specific antigen level ≤ 4.0 ng/mL. N Engl J Med 350:2239, 2004. Copyright © 2004 Massachusetts Medical Society. All rights reserved.

with PSA of less than 0.5 ng/mL at a rate of 6.2%.[12] One must wonder how many of these low-PSA, negative-DRE cancers would ever have become clinically significant during that man's lifetime. Does biopsying men with low PSA represent a quest for lethal cancers in a "haystack" of indolent disease?

Watchful Waiting

There is a body of published literature examining the outcomes of watchful waiting protocols. Watchful waiting, as used by these studies, examines the outcomes of men in whom there was no effort to cure prostate cancer, although many did receive palliation. This is contrasted with expectant management or active surveillance, in which men are initially left untreated but are closely followed, so that the decision to treat or not treat is revisited with regularity. The watchful waiting studies, mostly observing patients from the pre-PSA era, focus their attention on patients who are poor candidates for aggressive treatment. Most of these men are elderly or have significant comorbidity and thus have a relatively short life expectancy at the time of enrollment.

Early Retrospective Series

Establishing Equipoise

One of the first studies ever to examine the natural history of early prostate cancer came from Barnes and associates.[13] The authors examined 86 patients who were treated conservatively for prostate cancer. They noted that most of these men died of diseases other than prostate cancer. Their conclusion was that prostate cancer is rather more like a chronic disease that may be managed with conservative therapy. Although several other studies from the period supported the conclusion that men with localized prostate cancer had a long survival even if treated conservatively,[14,15] some studies described varied and sometimes unfavorable outcomes from delayed treatment.[16,17]

Another such study was published by Johansson and coworkers.[18] The authors examined a group of 223 patients from Sweden who were diagnosed with early-stage (T0-2) prostate cancer and did not undergo initial treatment. At the time of symptomatic progression, however, they did receive hormone therapy either in the form of orchiectomy or estrogen administration. Only 19 of a total of 124 deaths in this group were from prostate cancer. The 10-year prostate cancer-specific survival rate was 86.8% (95% confidence interval 80.7–92.9%), and the 10-year progression-free survival rate was 53% (95% CI 44.2–62.0%). Of 76 patients who demonstrated clinical progression, 50 had local-only progression. The researchers found similar results in a subgroup analysis examining men whom they felt would have met eligibility criteria for radical surgery. The authors concluded that clinical trials were necessary before any therapy could be recommended for patients with prostate cancer. This study is particularly significant because it spawned a randomized trial, the results of which have been extremely illuminating and influential in the field of urology.

Establishing Negative Prognostic Indicators

Chodak and associates[19] performed a meta-analysis of six pre-PSA era studies enrolling men who had clinically localized prostate cancer (clinical stage T1 or T2) and who did not receive initial treatment, but rather were observed and received delayed hormonal therapy. Eight hundred twenty-eight patients were reviewed. Similar to the results from the initial report from Johansson and coworkers,[18] 10-year prostate cancer-specific survival rate was 87% for men with grade 1 or 2 tumors, but only 34% for those with grade 3 tumors (Fig. 4-5); the initial report of Johansson and coworkers[18] did not evaluate the effects of tumor grade. They confirmed these findings in their 2004 update.[20] Prostate cancer-specific survival was not affected by early disease stage, patient age, comorbidity, or delayed intervention in the form of surgery or radiation. They also noted that further follow-up, in the interval from 15 to 20 years, demonstrated a substantial worsening in progression-free, metastasis-free, and prostate cancer-specific survival (from 77% at 15 years to 54% at 20 years), although these estimates were based on a limited number of patients and were reported with wide confidence intervals (Fig. 4-6). Based on their results, the authors suggested that watchful waiting was a reasonable strategy for patients with low-grade prostate cancer having a life expectancy of fewer than 10 years, but that radical treatment should be con-sidered for men with a life expectancy of more than 15 years and that novel strategies must be applied to those with grade 3 disease.

Adolfsson and coworkers[21] from the Karolinska Institute also performed a similar study of 172 patients with prostate cancer managed with deferred therapy until the onset of symptomatic progression. In contrast to the previously discussed papers, the Karolinska group included men with T3 lesions. Ten-year prostate cancer-specific survival rate was 80% for the entire patient cohort. However, subgroup analysis revealed an 84% 10-year prostate cancer-specific survival rate among the men with clinically localized (T1-T2) prostate tumors, whereas men with T3 lesions had only a 70% prostate cancer-specific survival rate at 9 years. This led to the researchers' recommendation that deferred therapy (essentially watchful waiting, since only 52% of patients ever received therapy) be considered for those with clinically localized disease.

McLaren and associates[22] describe a cohort of 113 patients with prostate cancer from the British Columbia Cancer Agency who were managed with watchful waiting. Forty percent of patients with T1 disease and 51% of those with T2 disease developed clinical progression by 2 years. The authors found that PSA doubling time (PSADT) correlated with clinical progression, stage progression, and time to treatment and that patients with PSADT of less than 18 months progressed within 6 months. They concluded that patients undergoing watchful waiting exhibit high rates of clinical progression and that PSADT rather than standard pathologic criteria gave a better prediction of this occurrence.

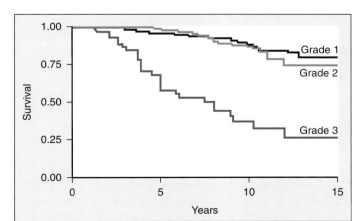

Figure 4-5. Disease-specific survival among untreated patients with localized prostate cancer, according to tumor grade. Data on patients who died of other causes were censored. (From Chodak GW, Thisted, RA, Gerber GS, et al: Results of conservative management of clinically localized prostate cancer. N Engl J Med 330:242, 1994. Copyright © 1994 Massachusetts Medical Society. All rights reserved.)

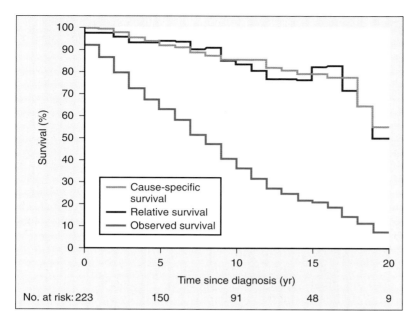

Figure 4-6. Survival of prostate cancer patients (n = 223). (From Johansson JE, Andren O, Andersson SO, et al: Natural history of early, localized prostate cancer. JAMA 291:2713, 2004, Figure 1.)

Other groups[23,24] have also examined PSADT as a predictor of delayed treatment. El-Geneidy and coworkers[23] examined 187 patients, 175 of whom had clinical stage T1 or T2 lesions. Patient age and percentage of biopsy cores involved with cancer were predictors on univariate analysis and independent predictors on multivariable analysis. PSADT, although not significant as a univariate predictor, became significant when added to a multivariable model.

Recent (Since 2000) Retrospective Series

Albertsen and others have published several studies looking at the long-term survival of men from a large population-based cohort with localized prostate cancer treated with immediate or delayed hormonal therapy.[25-27] Their most recent data examined 767 men 55 to 74 years of age, hoping to confirm or refute the long-term outcomes data from Johansson and coworkers[20] which demonstrated the decline in prostate cancer-specific survival after 15 years (more than 10 years)[28]; cases were identified from the Connecticut Tumor Registry and all patients had their pathology re-examined for the purposes of the study. A competing risks model demonstrated that there was not a statistically significant difference in the risk of death from prostate cancer in the first 15 years after diagnosis and the risk of death from prostate cancer

after 15 years of follow-up. The authors reaffirmed their previous findings[25,26] that men with low-grade, localized prostate cancer have a low risk of prostate cancer-specific mortality, whereas those with higher grades are at greater risk, even among older men (Fig. 4-7). They also concluded again that since the annual prostate cancer-specific mortality rate remains unchanged after 15 years from the time of diagnosis, aggressive treatment for low-grade, localized prostate cancer is not indicated.

Several other recent publications have demonstrated interesting insights into watchful waiting for prostate cancer. Patel and associates[29] have reported the Memorial Sloan-Kettering experience with deferred therapy for prostate cancer. Eighty-eight patients with clinical stage T1-2 who were eligible for, but elected not to be treated with, radical prostatectomy, were consecutively enrolled over the years 1984 to 2001. No specific enrollment criteria were established a priori. Patients were followed up with DRE and serum PSAs every 3 months for 1 year and every 6 months thereafter. Repeat biopsy was recommended at baseline, 1 year, then every 2 to 3 years. Biopsies were performed sooner if DRE, transrectal ultrasonography, or PSA suggested disease progression. However, there were no defined criteria to determine disease progression, since imaging and physical exam were considered subjective and PSA and

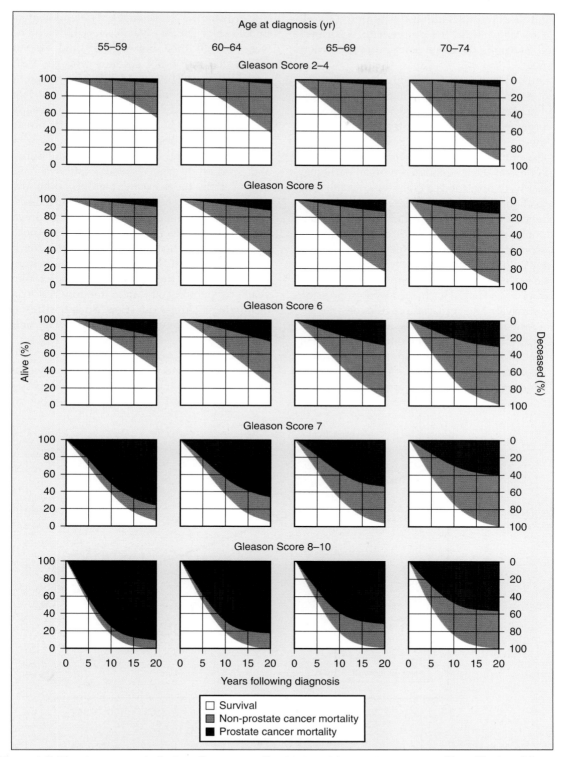

Figure 4-7. Twenty-year survival rates after conservative treatment for prostate cancer. (From Albertsen PC, Hanley JA, Fine J: 20-year outcomes following conservative management of clinically localized prostate cancer. JAMA 293:2095, 2005.)

repeat biopsy results are also considered unreliable. A point scale for progression was developed, assigning different point scores to various events.

Only 61% of men enrolled had cancer identified on a confirmatory biopsy. Twenty-two patients developed objective evidence of progression (defined as a point cut-off) during a median follow-up of 44 months. Seventeen patients underwent radical prostatectomy, of whom 15 had Gleason scores upgraded on final pathology; 7 cases were upgraded to Gleason 7. At the time, none of the 17 patients undergoing surgery had evidence of clinical or biochemical recurrence; the only patient to demonstrate biochemical recurrence had been treated with radiation therapy. Logistic regression revealed that absence of cancer on confirmatory biopsy and low initial PSA were associated with improved progression-free survival. The actuarial progression-free survival rate at 5 years was 67%, and at 10 years it was 55%. The authors conclude that active surveillance with deferred therapy is a feasible alternative in carefully selected patients.

Wong and associates[30] performed a retrospective analysis, examining men with prostate cancer from the Surveillance, Epidemiology, and End Results (SEER) Medicare database. There were 44,630 men between 65 and 80 years (older than the other studies) who were diagnosed between 1991 and 1999. The researchers found that 37% of the men in the watchful waiting group and 23.8% in the treatment group had died. The absolute difference in prostate cancer deaths, treated versus untreated, was 0.5% at 12 years. So although overall survival and prostate cancer-specific survival were improved in the treatment group, even when adjusted for patient age and for low-risk disease, the number needed to treat is 200 to prevent one prostate cancer death at 12 years. Another idiosyncrasy of the data was that the survival difference (Fig. 4-8) was evident almost immediately, whereas the survival difference took 10 years to demonstrate in a randomized trial[28] examining a similar question. Such a difference would be unlikely to occur so early unless the groups were unbalanced with respect to comorbidity.

Cuzick and associates[31] retrospectively examined a contemporary cohort of 2333 patients from the United Kingdom (diagnosed between

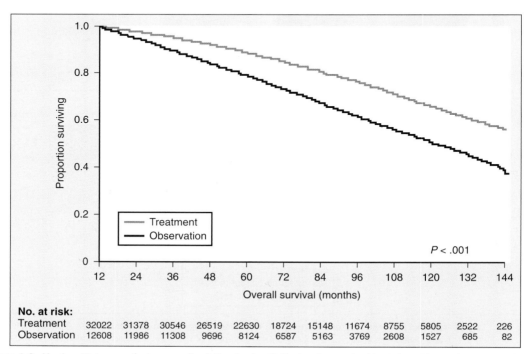

Figure 4-8. Kaplan-Meier survival curves for full cohort. Patients who survived less than 12 months were excluded from the analysis. (From Wong YN, Mitra N, Hudes G, et al: Survival associated with treatment vs observation of localized prostate cancer in elderly men. JAMA 296:2683, 2006.)

1990 and 1996) with available baseline PSA measurements and re-reviewed all pathologic (TURP [transurethral resection of prostate] chips [54%] or needle biopsy) specimens. Most patients did not receive initial treatment; however, 29% received hormonal therapy within 6 months of diagnosis. At 10 years, a competing risks analysis demonstrated 55% overall mortality, with 24% prostate cancer-specific and 31% representing death from other causes. However, using PSA and Gleason score, the authors were able to stratify patients into three groups with 10-year prostate cancer-specific mortalities of less than 10%, 10% to 30%, and greater than 30%. They conclude that new, better, biomarkers are necessary to predict the outcomes of men falling in the intermediate group.

Prospective Watchful Waiting

One of the most important studies on the subject of watchful waiting for prostate cancer (and, indeed, in all of urology) is the Scandinavian Prostate Cancer Study Group's prospective randomized trial originally published by Holmberg and coworkers[32] in 2002 and then updated by Bill-Axelson and associates[28] in 2005. This trial, in follow-up to the study performed by Johansson and coworkers,[18] compared radical prostatectomy with watchful waiting (followed by palliative rather than curative therapy) in men presenting with clinically localized prostate cancer. Would there really be no difference between the treated and untreated groups? One of the most important factors to consider when examining data from these studies is that approximately 75% of the men enrolled had palpable (T2) lesions and roughly 25% had Gleason grade greater than 6.

The first of the two reports[32] found that risk of prostate cancer-specific mortality was decreased in men treated with radical prostatectomy compared with the control arm (4.3% versus 8.9%, respectively). A statistically significant benefit held true with respect to the risk of developing metastases in the radical prostatectomy group. Overall survival, however, was not different between the two groups, and many investigators speculated as to what might be the ultimate outcome after more follow-up.[33] The results became clear in 2005, when Bill-Axelson and associates[28] published the 10-year follow-up data and demonstrated a benefit to radical pros-

tatectomy, compared with watchful waiting, with respect to relative risk of prostate cancer-specific mortality 0.56 (95% CI 0.36–0.88), distant metastasis 0.60 (95% CI 0.42–0.86), and local progression 0.33 (95% CI 0.25–0.44). Absolute mortality was lower in the surgery group (83 deaths) than the watchful waiting group (106 deaths), $P = .04$ (Fig. 4-9). An important point to consider when examining these results is that so many of the patients included in the study had palpable lesions on DRE (77.8% in the radical prostatectomy group and 74.4% in the watchful waiting group) and presented with symptoms of advanced prostate cancer (43.8% in the radical prostatectomy group and 39.7% in the watchful waiting group). As with T3 lesions with Adolfsson and co-workers[21] and higher-grade lesions in early work by Albertsen and associates,[25,26] this study demonstrated some of the limitations of simple watchful waiting in men having prostate cancer with adverse parameters. Further work on this patient cohort has been aimed at determining factors influencing progression.[34] Despite the clear statistically significant differences, the number needed to treat to prevent one prostate cancer death for men over 65 years of age is 330. The authors caution, however, that the survival estimates in older men are based on small numbers and should be treated as a hypothesis to investigate thoroughly in other studies.

Expectant Management of Prostate Cancer

Prediction

Most of the previously discussed studies examining watchful waiting as a treatment option come out in favor of watchful waiting, but only after identifying a subgroup of patients in whom watchful waiting would not be beneficial. Based on insights regarding the natural history of prostate cancer and the factors that influence the aggressiveness of disease, researchers set out to identify criteria that could determine which men could defer immediate therapy for prostate cancer and could be observed at least initially. Some of these criteria were derived from the early watchful waiting studies, whereas several others worked to determine novel, specific criteria to select for men who could be followed up expectantly.

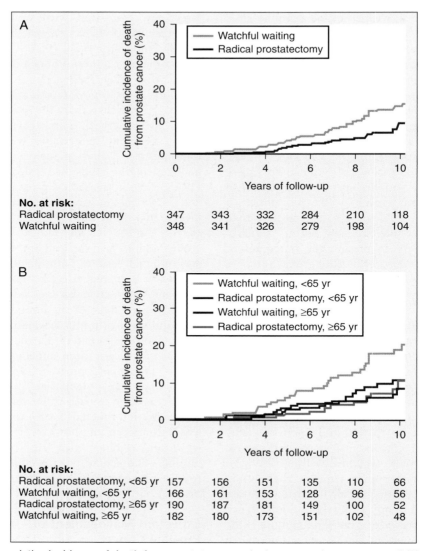

Figure 4-9. Cumulative incidence of death from prostate cancer in the two study groups overall (A) and according to age (B).   (From Bill-Axelson A, Holmberg L, Ruutu M, et al: Radical prostatectomy versus watchful waiting in early prostate cancer. N Engl J Med 352:1977, 2005. Copyright © 2005 Massachusetts Medical Society. All rights reserved.)

Epstein and coworkers[35] examined a series of 157 men with clinical stage T1c prostate cancer who had undergone radical prostatectomy for treatment of their disease. The authors created four classifications of pathologic outcomes: insignificant, minimal, moderate, and advanced. Pathologic criteria for the insignificant category, which comprised 16% of treated T1c tumors, were tumor volume less than 0.2 cm^3 and Gleason score less than 7. A model was created to predict "insignificant" tumor pathology based on presurgical criteria. Tumors having (1) preoperative PSA density (PSAD) less than or equal to 0.1 ng/mL/g and a lack of adverse findings

(defined as Gleason score greater than 6, more than two cores involved with cancer, or any core with more than 50% involvement with cancer) or (2) PSAD less than or equal to 0.15 ng/mL/g and less than 3 mm of tumor on a single biopsy core had a positive predictive value of 95%, a negative predictive value of 66%. The model correctly classified tumors as insignificant 73% of the time based on their preoperative information. The authors suggested that patients satisfying these criteria could possibly avoid treatment for prostate cancer.

The same investigators updated their findings and their model 4 years later.[36] Using a slightly different definition of insignificant disease (tumor volume changed from less than 0.2 cm^3 to less than 0.5 cm^3),[37] they found that 25% of treated T1c tumors were insignificant. One hundred sixty-three patients with clinical stage T1c prostate cancer were examined. These men had undergone radical prostatectomy and had information on preoperative biopsy and preoperative free and total PSA measurements. Of these 163 patients, 30.7% had insignificant disease. A model with criteria of preoperative free to total PSA fraction greater than or equal to 0.15 and the absence of adverse pathologic criteria[35] had a positive predictive value of 94.4%, a negative predictive value of 77.2%. Findings from these two studies laid the foundation for future prospective analyses.

Concurrent to the group at Johns Hopkins, Ohori and coworkers[37] examined whether preoperative information allowed clinicians to detect clinically significant prostate cancer more efficiently than simply what might be found incidentally. Three hundred and six cases were identified with prostate cancer treated with radical prostatectomy; 90 patients with incidental prostate cancer discovered by radical cystoprostatectomy for bladder cancer served as controls. This analysis revealed that cancer detected by DRE, PSA screening, or transrectal ultrasound was less likely to be advanced than cancer found incidentally during radical cystoprostatectomy. Also notable was that the fraction of "clinically unimportant" disease (defined as tumor volume less than or equal to 0.5 cm^3, Gleason grades 1 to 3, and organ confined) was not significantly different between groups.

Goto and associates[38] furthered the application of these data by specifically predicting clinically unimportant disease. The group examined 170 patients with prostate cancer, 10% of whom had clinically unimportant[37] disease. Logistic regression analysis determined that maximum length of cancer within any core and PSAD were the only statistically significant variables. Patients with PSAD less than or equal to 0.1 ng/mL/g and maximum cancer length of 2 mm or less had clinically unimportant cancer 75% of the time.

An additional step in the determination of which patients may be suited to a conservative management approach was the determination of a nomogram predicting indolent cancer (tumor volume less than or equal to 0.5 mL, pathologically organ confined, and no poorly differentiated elements) by Kattan and coworkers.[39] Data were used from 409 patients with T1c or T2a, N0 prostate cancers who were treated by radical prostatectomy, 20% of whom had indolent cancer. Logistic regression was used to construct nomograms, the best of which had an area under the receiver operator curve (AUC-ROC) of 0.79. Some of the models created, however, used variables not determined to be statistically significant by logistic regression.

Prospective Series

The previously discussed published case series demonstrating that at least in some cases prostate cancer could be managed conservatively, and the work of other groups attempting to identify a priori those patients who could be managed conservatively, laid the groundwork for prospectively assembled cohorts of patients undergoing the expectant management with curative intent of prostate cancer. Despite the interest in conservative management for prostate cancer and all the retrospective studies performed on the subject, there are very few prospectively assembled expectant management cohorts in the published literature. Expectant management studies differ from those described in the watchful waiting section because these use specific criteria to enroll select patients eligible for expectant management and actively follow those patients with the intention of treating those individuals who experience disease progression.

The University of Toronto has published the results of their series of a prospective, single-arm phase II study of a watchful waiting protocol with selective delayed intervention.[40,41] The initial report[40] laid out the enrollment criteria as well as the disease progression criteria necessitating a recommendation for treatment. Patients received a confirmatory biopsy at 12 or 18 months into the study. Patients were followed up with physical exam, PSA, and creatinine every 3 months for 2 years and every 6 months thereafter. Bone scan was performed yearly for 2 years and then biannually thereafter; bone scans were performed yearly when PSA reached 15 ng/mL. The study enrolled men with baseline PSA less than or equal to 15 ng/mL, Gleason score 7 or lower, and clinical stage T2b or lower. Disease progression resulting in therapeutic intervention was said to occur if patients met treatment criteria in any of three categories:

clinical (a doubling in lesion size in any DRE dimension, any requirement for transurethral resection, ureteral obstruction, or evidence of distant metastasis), histologic (Gleason score 8 or higher on repeat biopsy), and PSA (PSA doubling time of 2 years or less, PSA greater than 8 ng/mL, *and* statistically significant PSA progression from a regression analysis of ln(PSA) on time) progression. The initial report concluded that such a study was feasible based on the progression rates of 206 patients.

The series was updated several years afterward by Klotz.[41] At the time of this update, a total of 299 patients had been recruited with a median follow-up of 55 months. Through that time, 60% of those enrolled remained on active surveillance. At 8 years, overall survival rate was 85% (Fig. 4-10A) and prostate cancer-specific survival rate was 99% (Fig. 4-10B). Twelve percent of initially enrolled patients were treated because of PSA progression, 8% because of clinical progression, and 4% because of histologic progression. Of 24 men who underwent radical prostatectomy for PSA progression, only 42% had organ-confined disease and 8% had lymph node metastasis. The investigators conclude that men with favorable risk prostate cancer will die of other causes, but that longer-term follow-up is necessary to confirm these observations. Further follow-up was performed assessing

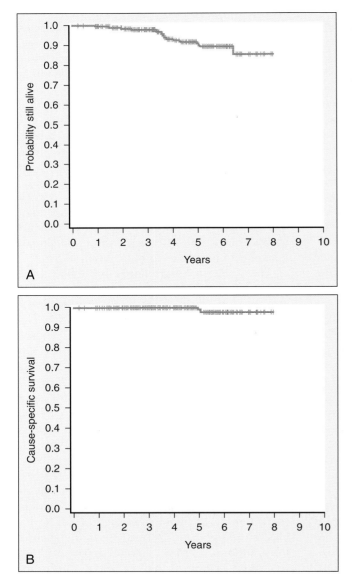

Figure 4-10. **A,** Overall survival in surveillance cohort of 299 men. **B,** Prostate cancer-specific survival in surveillance cohort of 299 men. (From Klotz L: Active surveillance with selective delayed intervention: using natural history to guide treatment in good risk prostate cancer. J Urol 172:S48–S51, 2004, Figures 1 and 2. Copyright © 2004, with permission from American Urological Association.)

Box 4-1. Enrollment Criteria for Inclusion in Johns Hopkins Expectant Management Cohort

---

Clinical stage T1c adenocarcinoma of the prostate
PSA density < 0.15 ng/mL/cm^3
Absence of any of the following on a minimum 12-core biopsy:
    Gleason score > 6
    Any Gleason pattern 4 or 5
    >2 cores involved with cancer
    >50% of any single core involved with cancer

Box 4-2. Surveillance Protocol for Men with Prostate Cancer on Protocol for Expectant Management with Curative Intent

---

Serum free and total PSA every 6 months
Digital rectal exam every 6 months
Transrectal ultrasound-guided prostate biopsy every year with:
    Minimum of 12 cores
    Mandatory sampling of far lateral peripheral zones and midsagittal regions from apex to base

---

Box 4-3. Criteria for the Recommendation of Treatment of Patients Followed on Expectant Management Protocol

---

Development of a palpable nodule on direct rectal exam
Gleason score > 6 on surveillance biopsy
Any Gleason pattern 4 or 5 on surveillance biopsy
> 2 cores involved with cancer on surveillance biopsy
> 50% of any single core involved with cancer on surveillance biopsy

---

PSADT as a predictive parameter in this cohort.[42] The group determined that patients could be stratified into low- and high-risk groups based on PSADT and repeat biopsy pathology. In an editorial comment by Carter from the same article, the important point was raised that it is problematic to use a variable as both a definition of failure and as a means of stratifying risk a priori.

The group from Johns Hopkins is currently evaluating a prospective strategy for the expectant management of prostate cancer based on the Epstein criteria[35,36] for the identification of insignificant tumors.[43,44] Patients with T1c prostate cancer satisfying pathologic and PSAD criteria were consecutively enrolled (Box 4-1). Patients were followed up with DRE and PSA every 6 months and a yearly prostate biopsy (Box 4-2). Included patients had all been followed for 1 year or more. Treatment was recommended for patients based on clinical stage progression or unfavorable criteria on follow-up biopsy (Box 4-3). Changes in serum levels of PSA or its isoforms were not used as criteria for the recommendation of treatment, since there was significant overlap in these values between men remaining on surveillance and those requiring treatment. Changes in these values may some-

times be erratic, perhaps because of trauma to the prostate during repeated biopsies.

The initial report described 81 patients, with a median follow-up of 23 months, of whom 25 (31%) were recommended to undergo treatment during the study period. Thirteen men underwent radical prostatectomy based on a recommendation for treatment. Of these, 12 had "curable" disease, as defined by any pure Gleason 6 tumor or any organ-confined tumor less than or equal to Gleason 7 or any tumor with Gleason 3 + 4 or less with negative surgical margins. Higher PSAD and lower percent free PSA were both significantly associated with those men who were recommended treatment; men who had at least one follow-up biopsy without cancer were more likely to remain on surveillance than those demonstrating cancer on all follow-up biopsies. These data were updated by Warlick and colleagues[44] in 2006. In the updated database, 320 men were enrolled in the program, 98 (31%) of whom underwent curative intervention. Out of this group of 98, 38 underwent radical prostatectomy without neoadjuvant therapy, and 29 (84%) had curable tumors on pathologic examination. Based on these observations, Carter and associates[43] concluded that expectant management is a reasonable alternative management plan for older men with low-stage and low-grade prostate cancer.

Delayed Therapy

Zietman and associates[45] retrospectively reviewed 199 patients with stage T1-2 (52% had nonpalpable lesions) prostate cancer and PSA of less than 20 ng/mL, who were followed up expectantly in their practice. With a median follow-up of 3.4 years, disease-specific survival rates at 5 and 7 years were 98% and 98%, whereas overall survival rates were 77% and 63%, respectively. Sixty-four patients underwent treatment;

treatment-free survival rate at 5 years was 56%. In a telephone interview, 81% of patients who had undergone treatment believed that treatment had been recommended by their physician because of a PSA elevation or the palpation of a nodule, whereas physicians had recorded only having advocated treatment in 24% of cases. The authors concluded that expectant management in the PSA era effectively becomes nothing more than a delayed form of radical therapy.

A similar conclusion was reached by Carter and coworkers[46] in their review of 313 men aged 70 years or younger with low-grade and low-stage prostate cancer who had initially selected watchful waiting as a management strategy. They found that 215 men proceeded to treatment; 57.3% by year 2 and 73.2% by year 4. The group concluded that younger men choosing watchful waiting as an initial management option are more likely to undergo secondary therapy than their older counterparts.

Two subsequent studies attempted to determine whether delaying surgery in men eligible for expectant management would adversely affect their outcome. The first study was performed by Khatami and associates[47] and examined 26 patients with T1-T2 disease managed by initial surveillance who ended up undergoing radical prostatectomy in a mean of 23.4 months. These men were compared with two controls each who underwent immediate radical prosta-

tectomy. These patients were matched for PSA, age, clinical stage, and biopsy Gleason score. The authors found that there were no statistically significant differences between groups with respect to tumor size, pathologic variables, and biochemical recurrence-free survival at 2 years.

Warlick and associates[44] performed a similar study, examining the outcomes of 38 men from the Johns Hopkins expectant management cohort who were recommended to undergo therapy for their prostate cancer and who underwent radical prostatectomy. These patients were compared with 150 matched patients, who would have been eligible for expectant management, but who elected to undergo immediate surgical therapy. The authors found that the men from the expectant management cohort underwent surgery at a median of 26.5 months after diagnosis and the men electing immediate surgery were actually operated on at a median of 3.0 months. "Noncurable cancer," defined as pathology associated with a less than 75% chance of remaining PSA-recurrence free at 10 years after surgery, was diagnosed in 9 (23%) of the 38 patients from the expectant management group and in 24 (16%) men in the immediate intervention group. Adjusting for age and PSAD, there was no significant difference in the risk of noncurable cancer between the delayed and immediate intervention groups (Table 4-2). The researchers concluded that delayed prostate

Table 4-2. Risk of Noncurable Prostate Cancer in the Delayed Intervention Cohort of Patients Initially Managed Expectantly and Then with Surgery Compared with the Immediate Surgery Cohort*

| Comparison | Nonadjusted | | Adjusted[†] | |
	RR (95% CI)[‡]	P Value[§]	RR (95% CI)[‡]	P Value[§]
Delayed versus immediate intervention	1.48 (0.75–2.92)	0.266	1.08 (0.55–2.12)	0.819
Age: 63–70 yr versus 52–62 yr	1.96 (1.06–3.63)	0.030	nd	nd
PSA density: ≥ 0.10 versus < 0.10 ng/mL/cm³	2.21 (1.16–4.24)	0.013	nd	nd
PSA: > 6.0 versus ≤ 6.0 ng/mL	2.27 (1.24–4.17)	0.008	nd	nd

*Noncurable cancer, defined as a less than 75% chance of biochemical freedom from disease at 10 years after surgery, was stage pT2 (organ confined) if the Gleason sum was ≥7 (4 + 3) and/or the surgical margins were positive, stage pT3aN0 (extraprostatic extension) if the Gleason sum was ≥7 and/or surgical margins were positive, and any stage higher than pT3a regardless of grade or margin status or any N+ stage.
[†]Adjusted for age and PSA density.
[‡]Proportion of men with noncurable tumors in the delayed intervention cohort divided by the proportion with noncurable tumors in the immediate intervention cohort. The Mantel–Haenszel procedure was used to obtain estimates of relative risks (RRs) and 95% confidence intervals (CIs), adjusted for potential confounding factors at diagnosis including age, PSA, PSA density, number of positive cores, maximum percentage of a core positive for cancer, year of diagnosis, and year of surgery.
[§]Two-sided P values were derived from Cochran–Mantel–Haenszel statistics.
PSA, prostate-specific antigen; nd, not done. Adjusted analyses were not performed for these risk factors because they were not the major focus of the study.
From Warlick C, Trock BJ, Landis P, et al.: Delayed versus immediate surgical intervention and prostate cancer outcome. J Natl Cancer Inst 98:355, 2006, Table 2. Reprinted with permission of Oxford University Press.

cancer surgery for patients with small, lower-grade prostate cancers followed up expectantly does not appear to compromise the surgical curability of these cancers. Therefore, at the very worst, expectant management delays the potential morbidity of surgery in a cohort of patients who are not adversely affected by deferring their treatment.

Prediction of Delayed Treatment

The best predictors of progression come from analyses of prospectively collected data. The Johns Hopkins group examined their data to determine whether there were any biomarkers obtained at the time of entrance into the expectant management algorithm that could predict a future change from favorable to unfavorable pathology status on routine follow-up biopsy.[48] Seventy-eight men who had serial biopsies were examined in the study. Seventeen of 67 (25.4%) men developed unfavorable biopsy criteria[35] on their first follow-up biopsy, 6 of 36 (16.7%) did so on a second follow-up biopsy, and none of 14 men had unfavorable biopsy criteria who had a third follow-up biopsy. Backward, stepwise logistic regression determined a model incorpo-

rating percent free PSA at a 20.5% or less cutoff, PSA velocity (PSAV) cutoff at 1.7 ng/mL/year or less, and gland volume cutoff at greater than 55.5 mL to separate favorable from unfavorable groups using information available at the time of enrollment with an AUC-ROC of 83.1%. The conclusion of the study was that quantitative biopsy pathology along with information provided by serum biomarkers can predict men who are likely to maintain future biopsy pathology, although new biomarkers would be able to improve upon our ability to make this prediction.

Work is also ongoing in the development of new biomarkers. Our group has been working on predicting favorable from unfavorable groups based on quantitative nuclear grading (QNG)[49] (Fig. 4-11). Seventy-five men with at least two biopsies demonstrating prostate cancer were examined; 30 developed an unfavorable biopsy requiring treatment,[35,43] and 45 maintained favorable biopsies throughout a median follow-up of 2.7 years. Logistic regression models were developed using demographic and clinical data as well as tissue histomorphometry. A QNG signature using 12 nuclear morphometric descriptors had an area under the receiver

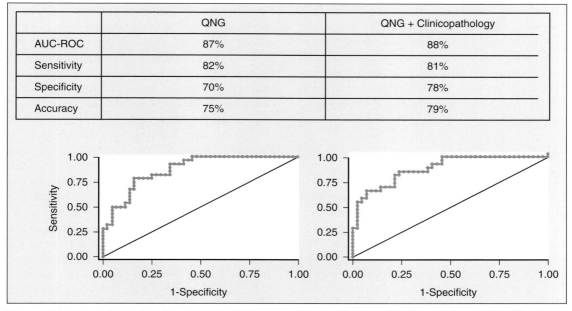

	QNG	QNG + Clinicopathology
AUC-ROC	87%	88%
Sensitivity	82%	81%
Specificity	70%	78%
Accuracy	75%	79%

Figure 4-11. Comparison of clinicopathology alone versus the combination of clinicopathology with QNG (quantitative nuclear grading). AUC-ROC, area under the receiver operator curve. (From Makarov DV, Marlow C, Epstein JI, et al: Predicting the need for treatment among men with low grade, low stage prostate cancer enrolled in a program of expectant management with curative intent [Abstract 91637]. Presented at the 102nd Annual Meeting of the American Urological Association, Anaheim, CA, May 19–24, 2007.)

operator characteristic curve (AUC-ROC) for the prediction of unfavorable biopsy status of 87%. A model based on traditional descriptors such as prostate volume, PSA density, and number of prediagnosis biopsies resulted in an AUC-ROC of 68%. A combined model containing QNG and clinicopathologic variables yielded an AUC-ROC of 88%. We found that QNG analysis of initial prostate biopsies improves the accuracy of models predicting unfavorable pathology. Although this technique demonstrates great promise for the ability to determine which men qualifying for expectant management are best suited for this therapeutic approach, further validation must be performed before this technique can be used to aid in clinical decision making.

Demichelis and associates[50] have looked for the TMPRSS2:ERF gene fusion in this cohort. TMPRSS2:ERF is a gene fusion product recently reported to be present in 79% of prostate cancers, which changes the normally androgen-insensitive ETS family of cell growth promoters to become androgen responsive.[51] Demichelis determined that the presence of the gene fusion predicted a more aggressive prostate cancer phenotype because patients who had the TMPRSS2:ERG fusion had a statistically significant elevated risk of prostate cancer-specific mortality (cumulative incidence ratio 2.7, $P < .01$). However, unlike other studies from the CaPSURE[52] and Department of Defense Center for Prostate Disease Research[53] databases, within this cohort it has also been demonstrated that researchers are only poorly able to classify individuals into high- and low-risk groups (ROC analysis).[54]

Consensus Criteria for Expectant Management and for Intervention

Clearly, one of the most important aspects of safely following up men with presumed low-grade, low-volume prostate cancer is the selection of the most appropriate men for this management strategy. One of the hurdles to the wider use of this management strategy has been the lack of consensus regarding the definition of what constitutes "insignificant" prostate cancer, and the best way, based on clinical and biopsy pathologic criteria, to identify men with such disease. In the future, improved biomarkers or

imaging may also help to stratify risk. Although no consensus as to the best selection criteria currently exists, the parameters to consider include patient age, clinical stage, tumor grade, PSA parameters, and biopsy characteristics. Several groups have defined "low-risk" prostate cancer in terms of clinical parameters such as the D'Amico criteria[55]; however, the goal in selecting men for expectant management is to identify the lowest-risk men among this already low-risk category.

Although there is no agreement on a specific age cut-off below which expectant management is contraindicated, most would agree that older patients are better suited to this strategy. As outlined earlier in this chapter, men observed for localized prostate cancer begin to show a decrease in metastasis-free and prostate cancer-specific survival rates after about 15 years.[19] Therefore, we have been most enthusiastic about expectant management in men over age 65. In addition, younger age has been shown to be a predictor of eventual treatment in watchful waiting studies.[46] However, as increasing numbers of younger men are being diagnosed with localized prostate cancer, this group may have the most to gain in terms of avoiding or delaying therapy. Once the timing of definitive intervention without the loss of the window of curability may be determined reliably, a delay in intervention may allow a younger man to enjoy several additional years at his current quality of life before risking a change by undergoing definitive therapy. Such a deferred therapeutic strategy may prove attractive to younger men concerned with maintaining their current level of potency, for instance.

Clinical stage has long been known to be an important predictor of outcome in prostate cancer. Its application in determining selection and treatment criteria has also proved to be one of the most controversial issues in expectant management. Should men with clinical stage T2 disease be included in expectant management protocols? It is the feeling of the authors of this book that until further evidence from prospective trials is available to confirm the safety of including men with T2 disease, only men with T1 disease should be routinely included. Not all researchers agree with this assessment. A prospective trial from the University of Toronto routinely follows up men with T2 disease conservatively. This approach is supported by data previously outlined from retrospective trials of observation of localized prostate cancer, including large numbers of men with T2 disease who demonstrate excellent prostate cancer-specific survival (up to 10 to 15 years).[19] However, the outcomes of the Toronto group's study demonstrated a significant number of men with advanced disease at prostatectomy, including 8% with positive lymph nodes. A higher actuarial progression rate at 4 years was noted among the men with T2 disease compared with T1, although this only approached statistical significance (44% versus 24% $P = .07$).[40]

Most researchers agree that a Gleason score of 3 + 3 or less is an appropriate grade for expectant management. However, some groups have included men with Gleason 7 disease. Albertsen and associates[27] demonstrated that at 20 years, 27% of the men with Gleason 6 disease at diagnosis who were treated conservatively or with hormonal therapy for localized prostate cancer had died from prostate cancer, whereas 67% had died from other causes. For men with Gleason 7 disease, 45% died from prostate cancer, whereas 51% died from other causes, suggesting increased risk of death from prostate cancer in Gleason 7 versus Gleason 6 disease. Thus, although controversial, the authors of this paper do not advocate the inclusion of men with Gleason 7 disease.

PSA kinetics has proved to be a contentious issue in expectant management. The group from Johns Hopkins uses only PSA density as an inclusion criterion (as outlined above) in reference to PSA. Other groups have advocated using PSA doubling time as a trigger for intervention, but not in the initial selection of patients.[40] D'Amico and colleagues[56] have shown an increased risk of death from prostate cancer in men with an increase in PSA of more than 2 ng/mL/year in the year before undergoing radical prostatectomy compared with those with a PSA increase of less than 2 ng/mL/year. Thus, it seems prudent to avoid expectant management in men with a rise in their PSA of more than 2 ng/mL/year in the year before diagnosis.

Pathologic analysis of biopsy specimens can be very helpful in identifying low-risk disease as evidenced by the Epstein criteria outlined above.[35] El-Geneidy and coworkers[23] and Panagiotou and coworkers[24] found that the percentage of cores positive for cancer were predictive of progression of men to therapy in their expectant management programs. However, this criterion also remains controversial both as a criterion for the selection of patients for expectant management and as a trigger for definitive management.

No single consensus exists for determining the best candidates for expectant management programs. Indeed, it is likely that several systems will ultimately demonstrate efficacy in this regard. The common goal of all these approaches is to pick the lowest-risk men out of the men with generally accepted "low-risk" prostate cancer. Toward this end, the Standard Treatment Against Restricted Treatment (START) trial, a prospective randomized trial of expectant management versus standard definitive therapy is currently underway. The trial is organized by the group from Toronto and is based on their protocol.[57] The endpoint is prostate cancer-specific mortality. This may prove to be an important trial for the field of expectant management, and we anxiously await its results. However, given its endpoint, it may be many years before the data become available; until then, common sense and the available data published in the literature will guide the expectant management with curative intent of prostate cancer.

Conclusion

Prostate cancer encompasses a wide variety of diseases with disparate outcomes. Some men with prostate cancer, either because of a short life expectancy or because of an indolent form of disease, are likely to die of diseases other than prostate cancer. A significant and expanding body of literature has documented, both prospectively and retrospectively, that conservative or expectant management of prostate cancer with curative intent may be an ideal strategy for some men with prostate cancer.

Many questions remain to be answered, such as "For whom is expectant management a safe option?" "What are the selection criteria to determine whom to enroll in an expectant management program?" "What should be the triggers for intervention in a person who is being followed up in an expectant management program?"

Work is ongoing to determine answers to these questions. The development of new biomarkers and the design and implementation of randomized trials will help to shape our understanding of prostate cancer in general and in the optimum parameters for its expectant management. We may then hope to be able to spare patients who would otherwise never be affected by prostate cancer in their lifetime from the morbidity of unnecessary treatment.

References

1. Jemal A, Siegel R, Ward E, et al: Cancer statistics, 2009. CA Cancer J Clin 59:225–249, 2009.
2. Sakr WA, Grignon DJ: Prostate cancer: indicators of aggressiveness. Eur Urol 32(Suppl 3):15, 1997.
3. Minino AM, Heron MP, Smith BL: Deaths: preliminary data for 2004. Natl Vital Stat Rep 54:1, 2006.
4. Scardino PT, Weaver R, Hudson MA: Early detection of prostate cancer. Hum Pathol 23:211, 1992.
5. Harlan SR, Cooperberg MR, Elkin EP, et al: Time trends and characteristics of men choosing watchful waiting for initial treatment of localized prostate cancer: results from CaPSURE. J Urol 170:1804, 2003.
6. Cooperberg MR, Lubeck DP, Meng MV, et al: The changing face of low-risk prostate cancer: trends in clinical presentation and primary management. J Clin Oncol 22:2141, 2004.
7. Treatment and survival of patients with cancer of the prostate. The Veterans Administration Co-operative Urological Research Group. Surg Gynecol Obstet 124:1011, 1967.
8. Creevy CD: The mortality of transurethral prostatic resection. J Urol 65:976, 1951.
9. Sakati IA, Marshall VF: Postoperative fatalities in urology. Trans Am Assoc Genitourin Surg 57:132, 1965.
10. Horan AH, McGehee M: Mean time to cancer-specific death of apparently clinically localized prostate cancer: policy implications for threshold ages in prostate-specific antigen screening and ablative therapy. BJU Int 85:1063, 2000.
11. Han M, Partin AW, Chan DY, et al: An evaluation of the decreasing incidence of positive surgical margins in a large retropubic prostatectomy series. J Urol 171:23, 2004.
12. Thompson IM, Pauler DK, Goodman PJ, et al: Prevalence of prostate cancer among men with a prostate-specific antigen level < or = 4.0 ng per milliliter. N Engl J Med 350:2239, 2004.
13. Barnes RW, Bergman RT, Hadley HL, et al: Early prostatic cancer: long-term results with conservative treatment. J Urol 102:88, 1969.
14. Goodman CM, Busuttil A, Chisholm GD: Age and size and grade of tumour predict prognosis in incidentally diagnosed carcinoma of the prostate. Br J Urol 62:576, 1988.
15. Jones GW: Prospective, conservative management of localized prostate cancer. Cancer 70:307, 1992.
16. Whitmore WF, Jr, Warner JA, Thompson IM, Jr: Expectant management of localized prostatic cancer. Cancer 67:1091, 1991.
17. Warner J, Whitmore WF, Jr: Expectant management of clinically localized prostatic cancer. J Urol 152:1761, 1994.
18. Johansson JE, Adami HO, Andersson SO, et al: High 10-year survival rate in patients with early, untreated prostatic cancer. JAMA 267:2191, 1992.
19. Chodak GW, Thisted RA, Gerber GS, et al: Results of conservative management of clinically localized prostate cancer. N Engl J Med 330:242, 1994.
20. Johansson JE, Andren O, Andersson SO, et al: Natural history of early, localized prostate cancer. JAMA 291:2713, 2004.
21. Adolfsson J, Ronstrom L, Lowhagen T, et al: Deferred treatment of clinically localized low grade prostate cancer: the experience from a prospective series at the Karolinska Hospital. J Urol 152:1757, 1994.
22. McLaren DB, McKenzie M, Duncan G, et al: Watchful waiting or watchful progression? Prostate specific antigen doubling times and clinical behavior in patients with early untreated prostate carcinoma. Cancer 82:342, 1998.
23. el-Geneidy M, Garzotto M, Panagiotou I, et al: Delayed therapy with curative intent in a contemporary prostate cancer watchful-waiting cohort. BJU Int 93:510, 2004.
24. Panagiotou I., Beer TM, Hsieh YC, et al: Predictors of delayed therapy after expectant management for localized prostate cancer in the era of prostate-specific antigen. Oncology 67:194, 2004.
25. Albertsen PC, Fryback DG, Storer, BE, et al: Long-term survival among men with conservatively treated localized prostate cancer. JAMA 274:626, 1995.
26. Albertsen PC, Hanley JA, Gleason DF, et al: Competing risk analysis of men aged 55 to 74 years at diagnosis managed conservatively for clinically localized prostate cancer. JAMA 280:975, 1998.
27. Albertsen PC, Hanley JA, Fine J: 20-year outcomes following conservative management of clinically localized prostate cancer. JAMA 293:2095, 2005.
28. Bill-Axelson A, Holmberg L, Ruutu M, et al: Radical prostatectomy versus watchful waiting in early prostate cancer. N Engl J Med 352:1977, 2005.
29. Patel MI, DeConcini DT, Lopez-Corona E, et al: An analysis of men with clinically localized prostate cancer who deferred definitive therapy. J Urol 171:1520, 2004.
30. Wong YN, Mitra N, Hudes G, et al: Survival associated with treatment vs observation of localized prostate cancer in elderly men. JAMA 296:2683, 2006.
31. Cuzick J, Fisher G, Kattan MW, et al: Long-term outcome among men with conservatively treated localised prostate cancer. Br J Cancer 95:1186, 2006.
32. Holmberg L, Bill-Axelson A, Helgesen F, et al: A randomized trial comparing radical prostatectomy with watchful waiting in early prostate cancer. N Engl J Med 347:781, 2002.
33. Allaf ME, Carter HB: Update on watchful waiting for prostate cancer. Curr Opin Urol 14:171, 2004.
34. Holmberg L, Bill-Axelson A, Garmo H, et al: Prognostic markers under watchful waiting and radical prostatectomy. Hematol Oncol Clin North Am 20:845, 2006.
35. Epstein JI, Walsh PC, Carmichael M, et al: Pathologic and clinical findings to predict tumor extent of nonpalpable (stage T1c) prostate cancer. JAMA 271:368, 1994.
36. Epstein JI, Chan DW, Sokoll LJ, et al: Nonpalpable stage T1c prostate cancer: prediction of insignificant disease using free/total prostate specific antigen levels and needle biopsy findings. J Urol 160:2407, 1998.
37. Ohori M, Wheeler TM, Dunn JK, et al: The pathological features and prognosis of prostate cancer detectable with current diagnostic tests. J Urol 152:1714, 1994.
38. Goto Y, Ohori M, Arakawa A, et al: Distinguishing clinically important from unimportant prostate cancers before treatment: value of systematic biopsies. J Urol 156:1059, 1996.
39. Kattan MW, Eastham JA, Wheeler TM, et al: Counseling men with prostate cancer: a nomogram for predicting the presence of small, moderately differentiated, confined tumors. J Urol 170:1792, 2003.
40. Choo R, Klotz L, Danjoux C, et al: Feasibility study: watchful waiting for localized low to intermediate grade prostate carcinoma with selective delayed intervention based on prostate specific antigen, histological and/or clinical progression. J Urol 167:1664, 2002.
41. Klotz L.: Active surveillance with selective delayed intervention: using natural history to guide treatment in good risk prostate cancer. J Urol 172:S48, 2004.
42. Zhang L, Loblaw A, Klotz L: Modeling prostate specific antigen kinetics in patients on active surveillance. J Urol 176:1392, 2006.
43. Carter HB, Walsh PC, Landis P, et al: Expectant management of nonpalpable prostate cancer with curative intent: preliminary results. J Urol 167:1231, 2002.
44. Warlick C, Trock BJ, Landis P, et al: Delayed versus immediate surgical intervention and prostate cancer outcome. J Natl Cancer Inst 98:355, 2006.
45. Zietman AL, Thakral HJ, Wilson L, et al: Conservative management of prostate cancer in the prostate specific antigen era: the incidence and time course of subsequent therapy. J Urol 166:1702, 2001.
46. Carter CA, Donahue T, Sun L, et al: Temporarily deferred therapy (watchful waiting) for men younger than 70 years and

with low-risk localized prostate cancer in the prostate-specific antigen era. J Clin Oncol 21:4001, 2003.

47. Khatami A, Damber JE., Lodding P, et al: Does initial surveillance in early prostate cancer reduce the chance of cure by radical prostatectomy? A case control study. Scand J Urol Nephrol 37:213, 2003.

48. Khan MA, Carter HB, Epstein JI, et al: Can prostate specific antigen derivatives and pathological parameters predict significant change in expectant management criteria for prostate cancer? J Urol 170:2274, 2003.

49. Makarov DV, Marlow C, Epstein JI, et al: Using nuclear morphometry to predict the need for treatment among men with low grade, low stage prostate cancer enrolled in a program of expectant management with curative intent. Prostate 68:183, 2008.

50. Demichelis F, Fall K, Perner S, et al: TMPRSS2:ERG gene fusion associated with lethal prostate cancer in a watchful waiting cohort. Oncogene 26:4596, 2007.

51. Tomlins SA, Rhodes DR, Perner S, et al: Recurrent fusion of TMPRSS2 and ETS transcription factor genes in prostate cancer. Science 310:644, 2005.

52. Meng MV, Elkin EP, Harlan SR, et al: Predictors of treatment after initial surveillance in men with prostate cancer: results from CaPSURE. J Urol 170:2279, 2003.

53. Wu H, Sun L, Moul JW, et al: Watchful waiting and factors predictive of secondary treatment of localized prostate cancer. J Urol 171:1111, 2004.

54. Fall K, Garmo H, Andren O, et al: Prostate-specific antigen levels as a predictor of lethal prostate cancer. J Natl Cancer Inst 99:526, 2007.

55. D'Amico AV, Whittington R, Malkowicz SB, et al: Predicting prostate specific antigen outcome preoperatively in the prostate specific antigen era. J Urol 166:2185, 2001.

56. D'Amico AV, Chen MH, Roehl KA, et al: Preoperative PSA velocity and the risk of death from prostate cancer after radical prostatectomy. N Engl J Med 351:125, 2004.

57. Klotz L: Active surveillance with selective delayed intervention using PSA doubling time for good risk prostate cancer. Eur Urol 47:16, 2005.

5 Open Radical Retropubic Prostatectomy: Technique and Outcomes

Misop Han and William J. Catalona

KEY POINTS

- Excellent long-term outcome data of open radical retropubic prostatectomy are available in cancer control as well as in the preservation of potency and continence.
- Many clinical and pathologic parameters are associated with cancer control and return of urinary continence and potency following surgery.
- Over the past two decades, widespread screening for prostate cancer and better patient selection have resulted in a favorable shift of these parameters and improved surgical outcomes.

Introduction

Since the early 1980s, the management of patients with clinically localized prostate cancer has changed dramatically. Widespread screening with serum prostate-specific antigen (PSA) and digital rectal examination has allowed much earlier detection of prostate cancer.[1,2] The modification of surgical technique of radical retropubic prostatectomy by Walsh and Donker[3] has allowed better hemostasis, improved visualization during dissection, and preservation of neurovascular bundles supplying corpora cavernosa. As a result, radical prostatectomy can be performed with a high cure rate while preserving urinary continence and erectile potency in the majority of patients. Thus, radical prostatectomy has become the most commonly performed treatment for clinically localized prostate cancer with abundant long-term data confirming its efficacy.[4] Recently, a prospective, randomized trial (the first to adequately test the effectiveness of radical prostatectomy) demonstrated that radical prostatectomy reduces the rates of metastases and death from prostate cancer.[5,6] Therefore, the rationale for surgical treatment of clinically localized prostate cancer is more compelling than ever.

Anatomic radical retropubic prostatectomy has become the gold standard surgical treatment for prostate cancer for the past 25 years. Excellent long-term outcome data of open radical retropubic prostatectomy are available in cancer control as well as in the preservation of potency and continence. In this chapter, we discuss the technique, outcomes, and complications of anatomic radical retropubic prostatectomy using the senior author's surgical series, now including more than 4800 anatomic radical prostatectomies as an example. It not only is representative of large modern prostatectomy series but also includes all men who underwent surgery in the analysis, even those with known adverse prognostic features.

Patient Selection

An ideal candidate for radical prostatectomy should have a life expectancy of at least 10 years, a completely resectable and biologically significant tumor, and no comorbidity that might make the operation unacceptably risky. Actuarial life tables can project the life expectancy of U.S. men,[7] and with appropriate adjustment for comorbidities, life expectancy can be estimated for the individual patient.

After confirming the likelihood of a sufficiently long life expectancy, the next step in patient selection is to identify those with potentially curable disease. Radical prostatectomy provides the best chance for cure in men whose tumor is confined to the prostate gland. As a result of widespread screening for prostate cancer and more restrictive preoperative patient selection, the proportion of men with organ- or specimen-confined disease has increased in recent years.[8] However, the accuracy of conventional radiographic imaging studies in staging prostate cancer has been limited. Therefore, nomograms predicting the pathologic stage based on preoperative clinical and pathologic parameters have been widely used to identify patients who are likely to benefit from the surgical resection and those who are not.[9,10] Alternatively, nomograms predicting postsurgical or post–radiation therapy recurrence-free survival probabilities also are sometimes useful for patients.[11-13] For patients with a low probability of resectable disease or a short life expectancy due to age or comorbidity, an alternative treatment to surgery should be recommended.

For the patient to have realistic expectations concerning postoperative potency and continence outcomes, the surgeon should provide the patient with relevant information on the nerve-sparing aspect of radical prostatectomy during the preoperative consultation. Anatomic nerve-sparing radical retropubic prostatectomy is a safe choice without compromising cancer control in appropriately selected patients. Nerve-sparing radical prostatectomy is inappropriate in men with locally advanced disease, especially if the primary goal of the surgery is cancer control. The feasibility of the nerve-sparing surgery is questionable when a patient has extensive involvement by cancer according to prostate biopsies, palpable evidence on digital rectal examination of possible extraprostatic extension, a serum PSA level greater than 10 ng/mL, a biopsy Gleason score greater than 7, poor-quality erections preoperatively, a lack of interest and/or willingness of a partner in restoring potency, or the presence of other medical conditions that may adversely affect potency, such as diabetes mellitus, hypertension, psychological or psychiatric diseases, and neurologic diseases and medications. Therefore, it is important to review the clinicopathologic features of the tumor and the patient's medical history and erectile function status before embarking on a nerve-sparing operation.

After discussing the prospects for preservation of potency, information on the treatment of erectile dysfunction should be imparted. This should include information on phosphodiester-ase inhibitors, intraurethral and intracorporal vasodilators, vacuum erection devices, venous flow constrictors, and artificial penile prostheses. The discussion should include the anticipated postoperative erectile rehabilitation program to be used and the timing of the return of erections, which usually begins 3 to 6 months postoperatively and lasts for up to 36 months. If erectile function is of paramount importance, the patient can be reassured that erections can be almost always restored, regardless of whether or not nerve-sparing surgery can be successfully performed.

Finally, the surgeon should discuss the possible need for and the potential side effects of adjuvant radiation therapy or hormonal therapy if the final pathology report reveals adverse prognostic features. At the end of the preoperative counseling session, if nerve-sparing radical retropubic prostatectomy is appropriate, the patient and spouse or partner should sign an informed consent form authorizing a surgeon to perform the procedure.

Surgical Technique

Before the operation, a first-generation cephalosporin (or appropriate substitute, if the patient is allergic to cephalosporins) antibiotic is given intravenously. After a general endotracheal or regional anesthesia is administered, thigh-high elastic hose are placed on the patient. Sequential compression devices are used only in patients with increased risk for thromboembolic complications. The patient is positioned with his legs on spreader bars, and the operating table is dorsiflexed with the break just above the patient's anterosuperior iliac spine (Fig. 5-1). The abdomen and genitalia are appropriately prepped and draped.

There are nine key steps in performing anatomic nerve-sparing radical prostatectomy: (1) a limited pelvic lymphadenectomy; (2) incision of the endopelvic fascia and the puboprostatic ligaments; (3) proximal and distal suture ligation and transection of the dorsal venous complex; (4) placement of hemostatic sutures in the neurovascular bundles and the prostatic pedicles; (5) dissection of the prostate from the neurovascular bundles; (6) vascular control and transection of the prostatic pedicles; (7) transection and reconstruction of the bladder neck; (8) dissection of the seminal vesicles and ampullary

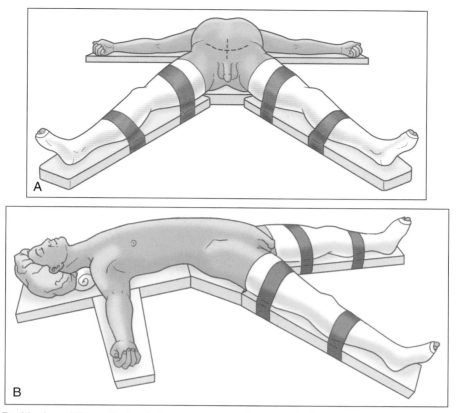

Figure 5-1. Positioning of the patient. **A,** Legs are separated on spreader bars. **B,** The operating table is flexed with the break just above the patient's anterosuperior iliac spine.

portions of the vasa deferentia; and (9) performance of the vesicourethral anastomosis. These steps are described in detail in the following text with corresponding illustrations.

Limited Pelvic Lymphadenectomy

A superficial midline (or transverse) lower abdominal incision is made with a scalpel. The linea alba is incised and the space of Retzius is entered. Anatomic radical retropubic prostatectomy performed in the extraperitoneal space is arguably less invasive than the laparoscopic and robotic prostatectomy in which a transperitoneal approach is frequently used. By avoiding any entry into the peritoneal cavity, anatomic radical retropubic prostatectomy can be performed while minimizing the risk of injury to bowel, major vascular structures, and other adjacent organs. In addition, the cosmetic results are not significantly different between a single infraumbilical incision for anatomic radical retropubic prostatectomy and multiple laparoscopic

ports site incisions and an incision for prostate removal during laparoscopic or robotic prostatectomy.

Taking care to avoid disrupting the lymphatic tissue lateral to the external iliac vein and to avoid compression of the vein itself, a Balfour retractor is placed. A modified pelvic lymphadenectomy is performed, removing only the lymph nodes medial to the external iliac vein. Care is taken during the lymphadenectomy to preserve any accessory arterial branches to the corpora cavernosa that arise from the distal external iliac or obturator arteries. The obturator nerve is identified and preserved. In most incidences, the patient elects to have the prostate gland removed, even if there are pelvic lymph node metastases. If the patient elects not to have the prostate removed and there are lymph node metastases, frozen-section examination of the lymph nodes is performed. If frozen sections reveal metastatic cancer, the operation is terminated. Lymphadenectomy is optional in patients who have a low risk for pelvic lymph node metastases by virtue of a low Gleason grade, low PSA, and low biopsy tumor volume.

After completing the lymphadenectomy, the adipose and areolar tissues are swept gently from the anterior surface of the prostate and the endopelvic fascia to expose the puboprostatic ligaments. Care is taken to avoid injury to the perforating branches of Santorini plexus that pierce the endopelvic fascia between the puboprostatic ligaments and pass cephalad on the anterior surface of the prostate gland and bladder.

Incision of the Endopelvic Fascia and the Puboprostatic Ligaments

The endopelvic fascia is incised in the groove between the levator ani muscles and the lateral border of the prostate (Fig. 5-2). Inside the endopelvic fascia, the lateral surface of the prostate is covered by a smooth, glistening membrane overlying the lateral portion of Santorini plexus. Strands of the levator ani muscles are gently dissected off the prostate to the level of the urogenital diaphragm. Often, venous tributaries pass from the levator ani muscles to the prostate just lateral to the puboprostatic liga-

ments. These vessels are either cauterized, secured with hemostatic clips, or ligated laterally, and then clamped medially with a delicate snub-nose right-angled clamp. After the vein is transected sharply, its medial portion is ligated. When the endopelvic fascia has been opened from the base to the apex of the prostate, the superficial branch of Santorini plexus is gently retracted medially, and the puboprostatic ligaments are placed on stretch and divided close to the pubic symphysis (Fig. 5-3). Care is taken not to divide the puboprostatic ligaments too medially or too far under the pubic symphysis to avoid injuring the dorsal venous complex.

Suture Ligation and Transection of the Dorsal Venous Complex

After the puboprostatic ligaments have been divided, the lateral surfaces of the urethra are palpated. The groove between the anterior surface of the urethra and the dorsal venous complex is developed with a pinching motion of the left index finger and thumb. The plane between the urethra and the dorsal venous complex is then developed gently, first with a large right-angle clamp. This facilitates tight ligation of the dorsal venous complex. After the

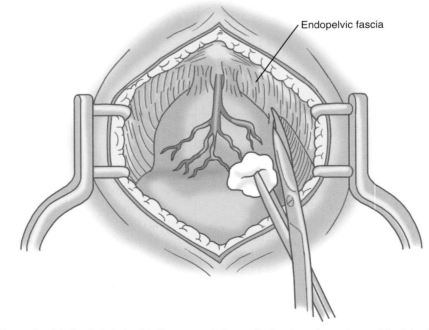

Endopelvic fascia

Figure 5-2. The endopelvic fascia is incised in the groove between the levator ani muscles and the lateral border of the prostate.

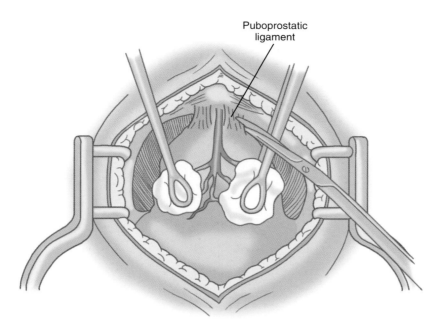

Figure 5-3. The puboprostatic ligaments are placed on stretch and incised.

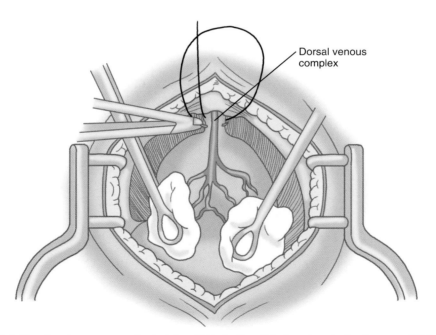

Figure 5-4. The dorsal venous complex is suture ligated with a 2-0 chromic catgut suture on a CT-1 needle.

dorsal venous complex has been ligated, it is also suture-ligated in a slightly more caudal site with a 2-0 chromic catgut suture on a CT-1 needle (Fig. 5-4). A suture ligature is also placed in the anterior surface of the prostate to reduce the back-bleeding from Santorini plexus (Fig. 5-5).

The right-angle clamp is then passed behind the dorsal venous complex, and the jaws of the clamp are spread. The dorsal venous complex is transected with electrocautery or a scalpel (Fig. 5-6). Back-bleeding from the dorsal venous complex is controlled with figure-of-eight 3-0

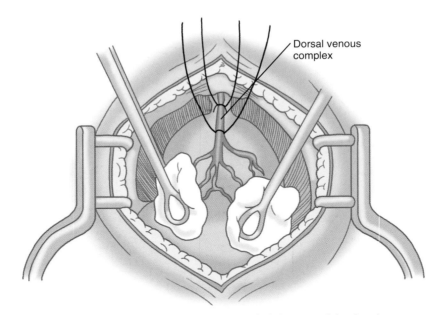

Figure 5-5. To reduce back-bleeding from Santorini plexus, the cephalad aspect of the dorsal venous complex is suture ligated.

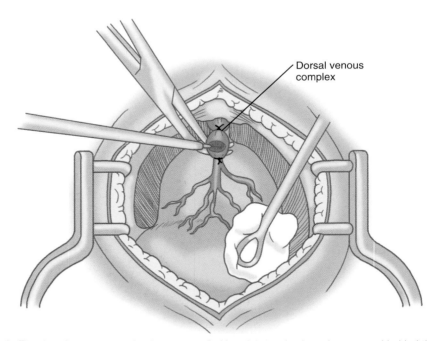

Figure 5-6. The dorsal venous complex is transected with a right-angle clamp jaws spread behind the complex.

sutures. It is important to obtain good hemostasis so that the apical dissection of the prostate may be performed in a relatively bloodless field. If the dorsal venous complex ligature slips off, the complex is oversewn using a 3-0 chromic catgut suture on a 5/8-circle needle.

The goal in oversewing the complex is to pass the suture just through the lateral borders of the complex itself in its anterior, middle, and posterior aspects, respectively. Wide, imprecisely placed sutures may damage the neurovascular bundles.

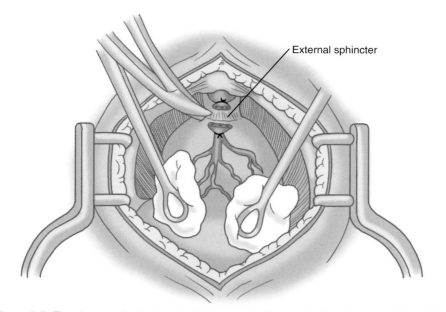

Figure 5-7. The circumurethral external sphincter muscle fibers are incised to expose the urethra.

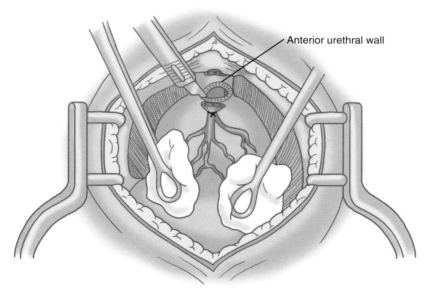

Figure 5-8. The anterior wall of the urethra is incised with a scalpel without dissecting around the lateral or posterior surfaces of the urethra.

The anterior surface of the urethra is palpated between the neurovascular bundles. The circumurethral sphincter muscle and the anterior wall of the urethra are incised with a scalpel just distal to the apex of the prostate without dissecting around the lateral or posterior surfaces of the urethra (Figs. 5-7 and 5-8). The incision should not be carried too far laterally, where it may injure the neurovascular bundles. The urethral catheter is exposed and carefully hooked with a delicate right-angle clamp. Gentle traction on the clamp in a cephalad direction exposes the posterior urethral wall. The catheter is divided and placed on cephalad traction; the posterior urethral wall is sharply transected. Fibromuscular bands tethering the apex of the prostate to the pelvic floor are incised using sharp dissection (Fig. 5-9). The rectourethralis muscle is incised, exposing the prerectal fat.

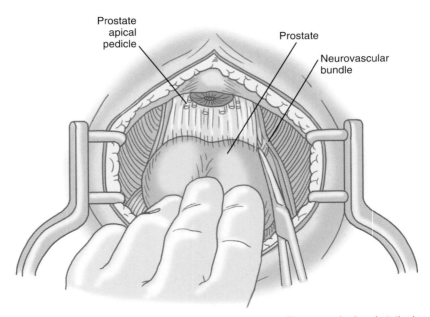

Prostate
apical
pedicle

Prostate

Neurovascular
bundle

Figure 5-9. The apical pedicles of the prostate may require suture ligation. Fibromuscular bands tethering the apex of the prostate to the pelvic floor are incised using sharp dissection. The prostate gland is dissected from neurovascular bundles.

Placement of Prophylactic Hemostatic Sutures in the Neurovascular Bundles and Prostatic Pedicles

To reduce bleeding during the dissection of the neurovascular bundles and prostatic pedicles in a manner similar to that achieved with the pneumoperitoneum during laparoscopic surgery, "prophylactic" hemostatic figure-of-eight suture ligatures of 4-0 plain catgut are placed in the neurovascular bundles lateral to the prostate. Similarly, 3-0 suture ligatures are placed in the prostatic pedicles. After these sutures have been placed on both sides of the prostate, sharp, energy-free dissection can be used to dissect the neurovascular bundles from the prostate. The prophylactic hemostatic sutures are tied "softly" to avoid crushing the nerve fibers in the neurovascular bundles, and the plain catgut sutures are quickly absorbed. Using this technique, the use of hemostatic clips and sutures that may permanently entrap the neurovascular bundles can be avoided.

Separation of the Prostate from the Neurovascular Bundles

The lateral pelvic fascia is incised from the apex of the prostate to the base. A delicate right-angle clamp may be used to elevate the lateral pelvic fascia from the underlying veins on the surface of the prostate. Small perforating bleeders not controlled by the prophylactic hemostatic sutures may be secured with hemoclips, ties, or ligatures to ensure adequate hemostasis. The posterolateral groove between the prostate and the neurovascular bundles is developed using sharp and blunt dissection, allowing the prostate to assume a more anterior position in the pelvis.

The lateral aspect of the prostate is then dissected from the neurovascular bundles, allowing the bundles to retract laterally. In a case of extensive fibrosis, the dissection is performed only sharply to avoid tearing into the rectum with blunt dissection. The dissection is carried cephalad until the portion of Denonvilliers fascia covering the ampullary portions of the vasa deferentia and the seminal vesicles is exposed (Fig. 5-10). Denonvilliers fascia is incised with the cautery. The Metzenbaum scissors are then used to develop the proper plane of dissection for the prostatic vascular pedicles. If there is continued bleeding from the periurethral tissues and apical pedicles of the prostate, hemostatic sutures should be placed at this juncture to avoid continued blood loss during the remainder of the procedure.

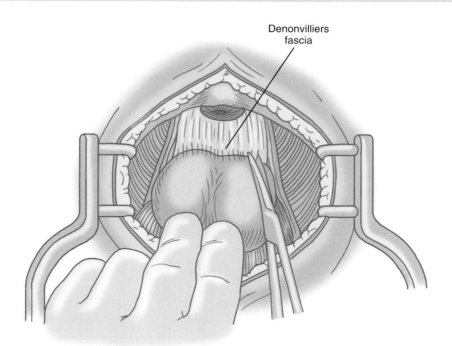

Denonvilliers
fascia

Figure 5-10. The dissection is carried cephalad until the portion of Denonvilliers fascia covering the ampullary portions of the vasa deferentia and the seminal vesicles is exposed. Denonvilliers fascia is incised with the cautery; it is incised to expose vascular pedicles at the prostate base.

Vascular Control and Transection of Prostatic Pedicles

The prostatic pedicles are divided by inserting the right-angled clamp medial to them, with the tip of the clamp directed almost parallel to the lateral surface of the prostate. The prostatic pedicle is ligated or hemoclipped laterally, taking care to place the tie or clip medial to the neurovascular bundle (Fig. 5-11). The pedicle is divided close to the prostate. This dissection is performed on both sides to a point just cephalad to the seminal vesicles. Care is taken when dissecting near the seminal vesicles to avoid injuring the neurovascular bundles that are situated just lateral to the seminal vesicles. The seminal vesicles are freed from the bladder base using sharp and blunt dissection, and a large right-angle clamp is used to further develop this plane. Two hemostatic sutures of 3-0 chromic catgut are placed in the lateral bladder pedicles cephalad to the seminal vesicles, one just lateral to the prostate and another just medial to the neurovascular bundles. The lateral bladder neck fibers are then partially incised with the cautery, but are not incised through their entire thickness.

Transection and Reconstruction of the Bladder Neck

The anterior bladder neck is transected with electrocautery in the natural groove between the bladder and the prostate. The bladder neck opening is enlarged with scissors, and the catheter is pulled through and used as a tractor on the prostate (Fig. 5-12). The posterior bladder neck is incised with the cautery. The muscular attachments between the bladder and the prostate are divided using electrocautery and/or hemostatic clips for hemostasis.

Dissection of Seminal Vesicles and Ampullary Portions of the Vasa Deferentia

The seminal vesicles are dissected first along their lateral edges, carrying the plane of dissection medially. Many small perforating arteries enter the lateral and terminal portions of the seminal vesicles. These are secured with small hemoclips. The ampullae are freed, using sharp and blunt dissection, and then are clipped and transected. After the seminal vesicles have been dissected to their tips and the hemoclips placed,

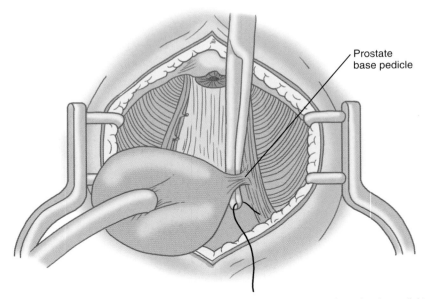

Figure 5-11. Prostate base pedicle is ligated or hemoclipped laterally, taking care to place the tie medial to the neurovascular bundle.

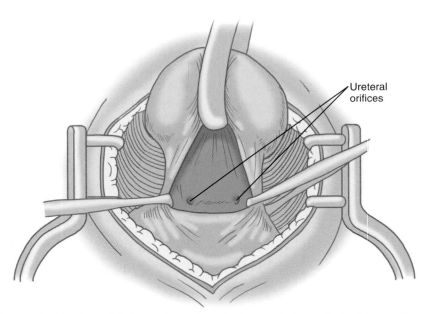

Figure 5-12. The anterior bladder neck is transected in the natural groove between the bladder and the prostate. The bladder neck opening is enlarged with scissors. The ureteral orifices are identified.

the surgical specimen is removed. At this point, the pelvis is carefully inspected for hemostasis. Small bleeders on the neurovascular bundles may require 4-0 absorbable suture ligatures. It is important not to use the cautery for hemostasis on the neurovascular bundles to avoid cautery injury to the cavernosal nerves. Suture ligatures of 3-0 or 4-0 absorbable material are placed in the "pockets" of the seminal vesicle pedicles on the medial aspects of the neurovascular bundles to ensure good hemostasis in this difficult-to-visualize region.

Vesico-Urethral Anastomosis

Reconstruction of the bladder neck begins by placing a continuous running everting suture of 3-0 chromic catgut that encompasses bladder mucosa and underlying muscle for a distance of nearly the entire anastomotic circumference (Fig. 5-13). The bladder neck is then reconstructed in a tennis racket fashion, with the handle of the racket directed posteriorly. The bladder neck closure is accomplished with a continuous 2-0 chromic catgut suture. Care should be taken to avoid compromising the ureteral orifices. The bladder neck is closed to a size of approximately 22 to 24F.

An 18F catheter is passed through the urethra. While an assistant exerts pressure on the perineum with a sponge forceps to better expose the cut end of the urethra (Fig. 5-14), double-armed 2-0 chromic catgut sutures are used for the vesicourethral anastomosis (Fig. 5-15). A 5/8-circle needle is used to place the sutures in the urethra from inside to outside, avoiding placing the suture into the neurovascular bundles. The tip of the catheter is grasped and brought out of the wound to expose the posterior lip of the cut end of the urethra. The posterior sutures are similarly placed. The anterior sutures are placed at the 10 o'clock and 2 o'clock positions, and the posterior sutures are placed at the 5 o'clock and 7 o'clock positions. In addition, a

stronger 2-0 monocryl suture is placed at the 6 o'clock position to secure the most posterior aspect of the reconstructed bladder neck to the urethral stump. The other ends of the sutures containing an SH 3/8-circle needle are placed in the corresponding positions of the bladder neck from inside to outside. These sutures encompass mucosa and muscle and exit at the edge of the mucosa. The catheter tip is placed in the bladder, and the bladder neck is guided gently toward the cut end of the urethra. The anastomotic sutures are tied carefully under direct vision. The bladder is then irrigated free of clots, and a single suction drain is placed in the pelvis and brought out the lower end of the wound. The incision is closed with #1 loop Maxon running sutures on the fascia, a 2-0 chromic catgut suture on the subcutaneous tissue, and a 4-0 polyglycolic acid subcuticular suture on the skin. The skin incision is covered with Steristrips.

Postoperative Care

Patients are ambulated with assistance once on the night of surgery, five times on the first postoperative day, and seven times on the second postoperative day. A clear liquid diet is given on the night of surgery, advancing to a regular diet as tolerated on the following days. A suction drain and dressing are removed on the second postoperative day. Intravenous antibiotics are

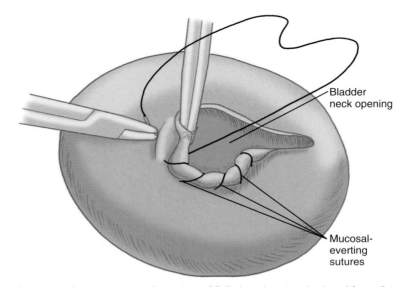

Bladder
neck opening

Mucosal-
everting
sutures

Figure 5-13. A continuous running mucosa-everting suture of 3-0 chromic catgut is placed for a distance of nearly the entire anastomotic circumference.

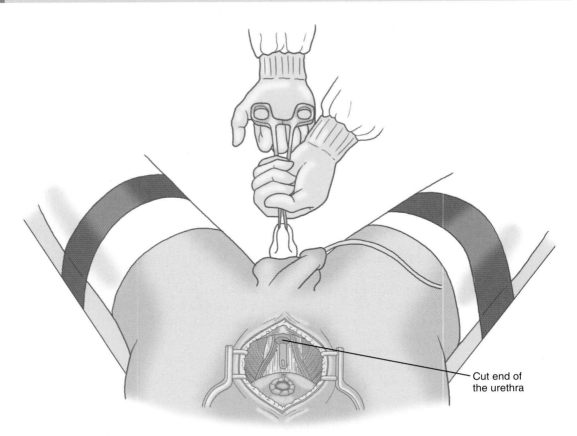

Figure 5-14. Perineal pressure is applied with a sponge forceps to better expose the cut end of the urethra.

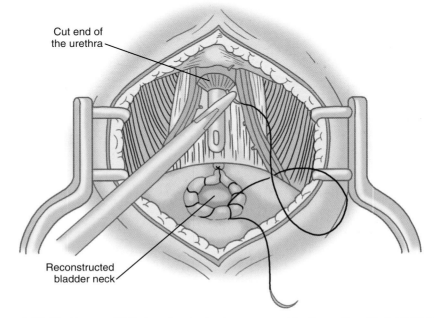

Figure 5-15. Double-armed 2-0 chromic catgut sutures are used for the vesicourethral anastomosis.

discontinued after the suction drain is removed. For analgesia, ketorolac (30–60 mg) is given intravenously every 6 hours for the first 48 hours. It may be supplemented sparingly with morphine, as needed.

Although some claim a quicker recovery after laparoscopic surgery compared with anatomic radical retropubic prostatectomy, a recent study has shown similar low narcotic usage and patient-reported pain scores regardless of which approach was used.[14] Therefore, the same clinical care pathway, without a significant difference in length of hospital stay, can be applied to patients treated by either open radical prostatectomy or laparoscopic/robot-assisted radical prostatectomy.[15] Most patients are discharged from the hospital on the second or third postoperative day after anatomic radical retropubic prostatectomy.

Antibiotic ointment is applied to the urethral meatus around the catheter four to six times a day until catheter removal. The catheter may be removed on either the seventh, tenth, or fourteenth postoperative day, depending on the perceived amount of tension on the vesicourethral anastomosis. A cystogram is not performed before removing the catheter unless an anastomotic leak is suspected. The catheter should not be removed before 7 days, since 10% to 15% of men may experience urinary retention from edema and require re-catheterization.[16,17] Oral fluoroquinolone is given 1 day before and 1 week after catheter removal. Daily Kegel exercises are performed in four sets of ten, before the surgery and after the catheter removal until continence returns. A protective pad or diaper is used until a complete urinary control is achieved. The first postoperative serum PSA level is measured 1 month after the operation.

Cancer Control Outcome

The most important objective of radical prostatectomy is cancer control. A rising serum PSA level is usually the earliest evidence of recurrence or progression following prostatectomy.[18] Because follow-up data are not sufficiently mature to effectively evaluate cancer-specific survival trends, biochemical recurrence (detectable serum PSA)-free survival has been used frequently as a surrogate in evaluating the treatment efficacy in radical retropubic prostatectomy series.[19–21]

Analyses of the first author's series recently have been reported.[21–23] They include almost 3500 men who underwent anatomic radical retropubic prostatectomy between 1983 and 2003, including those with adverse prognostic features. Cancer progression was defined as detectable serum PSA (more than 0.2 ng/mL), local recurrence, or distant metastases. With a mean follow-up of 65 months (range 0 to 233), actuarial 10-year cancer progression-free survival probability was 68%. Actuarial 10-year cancer-specific and overall survival rates were 97% and 83%, respectively. Other larger radical prostatectomy series have reported similar excellent results.[19,20] Similar long-term oncologic outcome results are not yet available in laparoscopic or robotic prostatectomy series.

Cancer progression after radical prostatectomy was strongly associated with clinical and pathologic parameters, including Gleason grade, clinical and pathologic tumor stage, era of treatment, and patient age. For example, the preoperative serum PSA level was inversely related to both the percentage of patients with organ-confined disease and the 10-year progression-free survival rate. Patient selection and the duration and frequency of follow-up monitoring are critical in determining outcomes as well. Therefore, factors other than treatment effectiveness can influence treatment outcomes. Accordingly, caution is indicated in comparing the results of contemporary radical prostatectomy series using different patient selection criteria and follow-up protocols.

Urinary Continence Outcome

The overall urinary continence outcome following nerve-sparing radical retropubic prostatectomy was excellent in the current series. More than 93% of men achieved complete urinary continence, defined as requiring no protection for daily activities.[22] The return of urinary continence was strongly associated with the age of the patient. For example, more than 95% of men younger than age 50 were continent following surgery. In contrast, 86% of men above age 70 were continent postoperatively. Only four men (0.2%) eventually required an artificial urinary sphincter placement for stress urinary incontinence. The relative long-term functional outcomes of laparoscopic and robotic prostatectomy methods are yet unknown.

6

Robotic and Laparoscopic Radical Prostatectomy

Desiderio Avila and Richard E. Link

KEY POINTS

- A steadily increasing proportion of radical prostatectomies in the United States and Europe are being performed using laparoscopic techniques.
- Laparoscopic radical prostatectomy (LRP) can be performed either transperitoneally or extraperitoneally with or without the assistance of the da Vinci surgical robot.
- Potential advantages of the da Vinci robot for prostatectomy include three-dimensional magnified vision, tremor filtering, and motion scaling and instruments with 7 degrees of freedom that more accurately replicate human wrist movements.
- Relative disadvantages of LRP include increased cost, lack of universal availability at all centers, and a steep learning curve for experienced urologic oncologic surgeons trained only in open surgical techniques. As LRP becomes more widely disseminated and integrated fully into residency training throughout urology, these disadvantages will likely become less significant.
- Cancer control using LRP appears to be equivalent to radical prostatectomy using either the traditional open retropubic or the perineal approach.
- LRP, and particularly its robotic variant, is an excellent technique for radical prostatectomy in obese patients, who may be more challenging candidates for open radical prostatectomy.
- Advantages of LRP over open retropubic radical prostatectomy include less blood loss and postoperative pain, as well as an earlier return to full activity.
- Health-related quality of life after LRP appears to be excellent. Reported outcomes are at least equivalent and perhaps superior to outcomes from open retropubic radical prostatectomy, particularly with respect to early return of urinary continence.

Over the past 15 years, advances in instrumentation, optics, and technique have transformed laparoscopy into a viable, safe and reliable option for treating urologic malignancies in the retroperitoneum and pelvis. The surgical management of prostate cancer, in particular, has been radically altered over the past decade through the application and widespread dissemination of laparoscopic techniques. The push toward laparoscopic radical prostatectomy (LRP) has been fueled in the United States by a complex relationship between surgeons seeking improved functional outcomes, patients seeking less morbid surgical options, and industry partners eager to promote applications for new technologies (i.e., surgical robotics). This tripartite relationship has been at times both extremely productive and somewhat controversial. It is also important to recognize that these new developments arose within the context of a rich history of more than 25 years of clinical and scientific experience with nerve-sparing open radical retropubic prostatectomy.

The goal of this chapter is to provide a general perspective on the role of laparoscopic and robotic-assisted approaches to radical prostatectomy in 2009.

History of Urologic Laparoscopy

Hans Jacobaeus coined the term "laparoscopy" in 1910 after using a cystoscope to inspect the peritoneal cavity. Laparoscopy has since taken on a broader meaning to include all endoscopic abdominal or pelvic procedures conducted by either an extra or intraperitoneal approach. Clayman and colleagues[1] first described the use of laparoscopy for genitourinary cancer in 1991 with the first report on laparoscopic radical nephrectomy. Schuessler and colleagues[2] performed the first human LRP in the early 1990s. This group reported in 1997, however, that although oncologic control was comparable to

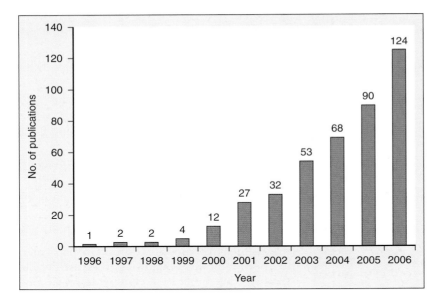

Figure 6-1. Publications relevant to laparoscopic or robotic-assisted laparoscopic prostatectomy by year of publication. Data derived from a Medline search using the terms "laparoscopic prostatectomy" or "robotic prostatectomy" in the title limited by year of publication.

open radical retropubic prostatectomy (RRP), LRP was burdened with longer operative times and hospital stay. They concluded that LRP offered no significant advantage over RRP.

Notwithstanding these observations, two centers in France refined the LRP procedure and built an extensive experience with the technique during the late 1990s.[3,4] These groups reported similar positive margin, continence, and potency rates and suggested that LRP was associated with decreased perioperative morbidity compared with RRP. The documented success of the French investigators with LRP combined with the rapid development of surgical robotics rekindled interest in laparoscopic approaches to radical prostatectomy in the United States. This trend is substantiated by the exponential rise in the number of publications relating to LRP from less than 5 in 1996 to over 120 in 2006 (Fig. 6-1).

LRP can be performed with or without a surgical robot. For the purposes of this chapter, LRP refers to any laparoscopic approach to radical prostatectomy including *or* excluding robotic assistance.

Patient Selection

The indications for LRP are generally identical with those for open radical prostatectomy. LRP should be reserved for men who are likely to be cured of prostate cancer by surgery and who will live long enough to benefit from that cure. Spe-

cifically, patients undergoing LRP should have biopsy-proven prostatic adenocarcinoma without clinical or radiographic evidence for metastatic disease. Moreover, during patient counseling, LRP should fit within a constellation of options for prostate cancer management that also includes observation, radiation therapy, androgen ablation, cryotherapy, and open surgical alternatives.

Absolute contraindications to LRP include uncorrectable coagulopathy, active urinary tract infection, and the inability to undergo a general anesthetic. Relative contraindications include prior radiation therapy, pelvic lipomatosis, and major medical comorbid disease. Numerous factors can also make LRP more technically difficult and should be factored into the clinical decision-making process, particularly early in a surgeon's experience. These include an extremely large prostate gland (more than 100 g); a large median prostatic lobe; a history of neoadjuvant hormonal therapy; prior pelvic, abdominal, or prostate surgery; prior pelvic trauma; or a history of documented severe prostatic infection.

When comparing LRP with open RRP, several patient characteristics may make the LRP approach more attractive. The most notable of these factors is obesity. More than 70% of men who are candidates for radical prostatectomy are classified as overweight or obese by body mass index.[5] Open retropubic approaches to prostatectomy can be significantly more challenging in the obese patient, necessitating a larger incision for operative exposure. RRP is also associated with greater intraoperative blood loss in patients with a higher body mass index.[6] In contrast, LRP can be performed in patients with moderate obesity with only minor modifications in technique.[7-9] LRP may also hold significant advantages in patients with a small retropubic prostate gland and a narrow pelvis. In these cases, exposure for dissection of the prostatic apex and the urethrovesical anastomosis can be challenging with the RRP approach. LRP, and particularly its robotic-assisted variant, provides substantially better visualization of the prostatic apex in these more challenging cases. Moreover, the small size of the long instruments used in robotic-assisted LRP allows precise suturing of the urethrovesical anastomosis even in the setting of a very narrow pelvis.

Technique

Radical prostatectomy involves the removal of the entire prostate within its investing fascia along with the seminal vesicles and transection of the vas deferens. By necessity, this requires the removal of the prostatic urethra and reconnection of the detached bladder neck to the urethra via a urethrovesical anastomosis (Fig. 6-2).

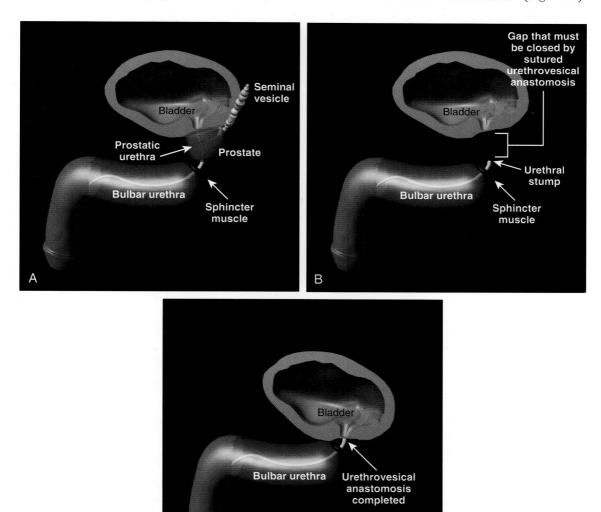

Figure 6-2. Simplified diagram showing critical anatomic landmarks during radical prostatectomy.   A, Prior to removal of the prostate. **B,** After prostate removal. **C,** After completion of the urethrovesical anastomosis.

Depending on the grade and stage of disease, radical prostatectomy may also include a bilateral pelvic lymphadenectomy.

The prostate gland is located in the deep pelvis in an extraperitoneal, retropubic potential space (the space of Retzius). Radical prostatectomy, therefore, can be performed using either an extraperitoneal or a transperitoneal approach to the gland. Open radical retropubic prostatectomy is generally performed extraperitoneally, whereas LRP has been described using both approaches.

Access and Trocar Placement

Laparoscopic surgery requires the development and maintenance of a surgical working space, usually by insufflation with carbon dioxide (CO_2) under pressure. How that space is developed differs for the transperitoneal and extraperitoneal approaches to LRP.

Transperitoneal access methods can be broken down into two broad categories termed "open" and "closed" techniques. During open access, an incision is made and the peritoneal cavity is entered under direct vision at which point a blunt trocar is introduced and the abdomen is insufflated. In the closed access technique, the abdomen is initially insufflated with carbon dioxide via a small needle puncture, and then the first trocar is placed. Although both approaches have advantages and disadvantages, the laparoscopic surgeon should be comfortable with either form of access.

Open access techniques are commonly referred to as Hasson techniques in reference to Dr. Hasson, a laparoscopic gynecologic surgeon who popularized this approach.[10] To perform open access for laparoscopic surgery, an incision is made through the skin and subcutaneous tissues until the abdominal wall fascia is exposed. The fascia and peritoneum are incised, and intraperitoneal access is confirmed by finger dissection. A blunt-tipped trocar, with or without a balloon retention mechanism, is then inserted under direct vision and the abdomen is insufflated through this trocar. The other working trocars are then inserted using standard techniques under surveillance with the laparoscope. The primary theoretical advantage of open access is that it obviates the need for blind placement of a Veress needle into the abdomen for abdominal

insufflation and subsequent insertion of the first trocar after establishment of pneumoperitoneum. There is a general perception among surgeons that open access techniques are associated with a lower incidence of inadvertent intra-abdominal organ injury (most notably bowel injury). The literature, however, is mixed on this issue with some reports documenting lower[11] and others higher rates of intra-abdominal organ injury with open techniques.[12]

Closed access techniques depend on the initial placement of a Veress needle into the peritoneal cavity to prepare a pneumoperitoneum. Traditionally, the first working trocar was then placed "blindly," counting on the pneumoperitoneum to protect abdominal organs during access. This approach can be a source of stress, particularly for the novice laparoscopic surgeon. Trocars suitable for closed access come in a wide variety of styles, which can be broken down into four general classes: bladed trocars, nonbladed trocars, radially dilating trocars, and visual trocars. Most bladed trocars have a guard mechanism that deploys and sheaths the blade once the trocar passes through the abdominal wall and there is a loss of resistance. This mechanism serves to protect underlying organs in case the surgeon pushes too far with the trocar. Nonbladed trocars have either a plastic ridge or a screw mechanism that helps to pass the trocar through the abdominal wall. Radially dilating trocars depend on a two-step process for access. Initially, a sheath is inserted over a Veress needle. The sheath is then dilated to accept blunt-tipped trocars of varying diameter. Optical trocars accept a zero degree laparoscope and allow the trocar to be passed under direct laparoscopic vision. These systems have either a plastic cutting ridge or a blade mechanism controlled by a pistol grip. They allow the surgeon to visualize structures during trocar placement and avoid organ injury.

Extraperitoneal access for LRP involves a modification of the open access approach described previously. An infraumbilical incision is made through the abdominal wall fascia and the space of Retzius is identified and developed digitally. The larger working space is then usually prepared by introducing an inflation balloon. These balloons are available in several types, some of which accommodate a zero degree laparoscope and allow the development of the working space to be monitored visually. The working trocars are then introduced under direct vision after removal of the balloon.

Trocar Positioning

Port placement is designed to maximize surgeon maneuverability, assistant participation, and unobstructed camera manipulation. The total number of ports ranges from four to six depending on whether robotic assistance is used (Fig. 6-3). The camera port is placed in the periumbilical area first and then used to visually guide the placement of the working ports. Ports are placed just lateral to the rectus abdominal musculature (pararectus) in a configuration that triangulates in relation to the camera port. The pararectus ports serve as the primary working ports for the surgeon. Additional ports are placed bilaterally bisecting an imaginary line between the pararectus trocars and the anterior superior iliac spine. These ports are used for retraction and assistant participation. Compared with traditional open RRP, a laparoscopic technique may have an advantage with respect to cosmesis. In general, the total length of an open incision can be up to twice the accumulated size of all port incisions required for laparoscopy. Since these small port incisions are spread throughout the abdominal skin they tend to fade away and become less obvious over time.

Robotic-assisted laparoscopic prostatectomy

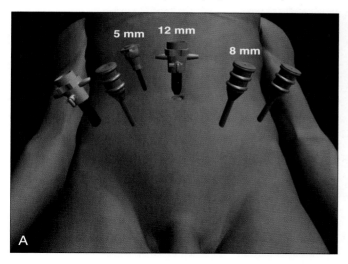

Laparoscopic prostatectomy

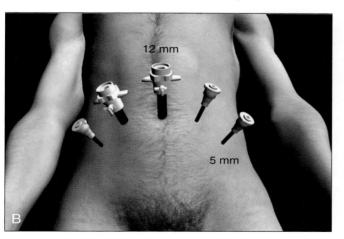

Figure 6-3. Standard trocar positions for laparoscopic radical prostatectomy with and without robotic assistance. During robotic surgery, the three robotic working arms are inserted through the 8-mm metallic trocars, and the fourth robotic arm holds the camera through the midline 12-mm port. The remaining two trocars are for the bedside assistant. Laparoscopic prostatectomy without robotic assistance is often performed with only a single bedside assistant, in which case the lateral 5-mm port on the patient's left is eliminated.

General Steps of LRP

In the original transperitoneal Montsouris technique for LRP, the procedure is begun by incising the peritoneum overlying the vas deferens bilaterally. Each vas deferens is dissected free of surrounding tissue, transected, and used to identify the corresponding seminal vesicle. The seminal vesicles are dissected free of surrounding tissue and Denonvilliers fascia is opened behind the prostate, exposing the perirectal fat plane. This plane is developed toward the prostatic apex. After completion of this posterior dissection, the peritoneum overlying the bladder is incised, and the space of Retzius is developed. A representative endoscopic view at this stage is shown in Figure 6-4. The endopelvic fascia is then entered bilaterally, and the dorsal vein complex is ligated using a suture ligature. If a nerve-sparing technique is used, the lateral prostatic fascia may be opened at this point to facilitate sweeping the nerves controlling erection off the posterolateral aspects of the prostate bilaterally. The bladder is then separated from the prostate by entering the bladder anteriorly and carrying this plane of dissection through the posterior bladder neck. Care must be taken during this step to avoid injury to the ureteral orifices. The seminal vesicles and vasa deferentia are elevated through the bladder neck, and the prostatic pedicles are transected using hemoclips, harmonic scalpel, or cautery for hemostasis.

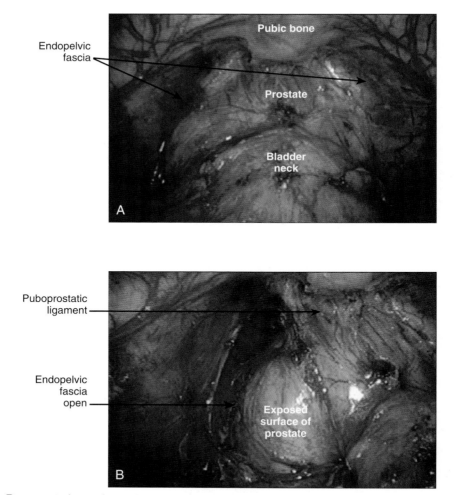

Figure 6-4. Representative endoscopic view after preparation of the space of Retzius.   A, Prior to opening the endopelvic fascia. **B,** After opening the left endopelvic fascia and sweeping the levator fibers off the lateral prostatic surface but before transecting the puboprostatic ligament. Note the fine level of detail with this view, which facilitates precise dissection.

Nerve sparing is then completed in an antegrade fashion toward the prostatic apex (Fig. 6-5). The dorsal vein complex is then divided and the urethra is defined and transected. The laparoscopic view during this phase of the operation is particularly advantageous because it allows for great precision during the critical dissection at the prostatic apex (Fig. 6-6). After releasing any residual posterior attachments to the rectum, the prostate is placed into an extraction bag and either removed immediately or placed into the peritoneal cavity for subsequent extraction. Figure 6-7 shows a view of the prostatic fossa after removal of the specimen, highlighting the position of the preserved neurovascular bundles after bilateral nerve sparing.

If a pelvic lymphadenectomy is planned, it is performed laparoscopically before moving on to the reconstructive phase of the procedure. After achieving hemostasis, the bladder neck is tailored (if necessary), and the urethrovesical anastomosis is performed using either a running or interrupted suture technique (Fig. 6-8). A new Foley catheter and pelvic drain are placed, and the trocar sites are closed to complete the procedure.

During an extraperitoneal LRP procedure, the space of Retzius has already been prepared during abdominal access, and the seminal vesicles are not accessible behind the prostate. The seminal vesicle and vas deferens dissections occur through the bladder neck after detaching the bladder from the prostate later in the case. Some surgeons skip the posterior dissection phase of the procedure and isolate the seminal vesicles through the bladder neck even in transperitoneal cases.

Many modifications of this basic technique have been described over the past 10 years. Notable modifications include the use of endovascular staplers to control the dorsal vein, techniques to preserve the endopelvic fascia and

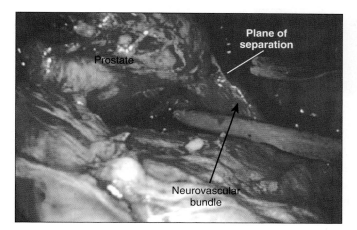

Figure 6-5. Antegrade nerve sparing. In this view, the prostate has been detached from the bladder neck, and the prostatic pedicle has been transected. Here, the right neurovascular bundle is being dissected off the posterolateral aspect of the prostate using cold shears.

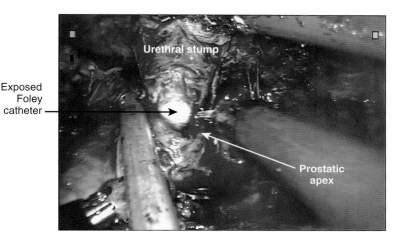

Figure 6-6. Apical dissection and urethral transection during robotic-assisted laparoscopic prostatectomy. These retropubic structures may be difficult to visualize during open prostatectomy in a deep and narrow pelvis. The laparoscopic approach provides magnification and proximity, which aid in dissection at the prostatic apex.

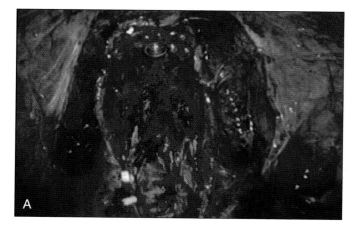

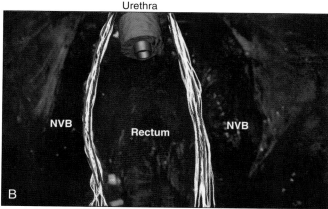

Figure 6-7. A view of the prostatic fossa after removal of the prostate specimen without (A) and with (B) a graphic anatomic overlay. Note the position of the urethral stump, rectum, bladder neck, and preserved neurovascular bundles (NVB).

puboprostatic ligaments during LRP, and myriad technical approaches to the urethrovesical anastomosis and nerve sparing. The specific details of these modifications are beyond the scope of this review. It is important to stress, however, that sound surgical principles refined over many years of open RRP experience should be applied to LRP. These include delicate tissue handling[1]; application of a knowledge of the patient's specific disease characteristics in planning prostatectomy dissection[2]; precise dissection at the prostatic apex to avoid positive margins and preserve continence mechanisms[3]; and minimization of nerve injury from stretch or energy sources during nerve sparing.[4]

Comparison of Transperitoneal and Extraperitoneal LRP Techniques

Advantages of the transperitoneal approach to LRP include (1) an ample working space (the peritoneal cavity, which allows more flexibility in port placement compared with the extraperitoneal approach), and (2) facilitation of the posterior approach to the seminal vesicles, which is favored by some prostate surgeons. A disadvantage of transperitoneal LRP is the impingement of bowel into the operative field and a potentially longer period of postoperative ileus. Bowel can be excluded through the use of steep Trendelenburg position or the addition of a second assistant instrument to serve as a retractor. Postoperative urine leakage from the urethrovesical anastomosis may also be more problematic after transperitoneal LRP because this urine is not limited to the extraperitoneal space.

The extraperitoneal LRP technique requires less steep Trendelenburg positioning and may be slightly faster owing to the elimination of the need to develop the space of Retzius as a separate step during prostatectomy. A relative advantage also is the ability to combine prostatectomy and hernia repairs with mesh without worry about adhesion to bowel or fistula formation.

Securing the posterior shelf of anastomosis

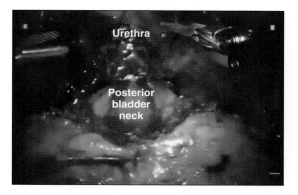

Closing the anterior portion of anastomosis

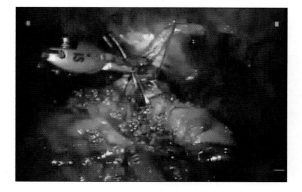

Completed urethrovesical anastomosis

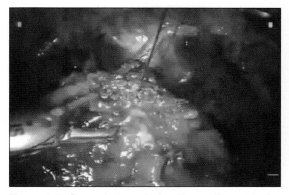

Figure 6-8. Several steps during the urethrovesical anastomosis during robotic-assisted laparoscopic prostatectomy. In this sequence, a running anastomosis was performed. The posterior "shelf" of the anastomosis is secured from the 4 to 8 o'clock position, and then the remainder of the anastomosis is sutured circumferentially. Wristed robotic instruments make this step of the procedure less technically demanding than that performed with standard laparoscopic needle drivers.

Similarly, the extraperitoneal approach would be preferred in patients with a history of multiple abdominal procedures that might make transperitoneal access more challenging or dangerous. Disadvantages to the extraperitoneal technique include a smaller working space that can collapse easily with suctioning during LRP and obscure visibility and the potential for increased tension at the urethrovesical anastomosis. This problem is rarely encountered with the transperitoneal approach because the urachus, which anchors the bladder to the anterior abdominal wall, is transected as part of the operation. Furthermore, increased CO_2 absorption has been reported with extraperitoneal insufflation, which can result in hypercarbia and associated acidosis requiring higher minute ventilation.

Although each technique offers its own modest advantages, no single technique has shown consistent superiority. Although initial comparative reports found the extraperitoneal approach to have decreased operative time, decreased hospital stay, and an earlier return of continence,[13] most studies have now established that there is essentially no substantive difference in outcome between intraperitioneal and extraperitoneal approaches. Therefore, deciding which approach to use for LRP is based on the surgeon's preference and operative experience.

Robotic-Assisted LRP

Robotic-assisted minimally invasive surgery has its origins in battlefield trauma surgery. It was first developed to allow a surgeon to operate from a safe distance by commanding the movement of automated surgical manipulators. The feasibility of robotic systems like the da Vinci surgical system (Intuitive Surgical, Inc., Sunnyvale, CA) has been established in cardiac, bariatric, endocrine, gynecologic, and urologic surgery. Currently, the da Vinci surgical system (Fig. 6-9) is the primary system used for robotic-assisted laparoscopic radical prostatectomy. Its popularity for radical prostatectomy in the United States has expanded tremendously over the past 5 years. In Europe, however, most of the LRP procedures continue to be performed without robotic assistance.

The potential advantages with robotic technology include a three-dimensional imaging system, 12-fold magnification, tremor filtering

Surgeon's console

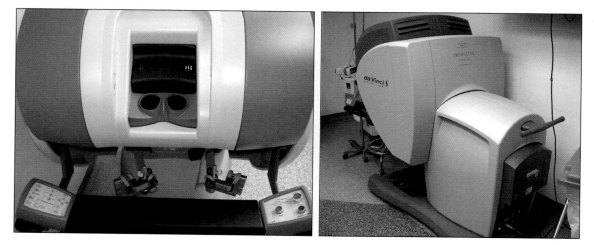

Robotic arms and monitor for bedside assistant

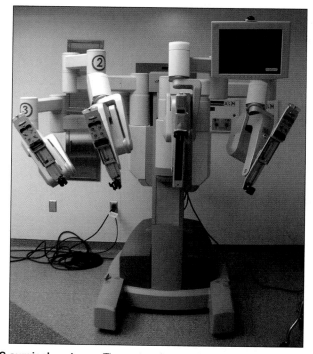

Figure 6-9. The da Vinci S surgical system.   The system has two components: a virtual-reality console, at which the surgeon sits to control the robot; and a unit composed of four robotic manipulator arms, which docks to trocars inserted into the patient's abdomen. The two components are connected by cables and serve as a master-slave system.

and motion scaling, and robotic instruments with 7 degrees of freedom that more accurately replicate human wrist movements. Three or four robotic arms are used to control working instruments and a camera, while a bedside assistant uses one or two additional trocars to retract, suction, pass sutures, or place hemoclips as needed. After mounting the robotic arms to the patient, the surgeon sits at a console physically separated from the operating table. The surgeon's hands are placed within manipulators and his or her hand motions are translated into movement of the robotic instruments using a master-slave system.

Robotic technology facilitates complex laparoscopic skills including intracorporeal suturing and knot tying, making LRP somewhat easier and less fatiguing for the surgeon. This is true especially during the early stages of a surgeon's laparoscopic experience. Indeed, in comparing learning curves for traditional LRP with robotic LRP, several studies have shown that the learning curve may be significantly reduced when applying robotic technology.[14,15] There is a very steep skills barrier for traditional LRP, particularly for experienced open prostate surgeons who have limited laparoscopic experience. The da Vinci robot has facilitated a smooth transition for many high-volume open-prostate surgeons to transition to laparoscopic prostatectomy over a relatively short time interval.[16,17]

Perhaps the biggest limitation of widespread use of robotic technology is its exorbitant cost. The da Vinci surgical system is priced at over $1 million not including a service agreement that costs more than $100,000 a year. In addition, several analyses have shown a significant cost disadvantage for robotic-assisted LRP compared with standard LRP or open approaches to prostatectomy.[18,19] In contrast, traditional LRP in the United States has been shown to approach the cost of open RRP owing to shorter hospitalization and lower transfusion rates.[19,20] These advantages are somewhat offset in the robotic-assisted cases by the higher cost of consumables and depreciation of the robotic equipment.[19] Despite these financial concerns, competitive market forces in the United States are pushing an increasing number of surgeons and hospitals to embrace robotic-assisted approaches to laparoscopic radical prostatectomy.

Results

Surgical Efficiency

Surgeon experience in LRP has been reported extensively in the literature, and the reader is referred to several exhaustive reviews for more details.[21,22] The first published series by Schuessler and colleagues[2] in 1997 reported operative times of over nine hours. With persistence and improvements in technique and technology, contemporary series now report LRP operative times that range between 2.5 and 5 hours, and as little as 1.9 hours for robotic-assisted LRP in high-volume centers.[23,24] For experienced laparoscopic and robotic surgeons, these results compare favorably with operative times for open RRP.

Blood Loss

During an open radical prostatectomy, most of the bleeding is due to low-pressure venous channels and divisions of the dorsal venous complex draining the penis. Blood loss is often closely linked to operative time, since this venous bleeding can be difficult to control until the prostate specimen is removed. During LRP, insufflation creates an effective tamponade mechanism that minimizes venous bleeding. Blood loss reported in most contemporary LRP series is only 100 to 500 mL.[3,17,23] The need for transfusion is also significantly decreased after LRP compared with that after open prostatectomy in most series.

Recovery

Minimally invasive approaches result in shorter hospital stays and reduced postoperative pain compared with open approaches for many surgical conditions.[25] These benefits have been particularly evident in urology with the application of laparoscopy to the treatment of renal disease. Through technical improvements and aggressive compliance with cost containment strategies, mean hospital stays following open radical prostatectomy have decreased to 2 to 3 days at most institutions in the United States. In addition, by making smaller infraumbilical incisions, postoperative pain following open radical prostatectomy is tolerable for most patients.[26] Early LRP series showed no clear advantage in length of hospitalization following LRP compared with that for open RRP.[27,28] However, with maturation of the technique and greater experience, an increasing number of institutions are discharging LRP patients on the first postoperative day.[23,29] Comparative analysis of postoperative pain between RRP and LRP is not extensive, and although some series show decreased pain scores following LRP,[29–31] others show no significant difference.[28,32,33] Perhaps an even more telling marker of recovery is the time required to return to baseline activity after prostatectomy. Several studies reported shorter times to full recovery for LRP (30 to 33 days) compared with that for open RRP (45 to 47 days).[29,31] In conclusion, although there appear to be some relative recovery advantages to LRP, these advantages are not nearly as dramatic as those observed when laparoscopy is applied to upper abdominal surgery such as nephrectomy or cholecystectomy.

Continence

In contemporary large series by established experts, continence after open RRP has been reported in more than 90% of patients with long-term follow-up.[34,35] Improvements in surgical technique and a better understanding of pelvic anatomy have contributed favorably to overall continence after open surgery. With improved instrumentation and magnified visualization, particularly during the dissection of the prostatic apex, laparoscopic approaches to radical prostatectomy have the potential to improve long-term outcomes and earlier return of continence. Indeed, published LRP series report similar 1-year continence rates (86–95%) and earlier return to continence compared with open approaches using validated questionnaires.[36–40] Caution should be exercised when interpreting outcome data, however, because of the variability in the method of information acquisition, questionnaire types, definitions of continence, timing of data collection, and investigator/patient biases.

Sexual Function

Comparison of sexual function after LRP and RRP is hindered by the same variability in methodology, acquisition, definitions, and bias that makes interpretation of continence difficult. Furthermore, preoperative potency, quality of nerve sparing during prostatectomy, and therapy for postoperative erectile dysfunction can influence sexual function outcomes. It is also important to recognize that the lack of available studies randomizing patients into either LRP or RRP groups hinders direct comparison between the two techniques. Nonetheless, preservation of cavernous nerves during prostatectomy is essential to maintain postoperative erectile function. Better visualization and improved instrument precision during LRP have the potential to positively affect erectile function postoperatively. Using validated questionnaires, several groups have reported that 40% to 64% of patients undergoing LRP return to preoperative baseline sexual function by 1 year.[37–39] This is comparable to reports of return to baseline sexual function after open techniques measured by similar instruments.[34,41,42]

Oncologic Outcome

Open prostatectomy remains the gold standard for the treatment of localized prostate cancer to which LRP must be compared. To date, results from LRP series show equivalent oncologic control compared with contemporary RRP series. Positive margin rates after LRP have been reported to be in the range of 9% to 22% for all stages of disease.[43–46] Biochemical recurrence-free survival has been reported in 83% to 90.5% of patients at 3 years' follow-up in three European series.[43,46,47] If only organ-confined disease is evaluated (pT2), margin-positive rate decreases to 4.5% to 16% and biochemical recurrence-free survival improves to 95%.[43]

Complications

The overall rate of perioperative complications for LRP range between 4% and 36%.[48,49] In descending order, the most common perioperative complications were anastomotic leak (10%), postoperative ileus (3.3%), anastomotic stricture (0–5%), bleeding (2.8%), rectal injury (0.7–2.4%), and deep venous thrombosis (0.4%).[27,50] Anastomotic stricture rates with LRP in particular compare favorably with the reported rates after open RRP (2.4–17.5%).[51–55] Most complications occurred during the early phase of the surgeon's experience and decreased substantially after the learning curve was achieved. Conversion rates to open RRP have also remained low (1–1.2%).

Obesity and Functional Outcomes

Significant obesity is associated with medical comorbidities such as diabetes mellitus and coronary artery disease. Moreover, obesity can significantly increase the degree of difficulty in performing open RRP, may require a larger incision for operative exposure, and may be associated with a higher complication rate. For this reason, many surgeons insist on weight loss before proceeding with radical prostatectomy, which may delay intervention significantly. LRP, and in particular its robotic-assisted variant, may offer some significant advantages when addressing prostate cancer in an obese patient. A wealth of experience with bariatric surgery has demonstrated that laparoscopy can be performed safely and effectively in even morbidly obese patients.[9] With only minor modifications in technique, LRP can be performed efficiently in patients with moderate obesity. Several studies report no difference in complications, blood loss, or functional outcomes between obese patients and normal controls following LRP.[7,8,56] However, in a study from University of California–Irvine, obese patients had significantly worse baseline urinary and sexual function, had more complications, and did not recover urinary function as quickly or as well as the nonobese controls after robotic-assisted LRP.[57] Several series have also shown an increase in operative time or open conversion rate for LRP in obese patients.[7,8,58,59] Clearly, more experience with LRP in obese patients is needed before we can truly quantify its advantages over RRP in this population.

Health Care Economics

Intraoperative costs for laparoscopic surgery are generally greater than for open surgery. This is mainly due to longer operative times and the expense of disposable laparoscopic equipment.[19,20] In particular, the large up-front investment in the da Vinci robot, its maintenance fees, and the high cost of disposable robotic instruments make robotic-assisted LRP less cost-effective than RRP. Several investigators have modeled these cost relationships in an effort to make LRP more cost-competitive with RRP. For traditional LRP, Link and colleagues[20] identified operative time, length of hospital stay, and consumable items (disposable equipment) to be the most influential factors affecting overall cost. These findings are supported by several studies.[19,60] By developing predictive models of cost, hospital charges, and professional fees, Link and colleagues determined that it would be equally costly to perform LRP as to perform open prostatectomy if disposable instruments were eliminated, only reusable instruments were used, and operative times for LRP were reduced to 3.4 hours.[20] To establish cost equivalence between robotic-assisted LRP and open prostatectomy, Scales and colleagues[61] developed a predictive model that accounted for parameters such as robotic surgical volume, length of hospital stay, and hospital cost. To achieve cost equivalence, a robotic surgical volume of at least 10 cases weekly was necessary, and a weekly caseload of 14 robotic LRPs was required to make robotic LRP less expensive compared with open prostatectomy. These results suggest that robotic LRP may be economically advantageous over RRP only in high-volume centers performing more than 500 surgeries per year. With the growing popularity of robotic-assisted LRP with both patients and surgeons, however, the costs for this technology are likely to drop substantially.

Conclusion

Over the past decade, LRP has developed into an accepted surgical approach for the treatment of localized prostate cancer. In many high-volume centers, LRP and robotic-assisted LRP have become the surgical therapy of choice. This trend has been fueled by both patient interest in minimally invasive surgery and surgeon enthusiasm for applying new technology to radical prostatectomy. Oncologic control and operative efficiency with LRP appear to be equivalent to RRP in experienced hands. Established advantages of LRP include slightly shorter hospital stays, less blood loss and postoperative pain, and potentially earlier return to full postoperative activity. Potential, but not yet fully proven, advantages of LRP include an earlier return to urinary continence, lower rates of bladder neck contracture, and applicability to obese patients. Whether LRP yields improvements in postoperative sexual function after nerve-sparing radical prostatectomy remains an open question and the subject of much ongoing research. Current disadvantages of LRP include a lack of availability at all centers and excess cost over open radical prostatectomy approaches—factors that should both improve over the next decade.

References

1. Clayman RV, Kavoussi LR, Soper NJ, et al: Laparoscopic nephrectomy: initial case report. J Urol 146:278, 1991.
2. Schuessler WW, Schulam PG, Clayman RV, Kavoussi LR: Laparoscopic radical prostatectomy: initial short-term experience. Urology 50:854, 1997.
3. Guillonneau B, Vallancien G: Laparoscopic radical prostatectomy: the Montsouris experience. J Urol 163:418, 2000.
4. Hoznek A, Salomon L, Olsson LE, et al: Laparoscopic radical prostatectomy. The Creteil experience. Eur Urol 40:38, 2001.

7 Perineal Prostatectomy

Timothy Y. Tseng and Philipp Dahm

KEY POINTS

- Radical perineal prostatectomy (RPP) represents the oldest form of radical prostatectomy and offers the most direct approach to the prostate.
- Appropriate candidates for RPP are patients with clinically organ-confined prostate cancer and an estimated life expectancy of more than 10 years.
- RPP is an excellent approach for many patients but offers distinct advantages over other approaches in patients who have undergone previous extensive abdominal surgery, those who have had renal transplants, and those who are morbidly obese.
- Advantages of the perineal approach include decreased blood loss, low transfusion requirements, infrequent postoperative ileus, and short hospital stay.
- RPP results in favorable long-term disease control comparable to other surgical techniques with 15-year cancer-associated survival rates approaching 86%.
- RPP demonstrates favorable urinary and sexual health-related quality-of-life outcomes, which appear comparable to those of other approaches such as radical retropubic and robot-assisted laparoscopic prostatectomy.

Introduction

Radical perineal prostatectomy (RPP) represents the oldest form of therapy offered for the treatment of clinically localized prostate cancer. First developed at the turn of the twentieth century, RPP was the mainstay of prostate cancer therapy until the development of ostensibly less morbid radiation therapy at mid-century.[1] Subsequently, radical retropubic prostatectomy (RRP) was introduced in 1945. At the time, this approach involved unacceptable morbidity, particularly with regard to blood loss.[2] As evidence for the significant morbidity associated with radiation therapy accumulated, RPP again became the treatment of choice for organ-confined disease. After the introduction of the anatomic RRP by Patrick Walsh in 1979 and further refinement of this technique to preserve erectile function, the open retropubic and robotic assisted laparoscopic approaches have become the more commonly performed forms of radical prostatectomy. Nevertheless, RPP is valued for its distinct advantages over the retropubic approach in appropriately selected patients.

Today, "modern" RPP accounts for only a small percentage of radical prostatectomies performed in the United States. However, recent developments continue to make the technique an attractive alternative to other surgical approaches. Notably, the introduction of nerve-sparing RPP and evidence supporting its effectiveness in preserving sexual function have demonstrated the technique's comparability to nerve-sparing RRP.[3] The downward stage migration in patients with newly diagnosed prostate cancer and the development of accurate predictive nomograms have also obviated the need for many staging lymph node dissections, which in RPP would have required a separate abdominal incision.[4-6] Furthermore, the long-term efficacy of RPP in treating clinically organ-confined disease has been well documented in large patient series with over a quarter-century of follow-up.[7-10] From a technical standpoint, the perineal approach allows for prostatic dissection in a relatively avascular field, provides good exposure for reconstruction of the urethrovesical anastomosis, and permits dependent postoperative drainage of the prostatic fossa. These features make RPP an attractive treatment option for patients with localized disease that is complementary to other surgical approaches.

maintain the cleanest possible surgical field in the event of rectal injury. In experienced hands, the rate of rectal injury for perineal prostatectomy ranges from 1% to 6%.[13,32] However, studies on the management of rectal injuries in retropubic prostatectomy have suggested that the lack of a thorough bowel preparation may not preclude successful immediate repair.[33] Because of the low incidence of this type of injury and the feasibility of immediate repair regardless of bowel preparation, no specific preoperative bowel preparation except a preoperative enema may be needed before surgery. Indeed, forgoing this step may eliminate preoperative gastrointestinal discomfort and may decrease the postoperative bowel dysfunction associated with mechanical bowel preparations. A well-designed randomized controlled trial to determine the usefulness of preoperative bowel preparation remains to be done, however. To date, many surgeons continue to make use of some type of bowel prep.

Positioning

Patient positioning is critically important and should be performed by someone who is adequately trained and experienced—ideally the surgeon himself. Traditionally, an exaggerated lithotomy position that places the perineum parallel with the floor is used (Fig. 7-1). However, such positioning, as well as the use of "candy cane" stirrups may increase the risk of lower-extremity neuropraxia. More recent experience has demonstrated that this operation can be successfully performed in a less exaggerated lithotomy position with decreased rates of this complication (Fig. 7-2). Allen stirrups are com-

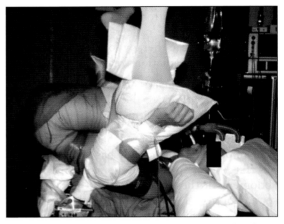

Figure 7-1. Patient positioning for radical perineal prostatectomy using the traditional Young table.   Note the highly exaggerated lithotomy position that places the perineum parallel with the floor. The Young table and the extreme lithotomy position demonstrated here have since been abandoned.

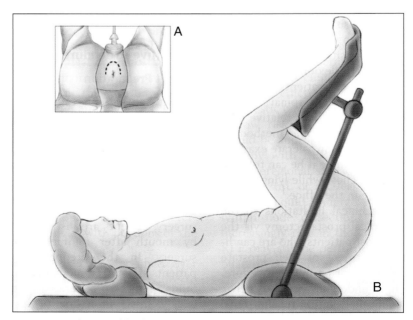

Figure 7-2. Contemporary patient positioning and draping for radical perineal prostatectomy.   A, The surgical field that includes the anus, perineum, scrotum, and penis is depicted. **B,** Patient positioning using Allen stirrups. Note the much less exaggerated lithotomy position.

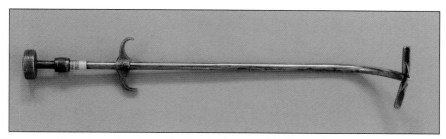

Figure 7-3. The curved Lowsley retractor. The Lowsley retractor is placed into the bladder where the prongs are opened (as shown). The Lowsley is the single most important instrument for this procedure because it allows intraoperative manipulation of the prostate.

monly used and ample padding is applied to all pressure points. The posterior scrotum and perineum are then shaved and a sterile skin preparation is applied from the umbilicus to the buttocks to include the inner thighs. Sterile drapes are applied leaving the genitalia and perineum exposed. A sterile towel is then fastened over the anus in such a way as to allow access to the rectum later during the operation. Positioning should further ensure that there is enough space to secure a perineal retractor device.

Classic RPP

Access to the Prostate

At this time, it is prudent to perform a digital rectal examination (DRE) to determine the size, location, and mobility of the prostate. A Lowsley retractor (Fig. 7-3) is placed through the urethra into the bladder to facilitate identification of landmarks and manipulation of the prostate during the procedure. The ability to manipulate the prostate in all three dimensions is an important prerequisite for this operation. If placement of the Lowsley retractor is difficult, digital guidance using a finger placed in the rectum may help. Sometimes, an overly exaggerated lithotomy position makes placement of the retractor difficult. In such cases, relaxing the stirrups and releasing tension on the lower extremities may be helpful. If Lowsley retractor placement is impossible, the operation can also be successfully performed with a Foley catheter in place. However, this makes the procedure significantly more challenging. Before proceeding with the operation, the surgeon should convince himself that the retractor is indeed in the bladder and not lodged in the prostatic urethra.

A curved skin incision is made 1.5 cm above the anal verge and extended posterolaterally on

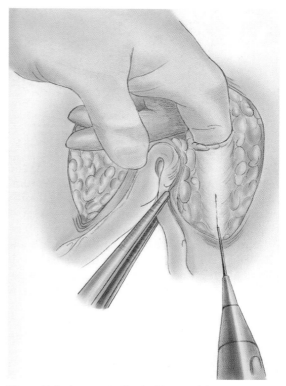

Figure 7-4. Access to the ischiorectal fossa.
Blunt dissection using a finger is used to develop the ischiorectal fossa bilaterally, here shown on the patient's left. The overlying fatty tissue is then transected using electrocautery.

either side medial to the ischial tuberosities. The superficial perineal fascia is incised using electrocautery dissection, and the ischiorectal fossae are developed bluntly (Fig. 7-4). Using two Allis clamps, the anal verge is retracted posteriorly to place the central tendon on traction. A finger is passed beneath the central tendon anterior to the rectum, and the central tendon is divided along the upper skin edge with cautery (Fig.

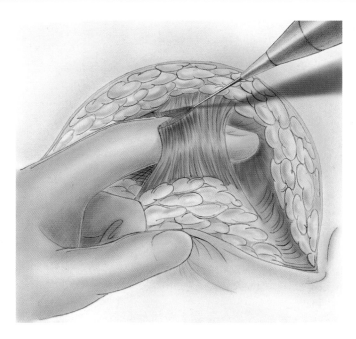

Figure 7-5. Division of the central tendon of the perineal body. The central tendon is divided at its superior aspect using electrocautery.

7-5). After division of the central tendon, the rectal sphincter is seen overlying the rectum. Manipulation of the Lowsley retractor facilitates orientation at this stage. An anterior retractor is then placed to retract the anal sphincter anteriorly. In the Belt approach, the rectourethralis muscle is identified as a band in the midline and, with a finger in the rectum to identify its course relative to the prostate, the rectourethralis is divided with Metzenbaum scissors in the midline (Fig. 7-6). At this point, the prostate is separated from the anterior surface of the rectum in the midline. Moist gauze is placed over the rectum to protect it from injury, and downward displacement is maintained by a posterior weighted retractor. Retractors are then placed to retract the divided rectourethralis and levator ani muscles superolaterally, allowing exposure of Denonvilliers fascia, colloquially known as "the Pearly Gates." Figure 7-7 illustrates the perineal anatomy.

Prostatic Dissection

Classically, RPP proceeds with a transverse incision of Denonvilliers fascia just below the apex of the prostate. Using blunt and sharp dissection, the posterior layer of Denonvilliers fascia is dissected away from the posterior prostatic surface beyond the seminal vesicles to the level of the bladder. The membranous urethra distal

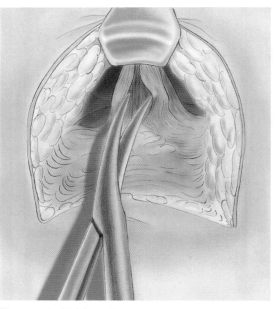

Figure 7-6. Division of the rectourethralis muscle. The medial aspect is divided. Lateral portions may be bluntly displaced laterally.

to the apex of the prostate and posterior to the puboprostatic dorsal venous complex is developed (Figs. 7-8 and 7-9). A right angle clamp is passed behind the urethra, the Lowsley retractor is removed, and the urethra is sharply divided. The urethral stump is then either tagged with a stitch to be discarded later or tagged with the first two urethrovesical anastomotic sutures (Fig. 7-10). A Young retractor is then passed through the prostatic urethra into the bladder and the wings are opened, allowing posterior displacement of the prostate. A plane on either side of the midline between the anterior surface of the prostate and the dorsal venous complex is developed, and the midline puboprostatic ligament is divided sharply. Dissection continues proximally until the bladder neck is reached. Once the prostatovesical junction is identified, the prostate is sharply dissected away from the

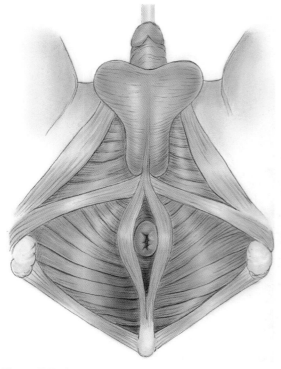

Figure 7-7. Anatomy of the perineum. This diagram shows the relationship of the external anal sphincter to the anus, levator anus, and ischiocavernosus muscle.

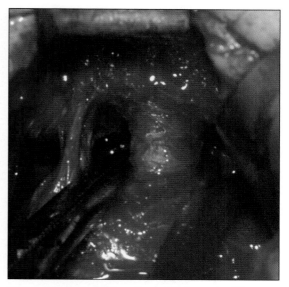

Figure 7-8. Apical dissection. Photograph of the prostatic apex. An anterior retractor and a Deaver blade are in place. Other instruments on either side of the urethra are a suction tip and the tip of a Tonsil clamp.

Figure 7-9. Apical dissection. This diagram depicts how the prostatic apex comes into view.

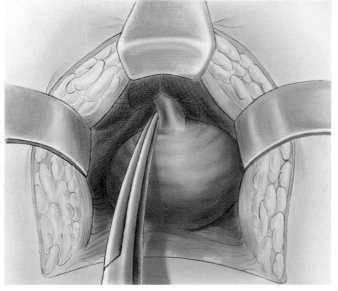

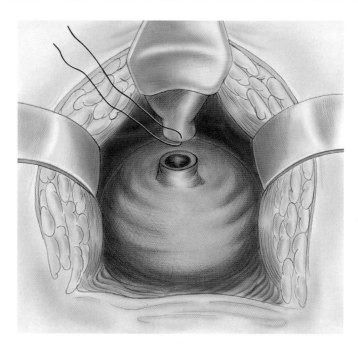

Figure 7-10. Division of the urethra.   The urethra has been divided and the urethral stump is tagged with a suture to prevent retraction into the perineal body.

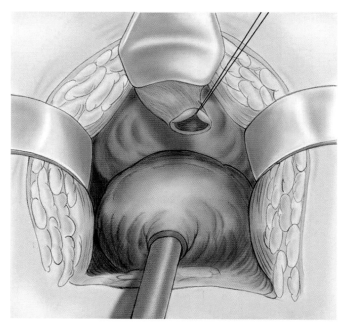

Figure 7-11. Placement of Young retractor. A straight Young retractor is placed to allow posterior retraction of the prostate.

circular fibers of the detrusor to spare the bladder neck to the greatest possible extent.

The anterior bladder neck is then incised sharply between the 10 and 2 o'clock positions. The Young retractor is removed, and a temporary Foley catheter is passed into the prostatic urethra and out through the anterior bladder incision to allow further manipulation of the prostate (Fig. 7-11). Traction on this catheter

allows sharp division of the bladder neck. Care is taken to divide the trigone distal to the ureteral orifices. Identification of the ureteral orifices can be aided by the routine use of intravenous indigo carmine. If in doubt, the patency of the ureters can be confirmed by catheterization with open-ended ureteral stents. Once the bladder neck has been divided completely, the seminal vesicles and ampullae of the

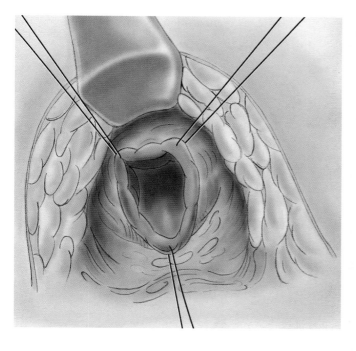

Figure 7-12. Bladder neck. Perspective of the bladder after removal of the prostate.

vasa deferentia are identified posterolateral to the prostate. The ampullae are isolated with a right angle clamp, ligated with right angle clips, and transected on the specimen side. Postero-lateral perforating arteries and veins at the 5 and 7 o'clock positions are controlled with surgical clips or absorbable sutures. The seminal vesicles are then dissected from their investing fascia bluntly. Arteries entering the apices of the seminal vesicles are ligated and the surgical specimen is removed.

Reconstruction

Reconstruction of the bladder neck is accomplished symmetrically using slow absorbable monofilament suture (Fig. 7-12). A running 4-0 suture is used on each side of the bladder neck to evert the mucosa (Fig. 7-13). Although abandoned as a routine part of RPP at many institutions, Vest sutures of 0-0 suture material may be placed at 11 and 1 o'clock in the anterior bladder neck in a horizontal mattress fashion to help align the vesicourethral anastomosis and relieve any potential tension. Two 2-0 sutures are then placed at 10 and 2 o'clock in the bladder neck and the urethral stump to become the anterior anastomotic sutures. The bladder neck is then reapproximated in a "racket handle" manner with interrupted 0-0 sutures from posterior to anterior with the last two sutures left

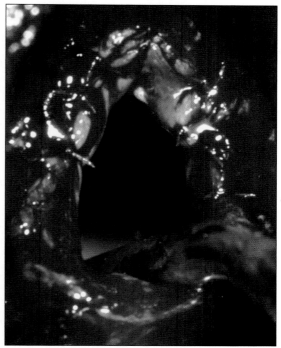

Figure 7-13. Eversion of bladder neck. Photograph of bladder neck after eversion of the mucosa with two fine running sutures on the anterior aspect of either side.

long enough to serve as posterior Vest sutures (Fig. 7-14). An 18F Foley catheter is passed through the urethra into the bladder and the balloon inflated. Another two 2-0 anastomotic sutures are then placed posteriorly at 4 and 6

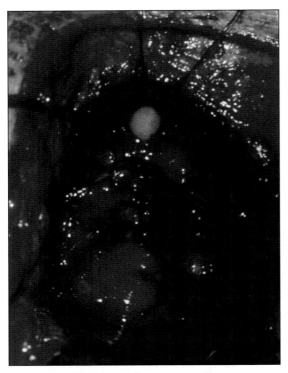

Figure 7-14. Bladder neck reconstruction.
Photograph of the bladder neck after racket-handle
approximation.

o'clock in the bladder neck and the urethral
stump. All retractors are then removed, and the
four 2-0 anastomotic sutures are tied down
under gentle traction of the Foley catheter under
direct vision. The presence of a watertight anastomosis may be tested by catheter irrigation.

Closure

The four Vest sutures are brought out through
the subcutaneous tissue of the perineal body
paralleling the urethra and gently tied down.
The incision is copiously irrigated, and the
rectum is inspected for signs of injury by DRE.
A Penrose drain is placed between the vesicourethral anastomosis and the rectum, brought
out through a separate stab incision, and secured
with a stitch. The rectourethralis, levator ani,
and central tendon are reapproximated in the
midline with absorbable suture. Subcutaneous
tissue is further reapproximated with absorbable
suture, and the skin is closed with interrupted
2-0 absorbable suture leaving the sutures long so
that they produce less discomfort postopera-

tively. A compression dressing is applied to the
perineum.

Nerve-Sparing RPP

In appropriately selected patients with small or
medium size glands (less than 100 g), nerve-
sparing RPP is feasible. Rather than a transverse
incision of Denonvilliers fascia, a vertical incision is made such that reflection of this layer
laterally and over the apex of the prostate allows
the development of a plane between the prostate and the neurovascular bundles. Given the
spatial constraints, nerve-sparing RPP requires a
variety of alternating maneuvers to displace the
prostate inward and/or laterally for dissection of
the neurovascular bundles. Hemostasis is
achieved with clips rather than electrocautery to
prevent thermal injury to the neurovascular
bundles. During dissection of the seminal vesicles, great care is taken not to inadvertently
injure the neurovascular bundles.

Wide-Field Dissection RPP

Patients considered to be at high risk for extracapsular disease may undergo wide-field RPP
that includes the lateral pelvic fascia en bloc
with the prostate specimen. This procedure
results in sacrifice of the neurovascular bundles
as the surgical margin includes the periprostatic
fascia. All fibrovascular pedicles are divided as
distantly from the prostate as possible. The
seminal vesicles are dissected and clipped to
include the neurovascular bundle in the specimen. Furthermore, wider bladder neck margins
may be taken as necessary.

Postoperative Care

The patient is transported to the recovery room
where serum electrolytes are routinely obtained.
Since average blood loss is less than 500 mL in
RPP, the need for blood transfusion is rare.
Because pain from this incision is low, pain
control is achieved with oral analgesics with
intravenous analgesics for breakthrough pain
starting in the recovery room. Patients are routinely started on clear liquids, and their diets are
advanced as tolerated. On the first postoperative
day, the compression dressing is replaced with
fluffed gauze, and the patient is encouraged to
ambulate. The Penrose drain is left in place until

the second postoperative day or until the patient's first bowel movement. At that time, the patient is taught to use antiseptic sitz baths or to clean himself with a hand-held shower-head. Prophylactic antibiotics are continued for 24 hours and suppressive oral antibiotics are continued until the patient's Foley catheter is removed in 10 to 14 days. Patients are typically discharged 1 to 2 days postoperatively when they demonstrate the ability to tolerate a regular diet, ambulate without assistance, and achieve good pain control with oral analgesics.

Complications

Major complications of RPP are infrequent. In a large retrospective analysis of 630 RPPs by Gillitzer and colleagues,[32] complications requiring surgical intervention occurred in only 1.7% of cases. The types of complications associated with RPP include those common to all forms of prostatectomy such as excess blood loss, rectal injury, and bladder neck contracture. Complications unique to RPP include lower extremity neuropraxia and rhabdomyolysis (Table 7-2).

Excess Blood Loss

Large-volume blood loss is less common in RPP compared with RRP because the dorsal venous

Table 7-2. Complications of Radical Perineal Prostatectomy (n = 630)

Complication	% (n)
Major (requiring open surgical intervention)	
Bleeding/hematoma	1.1 (7)
Urinary fistula	0.3 (2)
Stool fistula	0.3 (2)
Combined fistula	0.5 (3)
Perineal sinus	0.2 (1)
	Total 2.4 (15)
Minor (not requiring open surgical intervention)	
Rectal injury	5.1 (32)
Urinary fistula	3.5 (22)
Urinary retention	5.6 (35)
Bladder neck contracture	2.7 (17)
Epididymitis	2.2 (14)
Neuropraxia	0.6 (4)
	Total 20.0 (124)

From Gillitzer R, Melchior SW, Hampel C, et al: Specific complications of radical perineal prostatectomy: a single institution study of more than 600 cases. J Urol 172:124, 2004.

complex is not divided and venous pressure is decreased due to patient positioning.[34,35] Dissection in an incorrect plane leading to injury of the dorsal venous complex can result in significant venous bleeding. Such bleeding may be managed by tamponade with a narrow retractor or placement of a figure-of-eight stitch in the dorsal venous complex.

Rectal Injury

Rectal injury is a well-recognized risk of all prostatectomy approaches. Although older studies reported a risk of rectal injury with the perineal approach of up to 11%, more recent studies demonstrate an incidence of 1% to 6% in the hands of experienced surgeons.[32,35,36] The increased risk of rectal injury with RPP compared with RRP is attributed to the fact that the initial exposure of the prostate requires dissection in a plane between the rectum and the prostate. Rectal injuries most commonly occur at early stages of the operation during division of the rectourethralis muscle and placement of the posterior weighted retractor. With meticulous attention to the correct surgical plane and careful placement of retractors, such injury is avoidable in most cases. If a rectal injury is recognized, the surgical field should be copiously irrigated, and the defect closed in two to three nonoverlapping suture lines with an absorbable monofilament. Postoperatively, the patient is maintained on a clear liquid diet for 3 days and is treated with broad-spectrum antibiotics with anaerobic coverage. A rectal Penrose drain may be placed to help evacuate gas.

Alternatively, anal dilatation on a daily basis to prevent a build-up of pressure at the repair site has been recommended. The efficacy of such measures remains to be demonstrated, however. Usually, there are no adverse consequences as a result of a rectal injury identified and appropriately managed at the time of surgery. In patients with very large rectal tears, gross fecal spillage, prior pelvic irradiation, or a history of immunocompromise, a diverting colostomy is indicated to prevent a possible rectourinary fistula.

Ureteral Compromise

Reconstruction of the bladder neck may be difficult if the bladder neck incision is close to the ureteral orifices. In this situation, standard closure of the bladder neck may result in compromised ureteral drainage. In such cases, the ureteral orifices can be stented with open-ended ureteral catheters, and the posterior bladder neck closed with stitches incorporating only the detrusor musculature and excluding the bladder mucosa. The stents are brought out through separate perineal stab wounds and then typically left in place for 5 to 7 days. Alternatively, double-J ureteral stents may be placed and left in place for an extended period of time. Primary ureteral reimplantation from the perineal approach, though technically challenging, may also be performed.[37] If this procedure is infeasible from the perineal approach, patients may also be managed with placement of a percutaneous nephrostomy tube on postoperative day 1 when the affected collecting system has become somewhat dilated. This is then followed by delayed ureteral reimplantation from the abdominal approach in 6 to 12 weeks.

Transient Lower Extremity Neuropraxia

Exaggerated lithotomy positioning can result in lower extremity neuropraxia in the immediate postoperative period. Neuropraxia, defined as sensory or motor deficits of the lower extremity, occurred in up to 20% of patients in one series.[38] In most cases, neuropraxia was mild, limited to the area below the knee and primarily sensory. Management of this condition is expectant and conservative. Complete resolution of these symptoms, frequently before discharge from the hospital, reliably occurs in all patients. Attention to proper positioning and padding can reduce the incidence of this complication. To avoid unnecessary anxiety, patients should be made aware of this potential complication preoperatively.

Rhabdomyolysis

Rhabdomyolysis due to ischemic muscle necrosis has been reported with prolonged surgery in the exaggerated lithotomy position. Specifically, there have been four case reports of rhabdomyolysis progressing to acute renal failure in patients undergoing prolonged RPP.[39–42] Patients who develop rhabdomyolysis frequently complain of severe muscle pain. Early signs of rhabdomyolysis include decreased urine output, abnormal serum electrolytes, elevated serum creatine phosphokinase, and myoglobinuria. Treatment for rhabdomyolysis involves aggressive volume expansion and bicarbonate infusion to maintain urine pH greater than 6.5 to reduce the renal precipitation of heme. Proper padding of all pressure points and periodic lowering of the legs during prolonged procedures may decrease the occurrence of rhabdomyolysis. One of the main preventive measures is to keep the operative time as short as possible.[43]

Urinary Problems

Potential urinary problems include obstruction, persistent perineal leakage of urine, and urinary incontinence. Urinary obstruction evident in the immediate postoperative period after removal of the urinary catheter is relatively rare and is usually due to residual edema at the vesicourethral anastomosis. This can be treated with placement of a urethral catheter for an additional 1 to 2 weeks. Late urinary obstruction is usually the result of bladder neck contracture and can usually be treated with urethral dilation with filiforms and followers. If this is unsuccessful, direct-vision internal urethrotomy of the stricture may be indicated.

In up to 4% of patients, urinary extravasation through the perineal incision after removal of the urinary catheter may occur.[32] Extravasation that occurs only during voiding is indicative of a leak distal to the vesicourethral anastomosis and usually closes with time. Extravasation that occurs continuously is due to leakage from the anastomosis. In such cases, the urinary catheter is replaced carefully and left indwelling for an additional 1 to 2 weeks. A cystogram may then be performed to document healing.

As with all forms of prostatectomy, urinary control develops over the course of weeks to months after surgery. Persistent and severe urinary incontinence at 12 months after surgery is rare and suggests irreversible damage to the external urinary sphincter that may ultimately require placement of an artificial urinary sphincter.

Outcomes

Operative Outcomes

RPP demonstrates excellent operative outcomes. Operative time is generally similar to that for radical retropubic prostatectomy and ranges from a median time of 178 minutes to 200 minutes in recent series.[34,44] These operative times include the time required for lymph node dissection through a separate incision and are further shortened if node dissection is omitted in appropriately-selected, low-risk patients. Compared with the retropubic approach, perineal prostatectomy generally results in lower estimated blood loss and lower rates of blood transfusion. In a large, retrospective review, Salomon and colleagues[34] found that only 16% of RPP patients required blood transfusion compared with 26% of RRP patients. In the only randomized controlled trial published to date, Martis and colleagues[44] found that median estimated blood loss was 200 mL for RPP and 450 mL for RRP ($P < .001$), and the median number of

packed red blood cells transfused was none for RPP and two for RRP ($P < .001$). A study of matched controls of RPP and RRP patients from the Uniformed Services Urology Research Group found similar results[35] (Table 7-3).

Widespread anecdotal evidence suggests that the pain associated with perineal prostatectomy is significantly decreased compared with the pain due to the retropubic approach. Weizer and associates[43] investigated narcotic pain requirements after RPP and found that 84% and 98% of patients did not require parenteral narcotics by postoperative days 1 and 2, respectively. Similarly, a study by Sullivan and associates[45] found that the mean time for use of only oral analgesics was 1.7 days for RPP and 3.8 days for RRP. In a study by Weizer and associates, the

Table 7-3. Comparison of Operative Outcomes Between Radical Perineal and Radical Retropubic Prostatectomy

Outcome	RPP	RRP	P Value
	Median (Range)		
	(n = 100)	(n = 100)	
Martis et al[44] (2007)			
Operative time (min)	130 (100–180)	125 (110–180)	NS
Estimated blood loss (mL)	200 (100–600)	450 (200–900)	<.01
Transfusion rate (no. units)	0 (0–2)	2 (1–5)	<.01
Length of bladder catheterization (days)	7 (5–21)	13 (10–21)	<.01
Length of hospital stay (days)	8 (7–20)	13 (10–21)	<.01
	Mean ± SD		
	(n = 119)	(n = 145)	
Salomon et al[34] (2002)			
Operative time (min)	178 ± 69	197 ± 56	
Transfusion rate (% patients)	15.9%	26.2%	
Length of bladder catheterization (days)	11.7 ± 4.4	15.9 ± 7.7	
Length of hospital stay (days)	8.5 ± 4.8	15.2 ± 8.3	
	Mean		
	(n = 100)	(n = 190)	
Lance et al[35] (2001)			
Estimated blood loss (mL)	802	1575	<.01
Autologous transfusion rate (no. units)	0.3	1.7	<.01
Homologous transfusion rate (no. units)	0.1	0.2	.32
	Mean ± SD		
	(n = 79)	(n = 59)	
Sullivan et al[45] (1999)			
Operative time (min)	120 ± 24	126 ± 27	NS
Estimated blood loss (mL)	416 ± 288	1138 ± 607	<.01
Length of hospital stay (days)	4.5 ± 2.3	6.7 ± 1.7	<.01
Time to regular diet (days)	2.3 ± 1.5	5.1 ± 1.6	<.01
Duration of parenteral analgesics (days)	1.7 ± 1.2	3.8 ± 1.5	<.01

RPP, radical perineal prostatectomy; RRP, radical retropubic prostatectomy.

was not reached by 5 years in all Gleason score categories, suggesting that low-volume, high-grade disease can be successfully treated by RPP. For patients with specimen-confined and margin-positive disease, long-term survival rates were lower, but were nevertheless extended (Fig. 7-17).

In the era of PSA screening, most studies now use biochemical recurrence as a surrogate marker for disease recurrence. Median time to PSA recurrence occurred at approximately 80 months after RPP in the Uniformed Services Urology Research Group study and was not significantly different from the recurrence rate for RRP.[35] Similarly, there were no statistical differences in biochemical recurrence-free survival in the randomized controlled trial by Martis and researchers[44] at 60 months.

Functional Outcomes

Postprocedural health-related quality of life is increasingly recognized as an important determinant in the selection of a treatment modality. After radical prostatectomy, the primary health-related quality of life (HRQOL) issues include urinary, sexual, and bowel function. Such

HRQOL data are now being collected in large prospective, longitudinal studies using validated patient self-assessment instruments such as the Expanded Prostate Cancer Index Composite (EPIC) questionnaire. At Duke University, long-term data on the recovery of RPP patients' individual baseline HRQOL are now available. Figure 7-18 summarizes the time course to recovery of mental, physical, urinary, sexual, and bowel HRQOL in this cohort of patients.[51]

In the urinary domain, RPP demonstrates excellent outcomes. Variously defined and variously assessed, total urinary continence rates for those with RPP have ranged from 86% to 96% at 1 year.[44,45,48,52] Return of continence for the perineal approach has been suggested to occur earlier than for RRP. In particular, Bishoff and associates[53] found in a single time point mail survey of 784 RRPs and 123 RPPs that 79% of RPP patients versus 85% of RRP patients reported incontinence immediately after surgery ($P = .043$). In a prospective comparison of RPP to the newer technique of robot-assisted laparoscopic prostatectomy (RALP), no statistically significant differences in urinary outcomes were seen, with median time to social continence, defined as the use of 0–1 pads per day, being 3.3 months for RPP and 3.7 months for RALP ($P = .175$)[51] (Fig. 7-19). In addition, in studies using validated patient self-assessment instruments such as the EPIC questionnaire and the UCLA-Prostate Cancer Index (UCLA-PCI), RPP appears to offer an advantage over RRP in terms of recovery of urinary function and bother scores[54–56] (Table 7-6). However, well-designed, multi-institutional prospective studies that compare the various surgical approaches are lacking.

Owing to the location of the neurovascular bundles along the prostatic capsule, all forms of prostatectomy have detrimental effects on erectile function. Because of the earlier adoption of a nerve-sparing technique for retropubic prostatectomy, patients with good erectile function historically have been preferentially selected for retropubic prostatectomy. Using physician-reported data, Weldon and colleagues[3,52] found that potency after bilateral nerve-sparing RPP was 50% at 1 year and 70% at 2 years. Frazier and colleagues[48] also found 77% of RPP patients to be potent 12 months after surgery. In a comparison between RPP and RRP that did not control for nerve-sparing technique, Sullivan

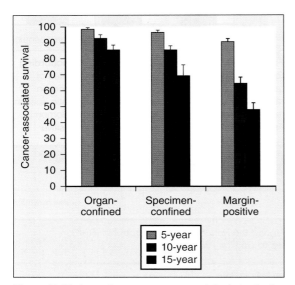

Figure 7-17. Long-term cancer-associated survival. This study of long-term cancer-associated survival in 1230 Duke University Medical Center patients over a 20-year time period is grouped by pathologic stage. (Data from Iselin CE, Robertson JE, Paulson DF: Radical perineal prostatectomy: oncological outcome during a 20-year period. J Urol 161:163, 1999.)

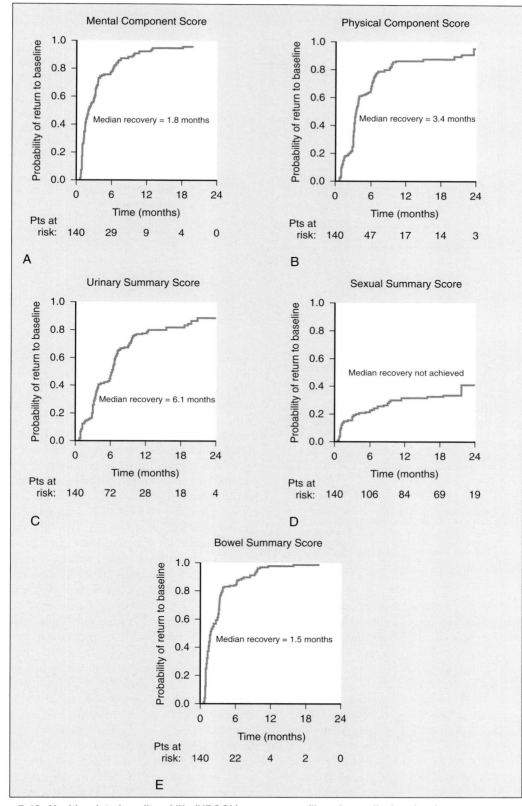

Figure 7-18. Health-related quality of life (HRQOL) recovery profiles after radical perineal prostatectomy.
Recovery of patients' individual baseline HRQOL was assessed in a prospective, longitudinal study of 140 radical perineural prostatectomy patients between 2001 and 2006 using the EPIC questionnaire. (Data from Tseng TY, Albala DM, Dahm P: Prospective Comparison of the Health-Related Quality of Life Outcomes of Robotic Prostatectomy and Radical Perineal Prostatectomy. Unpublished data, Duke University Medical Center, 2006.)

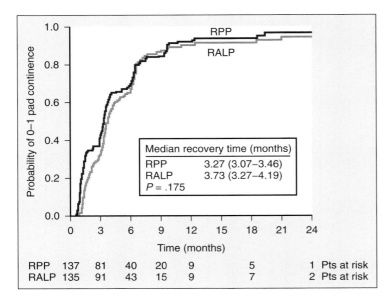

Figure 7-19. Comparison of time course for recovery of 0–1 pad social continence after radical perineural prostatectomy (RPP) and robot-assisted laparoscopic prostatectomy (RALP). Data were prospectively accrued using the EPIC questionnaire in 137 RPP and 135 RALP patients with no preoperative incontinence between 2001 and 2006. (Data from Tseng TY, Albala DM, Dahm P: Prospective Comparison of the Health-Related Quality of Life Outcomes of Robotic Prostatectomy and Radical Perineal Prostatectomy. Unpublished data, Duke University Medical Center, 2006.)

Table 7-6. Percent of Patients Returning to Their Individual Baseline Urinary HRQOL by 12 Months Using the EPIC and UCLA-PCI Questionnaires

HRQOL Domain	RPP[*] (%)	RRP[†] (%)	RALP[‡] (%)
Urinary function	73	56	71
Urinary bother	80	71	87

[*]Yang et al[65] (2004).
[†]Litwin et al[64] (2001).
[‡]Tseng et al[66] (2006).
RPP and RALP were assessed using the EPIC questionnaire. RRP was assessed using the UCLA-PCI. The urinary HRQOL assessment questions and scoring systems are the same for both questionnaires. HRQOL, health-related quality of life; RALP, robot-assisted laparoscopic prostatectomy; RPP, radical perineal prostatectomy; RRP, radical retropubic prostatectomy.

and associates[45] found patient-reported UCLA-PCI sexual function scores to be similar between the two groups at 21.2/100 and 21.9/100. Sexual bother scores were in fact higher in the perineal group at 35.8/100 and 26.6/100, respectively. In the randomized trial by Martis and associates[44] in which all patients underwent bilateral nerve-sparing procedures, mean (International Index of Erectile Function (IIEF) scores at 6 months were 18.5 ± 0.5 for RPP and 21.7 ± 1.9 for RRP. At 24 months, mean IIEF scores were 19.7 ± 1.1 and 23.1 ± 2.5, respectively. No significant differences in potency, as defined by the patient's subjective ability to "reach an erection capable of completing sexual intercourse in a satisfying way" were noted at 6 months. At 24 months, however, this group noted a statistically

significant difference in potency rates of 42% for RPP and 60% for RRP. Nevertheless, the efficacy of the nerve-sparing technique for RPP is evident in a recent study using the EPIC patient self-assessment questionnaire. In this study, median time to return of erectile function as defined by erections firm enough for intercourse was 23.8 months in patients undergoing nerve sparing and not achieved in those not undergoing nerve sparing[57] (Fig. 7-20).

A study by Bishoff and colleagues[53] suggested that RPP is associated with high rates of postoperative fecal incontinence. In a cross-sectional study using a mailed survey, they found that 17% of RPP patients had fecal incontinence more than once per month compared with 10% of RRP patients. However, two subsequent prospective studies have countered this finding.[58,59] Specifically, a longitudinal study of bowel-related quality of life found the incidence of new-onset fecal incontinence of any degree to be less than 4%. Furthermore, 92% of RPP patients recovered their individual baseline EPIC bowel domain scores by 6 months[59] (Fig. 7-21). These data suggest that bowel dysfunction after RPP is a real, but rare, event that resolves in most patients in the early postoperative period. In addition, there may be a high rate of unrecognized preoperative bowel dysfunction among radical prostatectomy candidates, which should be accounted for with the use of routinely administered, validated questionnaires prior to surgery.

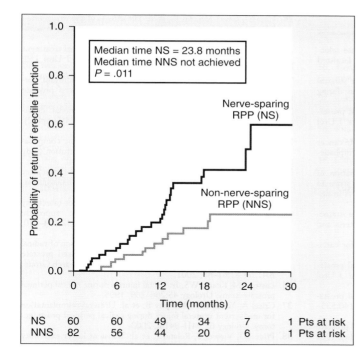

Figure 7-20. Comparison of time course for recovery of erectile function in radical perineal prostatectomy (RPP) patients undergoing nerve-sparing and non–nerve-sparing procedures. Data were prospectively accrued using the EPIC questionnaire between 2001 and 2004. Sixty-nine patients underwent nerve-sparing (NS) and 89 patients underwent non–nerve-sparing (NNS) procedures. All patients reported being sexually active before surgery. (From Kuebler HR, Tseng TY, Sun L, et al: Impact of nerve-sparing technique on patients' self-assessed outcomes in radical perineal prostatectomy. J Urol 178:488, 2007.)

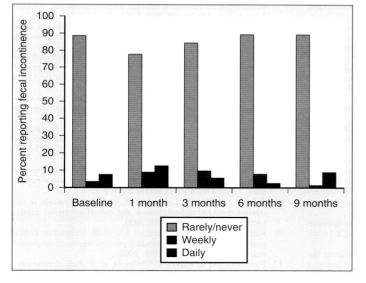

Figure 7-21. Prevalence of varying degrees of fecal incontinence at baseline before surgery and up to 9 months after radical perineal prostatectomy. Data were prospectively collected using the EPIC questionnaire. (Data from Dahm P, Silverstein AD, Weizer AZ, et al: A longitudinal assessment of bowel related symptoms and fecal incontinence following radical perineal prostatectomy. J Urol 169:2220, 2003.)

Conclusions

Radical perineal prostatectomy provides a number of advantages in the treatment of clinically organ-confined prostate cancer, including good long-term disease control, a relatively short convalescence period, and early return of urinary control. Nerve-sparing techniques have also demonstrated significant effi-cacy in the preservation of erectile function. Because of the decreased morbidity associated with the procedure, RPP remains an attractive treatment option for many appropriately selected patients.

Acknowledgments. The authors thank Diana Dai, M.D., M.Sc.BMC, for creating the drawings.

8

Basic Terms and Concepts of Radiation

*John Christodouleas, Jana Fox,
Danny Song, and Theodore DeWeese*

KEY POINTS

- Radiation therapy involves the use of high-energy x-rays or subatomic particles to kill tumor cells.
- Radiation is the most common initial treatment for localized prostate cancer in the United States.
- External-beam radiation and low dose rate brachytherapy are the most common radiation modalities for localized prostate cancer; other less commonly used radiation modalities are high dose rate brachytherapy, proton therapy, and neutron therapy.
- The choice of radiation treatment method and the decision to combine this with androgen ablation depend on a patient's risk stratification and baseline urinary and rectal symptoms.
- External-beam radiation may be appropriate after prostatectomy in the setting of adverse pathologic features or prostate-specific antigen (PSA) recurrence.
- Radiation is as effective as surgery for low-risk disease and is the preferred modality, when combined with androgen ablation, for locally advanced disease.
- Intensity-modulated radiation therapy (IMRT) is the most commonly used modern technique of external-beam radiation that allows for highly conformal dose distribution.
- The most important potential side effects of external-beam radiation therapy (EBRT) and brachytherapy are urethral irritation/stricture, proctitis, and erectile dysfunction.

Introduction

Radiation therapy involves the use of high-energy x-rays or subatomic particles to kill tumor cells. Radiation causes cell death by direct interaction with DNA or, more commonly, by initiating a secondary DNA damaging process. Radiation can be safely used to treat tumors for two important reasons: Normal cells are more adept than tumor cells at repairing radiation-induced DNA damage, and imaging and other technolo-

gies allow us to preferentially target tumors and limit normal tissue exposure.

Externally applied radiation, also known as external-beam radiation therapy (EBRT), is usually administered over a protracted course of many doses, commonly referred to as fractions. The use of multiple smaller fractions allows one to take repeated advantage of the superior repair ability of normal cells over tumor cells.

Radiation can also be internally applied by directly implanting radiation sources into tumors or cavities. This kind of treatment is referred to as brachytherapy (*brachy* means "short distance" in Greek). The radiation from brachytherapy sources usually travels only over very short distances, allowing for the delivery of high doses of radiation to tumors with minimal dose to normal surrounding tissues.

The SI unit of radiation measurement is the gray (Gy), which is defined as energy absorbed from ionizing radiation equivalent to 1 joule per kilogram. For clinical purposes, radiation dose is often described in terms of centigray (cGy). The older term was the rad; 1 rad is equal to 1 cGy. Treatment with heavy particles such as protons or neutrons is described in terms of centigray-equivalents. Contemporary treatments typically use linear accelerators that deliver high-energy photons and electrons in the megavoltage range. The methods of EBRT delivery vary in nature and are discussed in further detail in the following text.

The Role of Radiation Therapy in the Treatment of Prostate Cancer

Of all patients diagnosed with prostate cancer between 1998 and 2003, an estimated 40%

3D Plan   IMRT Plan

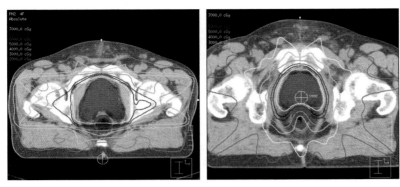

Figure 8-2. Comparison of 3D-CRT (conformal radiation therapy) and IMRT (intensity-modulated radiation therapy) for definitive radiation to the prostate. Dose levels are represented by different colored lines (isodose lines), with the higher dose lines closer to the target. Note the more highly conformal isodose lines in the IMRT plan compared with the 3D-CRT plan.

months, killing prostate cancer cells in the process. This approach is an attractive option for many patients in terms of convenience and minimal interference with daily activity and lifestyle.

Before the actual procedure, the patient undergoes a transrectal ultrasound or a CT-based volume study. This information allows the physician to pre-plan the 3D seed distribution required to deliver the prescribed dose to the prostate and periprostatic margin. Seeds are preferentially placed in a peripheral distribution to avoid overdosing the urethra. In the operating room, patients are placed in the dorsal lithotomy position, a Foley catheter is inserted, and a template is positioned against the perineum. Using transrectal ultrasound guidance, hollow needles are guided into the prostate using the template, and the seeds are deposited according to the plan (which is often modified in the operating room to account for possible changes in prostate size) (Figs. 8-3 and 8-4). Seeds can be placed either using a device called a Mick applicator, with needles preloaded with seeds, or using seeds strewn on ribbon at spaced intervals. Most commonly, iodine-125 (^{125}I or I-125) or palladium-103 (^{103}Pd or Pd-103) seeds are used. They measure approximately 4.5 × 0.8 mm, and generally 60 to 100 seeds may be placed, depending on the size of the prostate. A CT scan is typically obtained at some point following the implant to verify seed positioning.[11]

Relative contraindications to the use of prostate brachytherapy include large prostate size (more than 60 g), history of transurethral resection of the prostate (TURP), and irritative or obstructive urinary symptoms. These factors

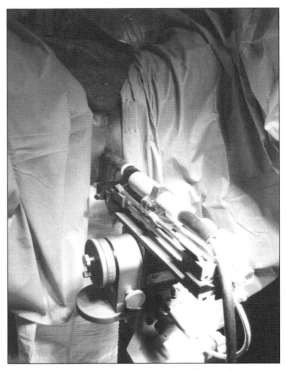

Figure 8-3. Patient in lithotomy position before placement of brachytherapy seeds. An ultrasound is inserted into the rectum before the placement of brachytherapy seeds in order to verify the position of the prostate and to help guide seed placement.

predispose the patient to an increased risk of complications. A history of TURP may increase the rates of urinary incontinence, and a high International Prostate Symptom Score (IPSS), a measure of urinary symptoms, has been found to predict for postimplantation urinary retention. A patient with a large prostate may be placed on a trial of androgen deprivation in an attempt to shrink the gland to an adequate size

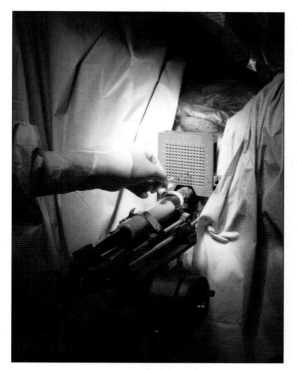

Figure 8-4. Patient in lithotomy position during placement of brachytherapy seeds. Brachytherapy seeds are inserted by a needle as shown in the photo. The position of seed placement is then verified by a rectal ultrasound that remains in position throughout the procedure.

for implantation, although controversy exists as to whether this reduces postimplantation urinary symptoms.[12,13] Other factors to consider are the presence of a large median prostate lobe, previous pelvic surgeries, and severe diabetes.[14]

Patient Stratification

The workup of patients with newly diagnosed prostate cancer is discussed in Chapter 2. The three most important factors used to risk stratify a patient are clinical stage, PSA, and Gleason score. The most common risk classification scheme was developed by D'Amico and colleagues.[15,16] This scheme classifies patients with a Gleason score of 2–6, PSA less than 10 ng/mL, and clinical stage of T1c-T2a as low-risk, patients with a Gleason score of 7 or PSA 10 to 20 ng/mL or stage T2b as intermediate-risk, and patients with Gleason score of 8–10 or PSA higher than 20 ng/mL or clinical stage T2c and above as high-risk. The risk of PSA failure at 5 years after single-modality treatment with

radical prostatectomy, EBRT, or brachytherapy was reported by D'Amico and associates[16] in a large retrospective analysis as less than 25%, 25% to 50%, and more than 50% for low-, intermediate-, and high-risk patients, respectively. This model has subsequently been validated in other series and is frequently used to guide current management decisions.

Outside of this formal risk stratification, other pathologic factors are taken into account as well when advising patients of their treatment options. These include, but are not limited to, the presence of perineural invasion, the relative percentage of involved tissue on biopsy, pretreatment PSA kinetics, and the size of the prostate.

The presence of perineural invasion (PNI) on biopsy has been found to have prognostic significance. A number of surgical series have reported that PNI seen on preoperative biopsy specimens has been associated with an increased likelihood of extraprostatic extension (EPE), worse final pathologic stage, higher grade, and/or the presence of seminal vesicle or lymph node involvement.[17–24] PNI was reported to have a significant adverse effect on biochemical disease-free survival for patients with a PSA of less than 20 ng/mL treated with EBRT, as well as on prostate cancer-specific mortality in patients with low- and intermediate-risk disease treated with radiation.[25,26] Given these data, some practitioners classify patients with PNI who would otherwise qualify as low-risk into the intermediate-risk category, thus altering their recommended treatment options.

The percent of positive biopsy cores has also been found to be predictive of outcome for patients with low- to intermediate-risk disease. D'Amico and associates[27] reported that patients with greater than half of sampled cores involved with disease had a significantly worse disease-specific mortality rate at 4.5 years. However, this factor influences management decisions only in patients with low-risk disease who might otherwise qualify for expectant management. The watchful-waiting paradigm set forth by Carter[28] at Johns Hopkins limits the number of positive cores to 2 or less for eligibility.

PSA kinetics has also been found to have prognostic significance. D'Amico and associates[29] have reported that men with localized prostate cancer and a preoperative PSA increase of greater than 2.0 ng/mL per year experience a

10-fold increase in prostate cancer-specific mortality despite radical prostatectomy. This was followed by an investigation for the same trend in patients treated with EBRT. Similarly, a greater than 2.0 ng/mL increase in PSA level during the year before diagnosis was found to be associated with a significantly higher cancer-specific mortality, even in patients with otherwise low-risk disease. They concluded that it would be reasonable to treat men with low-risk disease and a PSA rise of 2.0 ng/mL or more in the year before diagnosis with androgen suppression along with RT.[30] Studies of PSA doubling time (PSADT) have found that patients who undergo observation are more likely to require treatment if their PSADT is less than 4 years and are more likely to experience PSA relapse if their pre-treatment PSADT was less than 2 years.[31,32]

Treatment by Risk Group

Low Risk

Patients in the low-risk category have the most options available to them for treatment, including expectant management, surgery, EBRT, and brachytherapy. Expectant management and surgical options are discussed in Chapters 7 through 10 of this book. This section focuses on the results of EBRT and brachytherapy in low-risk patients.

The efficacy of EBRT compared with radical prostatectomy for low-risk patients has not been directly compared in a randomized controlled trial. Retrospective comparisons are complicated by the fact that EBRT patients tend to be older and less healthy and have more advanced disease. Moreover, radiation techniques and doses used in these patients have changed dramatically over the past 20 years, making the efficacy of radiation treatment a moving target. The same can be said for surgery, though probably to a lesser extent. Nonetheless, retrospective attempts at comparing EBRT and surgery have been made, and the results suggest that at contemporary doses of radiation (more than 72 Gy), EBRT and surgery have similar outcomes. For example, RTOG 77-06 reported on patients with organ-confined disease treated with conventional RT. The 5- and 10-year survival rates were 87% and 63%, respectively, comparable to age-matched controls without prostate cancer.[33] Disease-specific survival was 86%, similar to reports from surgical series.[34,35] Kupelian and colleagues[36] showed equivalent 8-year biochemical disease-free survival among patients treated with either surgery or doses of 72 Gy (86%) but showed inferior results when the radiation doses were less than 72 Gy (48%). At our institution, for patients not on a clinical trial, EBRT is delivered to the prostate and seminal vesicles plus a margin for the first 46 Gy, followed by a cone-down to the prostate plus a margin, to a total dose of 78 Gy. The entire prescription is delivered over 39 treatments.

Brachytherapy alone can be offered to men with a prostate measuring less than 50 mL, either at presentation or after a course of androgen ablation in an attempt to downsize the gland. The use of brachytherapy alone has also not been directly compared to either surgery or EBRT in a randomized trial. However, 10-year biochemical disease-free survival rates of 87% to 94% have been reported in patients with low-risk disease.[37,38] Blasko and associates[39] reported a 5-year biochemical disease-free survival rate of 94% in low-risk patients treated with Pd-103. Zelefsky and associates[40] reported similar 5-year biochemical disease-free survival rates in patients with low-risk disease treated with either 70.2 Gy of 3D-CRT or 150 Gy of brachytherapy with I-125 (86%, 82%). D'Amico looked at outcomes of prostatectomy, brachytherapy and EBRT and found equivalent biochemical disease-free survival rates among all three modalities at 5 years in low-risk patients.[16] Review of data from 13 case series and three cohort studies confirmed that brachytherapy is comparable to EBRT and prostatectomy for patients with low-risk disease.[41]

Intermediate Risk

Patients who fall into the intermediate risk category do not fare as well with surgery because of the higher risk of disease spread beyond the prostate. Gleason score of 7 or greater has been found to correlate with higher risk of disease recurrence after radical prostatectomy, as has PSA over 10.[42,43] Therefore, options that include radiation therapy become increasingly attractive. These include EBRT with hormone ablation or a combination of brachytherapy and EBRT. Despite a large body of research, it is difficult to draw definitive conclusions from the literature as to the best treatment strategy for this heterogeneous group of patients.

A number of trials have examined the role of androgen ablation therapy in conjunction with radiation therapy in patients with high-risk features. Initially, androgen blockade was used for cytoreduction in patients with clinical T3 disease. Later, it was noted in RTOG 75-06 that patients with unfavorable histology who received androgen suppression along with EBRT fared as well as those with favorable histology treated with EBRT alone.[44] It is now believed that androgen blockade results in apoptosis of hormone-responsive prostate cancer cells and may have a synergistic killing effect when combined with radiation.

RTOG 86-10 was a phase III randomized study that evaluated the role of neoadjuvant and concomitant androgen ablation using goserelin, a luteinizing hormone-releasing hormone (LHRH) agonist, and flutamide, an antiandrogen, in patients with bulky T2-4 disease. The results showed a biochemical disease-free survival benefit for patients treated with hormone therapy. However, an overall survival benefit was seen only in patients with Gleason scores of 6 or less.[45] D'Amico and colleagues[46] evaluated 6 months of adjuvant androgen ablation following definitive radiation in patients with localized disease, many of whom had intermediate-risk disease. An overall survival benefit was seen in this trial as well. These data, taken together, have led to our current paradigm, which is to incorporate 2 months of neoadjuvant and 2 months of concurrent androgen ablation with EBRT for patients with intermediate-risk disease. EBRT for intermediate-risk men is similar in dose and technique to that given to men with low-risk disease with a total dose of 78 Gy delivered over 39 treatments.

Patients with intermediate-risk disease have a higher likelihood of extraprostatic extension. Brachytherapy as monotherapy does not deliver what are felt to be adequate doses to periprostatic tissues. Therefore, if brachytherapy is used, the American Brachytherapy Society (ABS) recommends that supplemental EBRT be delivered in patients with intermediate- and high-risk disease. EBRT is directed to the prostate and periprostatic area for a dose of 40 to 50 Gy. The I-125 brachytherapy dose when combined with EBRT ranges from 100 to 110 Gy, and that of Pd-103 ranges from 80 to 90 Gy.[14] However,

significant controversy exists as to the value of adding EBRT to brachytherapy for this group of patients, and the most appropriate sequence of treatments is not well established.[47] At Johns Hopkins, we prefer to treat patients with EBRT to a dose of 40 to 45 Gy approximately 1 month after implantation. Recently, the Seattle Prostate Institute reported their long-term results on patients treated with combined brachytherapy and EBRT. Patients with intermediate-risk disease fared nearly as well as those with low-risk disease, with an 80% rate of biochemical disease-free survival at 15 years.[48] Others have reported similar long-term rates at 10 years with this approach.[49-51]

High Risk

The treatment of patients with high-risk disease requires a multimodality approach. Radical prostatectomy alone yields inferior results, as does brachytherapy or EBRT alone. Much data support the use of combined androgen blockade with definitive EBRT, some of which have already been discussed in the context of intermediate-risk disease. A pivotal study performed by the EORTC randomized patients with locally advanced or high-grade cancers to radiation alone or radiation with concurrent goserelin followed by 3 years of adjuvant goserelin. In addition to biochemical and clinical disease-free survival advantage, an overall survival advantage was shown in the men who received combined therapy.[52] Two other important studies that included men with high-risk disease were RTOG 85-31 and RTOG 92-02. RTOG 85-31 enrolled men with high-risk features and found a survival benefit from treatment with adjuvant hormone therapy. However, this trial treated men with hormone therapy indefinitely, leaving the optimum duration of treatment uncertain.[53] RTOG 92-02 examined the role of neoadjuvant and concomitant androgen ablation with or without an additional 2 years of treatment for locally advanced disease. An overall survival advantage was seen among patients with Gleason 8-10 disease.[54] This trial established the use of protracted androgen ablation in patients with high-risk disease.

Radiation therapy for patients with high-risk disease differs from that administered to patients with intermediate- and low-risk features. Given the higher risk of lymph node involvement, the initial 45 Gy are delivered to a whole pelvic field, which encompasses the internal and external iliac lymph nodes. Alternatively, if the patient is treated with IMRT, these lymph nodes are specifically targeted with an appropriate margin while minimizing dose to the rectum and bladder. Support for the use of a whole pelvic field in patients with high-risk disease is seen in RTOG 94-13. This trial used a 2 × 2 factorial design, comparing the use of neoadjuvant and concomitant androgen ablation with adjuvant androgen ablation and also comparing irradiation to a whole pelvic field with a prostate-only field. Most of the patients enrolled had high-risk disease, and all had a calculated risk of lymph node involvement of at least 15%. Progression-free survival was superior with the use of whole pelvic fields when combined with neoadjuvant and concomitant androgen ablation.[55]

At our institution, we treat men with high-risk disease with IMRT. For patients not on clinical trial we treat an initial volume, which includes the pelvic nodes to 46 Gy. The remainder of the dose is delivered to a cone-down volume to a total of 78 Gy. If the seminal vesicles are known to be involved, the cone-down volume includes this structure. Otherwise, the cone-down volume encompasses the prostate only, with an appropriate margin. As with the EBRT treatments for low- and intermediate-risk men, total dose is given over 39 treatments.

Other treatment approaches for intermediate- and high-risk disease have been reported in the literature. These include combining androgen ablation with prostatectomy or with brachytherapy, with or without EBRT. However, EBRT combined with neoadjuvant, concomitant and adjuvant androgen ablation remains the most widely used approach in this group of patients.

Adjuvant and Salvage Radiation after Radical Prostatectomy

After radical prostatectomy, we recommend radiation to the prostate bed if the patient is found to have adverse pathologic features at the time of surgery or if the patient develops a subsequent PSA recurrence in the course of follow-up. When a patient is treated because of adverse pathologic features, this is termed adjuvant radiation. The specific pathologic features that are an indication for adjuvant radiation are controversial. This controversy is discussed in the following section. When a patient is treated because of a persistent or recurrent PSA, this is termed salvage radiation. At Johns Hopkins, we consider a PSA persistent or recurrent if it remains or becomes greater than 0.1 ng/mL after prostatectomy. Other clinicians and researchers have used higher thresholds, 0.2 to 0.4 ng/mL, to define PSA recurrence.[56,57]

Until recently, radiation oncologists used a conventional four-field technique for adjuvant or salvage radiation. This technique necessarily encompasses part of a patient's rectum and bladder. In the last several years, we have begun using IMRT in the setting of postprostatectomy radiation to more closely conform to the prostate bed and thus better spare rectal and bladder tissue. Figure 8-5 shows a typical dose-distribution for a postprostatectomy IMRT plan.

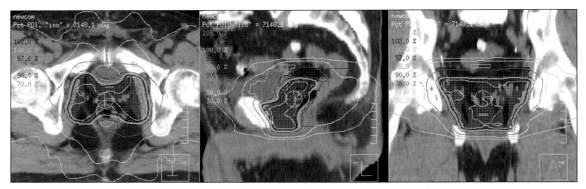

Figure 8-5. Dose distribution of an IMRT (intensity-modulated radiation therapy) plan for postprostatectomy radiation. Dose levels are represented by different colored lines (isodose lines), with the higher dose lines closer to the target. The area within the red line is the area receiving 100% of the prescribed dose. The postprostatectomy bed is contoured in blue in this plan.

3D Plan   IMRT Plan

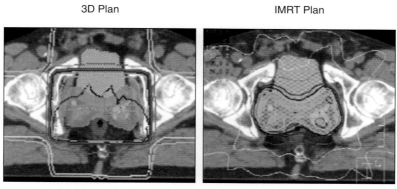

Figure 8-6. Comparison of 3D-CRT and IMRT for postprostatectomy radiation to the prostate bed.   Dose levels are represented by different colored lines (isodose lines), with the higher dose lines closer to the target. The area within the red line is the area receiving 100% of the prescribed dose. The postprostatectomy bed is contoured in green in this plan. Note how less of the bladder (in yellow) and the rectum (in purple) are encompassed within the red line in the IMRT plan. 3D-CRT, three-dimensional conformal radiation therapy; IMRT, intensity-modulated radiation therapy.

Postprostatectomy patients treated with adjuvant or salvage radiation are simulated and treated similarly to patients undergoing definitive radiation. These patients are generally prescribed total doses of 66.6 to 70.2 Gy in 37 to 39 treatments, depending on the features of their pathology. Dose is prescribed to the periphery of the prostatectomy bed, thereby delivering a slightly higher dose to central portions of this volume. Figure 8-6 shows the difference in dose distribution for a postprostatectomy patient planned by conventional technique compared with IMRT.

Adjuvant Radiation

The indications for adjuvant radiation to the prostate bed constitute an area of major controversy in the field of radiation oncology. Although there is broad agreement about how to manage patients with completely resected T1/T2 disease (no adjuvant treatment recommended) and gross residual tumor (adjuvant treatment recommended), there is disagreement with respect to the significant proportion of patients who are found to have positive surgical margins, extracapsular involvement, or seminal vesicle invasion. This issue has been explored in large retrospective studies, with differing conclusions.[58–61]

To date, there have been three randomized trials evaluating the role of adjuvant radiation in postprostatectomy patients with poor pathologic features. In 2005, the EORTC published a randomized trial comparing adjuvant radiation

to observation for postprostatectomy patients with pathologic T3 (pT3) tumors or pT2/T3 tumors and positive surgical margins.[62] This trial showed a superior biochemical failure-free survival and locoregional failure-free survival for the group treated with adjuvant radiation therapy (Table 8-1). No difference in distant failure rates or overall survival between the two groups has been seen, although the study has a median follow-up of only 5 years.

Another study from Southwest Oncology Group (SWOG), which included the same patient cohort and had the same trial design, found similar results.[63,64] This study showed significantly improved biochemical and local control rates with adjuvant radiation. In addition, men who were treated with adjuvant radiation had superior distant metastases-free survival (43.1% vs. 35.5%, $P = .06$) and overall survival (74% vs. 66%, $P = .16$), although these differences were not statistically significant even at a median follow-up of 10 years. Moreover, this study showed a superior 5-year freedom from initiation of hormone therapy for the adjuvant group (90% versus 79%, $P < .001$). Avoidance of total androgen suppression is important because it confers significant morbidity including hot flashes, diminished bone density, sexual dysfunction, cognitive dysfunction, and overall reduced quality of life.[65,66]

The third randomized trial comparing adjuvant radiation and observation conducted by the German Cancer Study Group included only postprostatectomy patients with pT3 disease,

Table 8-1. Randomized Adjuvant Radiation Trials

Trial	Patients	Biochemical Progress-Free Survival (Adj vs Obs)	Clinical Failure-Free Survival (Adj vs Obs)	Overall Survival (Adj vs Obs)
EORTC 22911	pT3 or positive margins	5 years (74.0% vs 52.6%) (SS)	5 years (91.2% vs 81%) (SS)	5 years (92.3% vs 93.1%) (NS)
SWOG 8794	pT3 or positive margins	10 years (52% vs 26%) (SS)	10 years (68% vs 49%) (SS)	10 years (74% vs 68%) (NS)
Germany Cancer Study Group	pT3	5 years (81% vs 60%) (SS)	NA	NA

Adj, adjuvant; NA, not available; NS, not statistically significant; Obs, observation; SS, statistically significant.

regardless of margin status. As with the EORTC and the SWOG studies, patients in this study who were treated with adjuvant radiation have already shown a superior biochemical failure-free survival with median follow-up of only 3.3 years.[67]

These studies make it clear that biochemical failure-free survival and locoregional failure-free survival are improved in selected patients who receive adjuvant radiotherapy after prostatectomy. However, it remains unclear whether overall survival is improved with immediate radiation treatment. Some of the patients in the observation arms of these studies who had biochemical failure ultimately underwent salvage radiation, which is known to be an effective strategy for controlling local recurrences. Therefore, salvage radiation may eliminate any overall survival difference or, perhaps, make the difference small and thus difficult to detect without a very large study. Moreover, the ability to detect an overall survival benefit in a relatively slowly progressive disease like prostate cancer likely requires very long median follow-up times.

As previously noted, the role of adjuvant radiation is a major controversy in urologic oncology. In fact, we do not have complete agreement on its role even within our own institution. At the very least, however, a patient who has positive margins or pT3 disease after prostatectomy should have a frank discussion with a radiation oncologist about the pros and cons of adjuvant radiation in his particular situation.

Salvage Radiation

Even men who had favorable pathologic findings at the time of prostatectomy may eventually require radiation to the prostate bed owing to a recurrence of their PSA. The rate of PSA recurrence after radical prostatectomy has been estimated to range from 20% to 53% in modern surgical series.[68–71] These values vary as a result of differences in definitions of recurrences as well as differences in inclusion criteria. Study results that use higher PSA thresholds to define recurrence or that consider men with only low-risk disease are likely to show relatively low rates of PSA recurrence. Furthermore, modern surgical series appear to have superior pathologic and biochemical failure results when compared with older series.[72]

A large proportion of men who experience PSA recurrence eventually develop clinically evident metastatic disease if left untreated.[73] Invariably, some of these men already have subclinical metastatic disease at the time biochemical recurrence is determined. It is important to determine which subset of patients would benefit from additional local therapy in the form of salvage radiation. Given the data that are currently available, it appears that even in subgroups of men with a high likelihood of already having metastatic disease, a significant proportion can be salvaged with additional local therapy.

Stephenson and associates[74] explored clinical and pathologic features that predicted a favorable response to salvage radiation. In this study of 501 men, the following pathologic and clinical features were associated with inferior response to salvage radiation: Gleason score of 8–10, preradiation PSA level higher than 2 ng/mL, PSA doubling time after prostatectomy of 10 months or less, negative surgical margins, and seminal vesicle invasion. However, a significant percentage of patients with one or more of these negative prognostic features had a durable response to salvage radiation, particularly if the radiation was given prior to a PSA level of 2 ng/mL. Even in a group of patients with the worst combination of prognostic features, a Gleason score of 8–10 and a preradiation PSA of 2 ng/mL, a progression-free survival rate of 12% at 4 years was achieved after salvage treatment.

Although the Stephenson data are some of the most persuasive data available to guide salvage radiation recommendations, it is important to emphasize that the study was retrospective and may suffer from selection bias. Prospective studies are needed to definitively determine whether patients with one or more poor prognostic features derive benefit from salvage radiation. However, given the available data and considering the limited morbidity of this treatment, especially with IMRT, it is reasonable to consider salvage radiation for postprostatectomy patients with PSA recurrence regardless of prognostic factors.

Treatment Toxicities

Toxicity due to radiation treatment is typically divided into two categories: acute toxicity, which refers to signs and symptoms that resolve within 3 months after the end of treatment, and late toxicity, which refers to signs and symptoms whose onset or duration is at least 3 months after the end of treatment. Acute and late toxicity reflects biologically different processes. Acute toxicity is usually the result of the relatively early injury to radiation-sensitive cells, such as cells of the mucosa, and of secondary acute inflammation and edema. In contrast, late toxicity is the result of injury to slowly dividing cells, such as neurons, as well secondary chronic inflammation and fibrosis.

In the setting of prostate cancer treatment, the most important side effects are acute and late genitourinary (GU), gastrointestinal (GI), and sexual side effects. The frequency of occurrence of these toxicities by treatment modality is summarized in the following paragraphs. Direct comparison of the toxicity profiles of the various radiation modalities is difficult, given that these treatments are not directly compared in prospective studies. Moreover, reports that describe toxicity often use different toxicity scoring criteria, further complicating comparisons. The two most commonly used toxicity criteria are the RTOG criteria and the National

Cancer Institute Common Toxicity Criteria for Adverse Events (CTCAE).[75,76] These criteria are extensive and are not reproduced here. For purposes of the discussion that follows, the following general definitions apply for both toxicity grading systems: grade 1 refers to a mild adverse event, grade 2 refers to a moderate adverse event, grade 3 refers to a severe adverse event, grade 4 refers to a life-threatening or disabling adverse event, and grade 5 refers to death as a result of an adverse event.

Toxicity of Radiation Therapy Alone

The use of IMRT has allowed radiation oncologists to treat localized prostate cancer to higher total doses without an increase in acute or late toxicity.[77] A recent review of our own institution's IMRT experience found that severe acute GI and GU toxicities are rare.[78] Of the first 100 men treated with IMRT at Johns Hopkins, none experienced diarrhea requiring parenteral support or rectal bleeding requiring the use of a pad (acute grade 3 or higher GI toxicity). Only 3% of men experienced hematuria or urinary frequency of at least every hour (acute grade 3 GU toxicity) with no cases of grade 4–5 acute GU toxicity.

Late toxicity results for patients treated by IMRT alone have recently been published by Zelefsky and associates.[79] Less than 1% of men experienced rectal bleeding requiring active intervention such as laser cauterization procedure or blood transfusion (late grade 3 GI toxicity). Only 3% of men developed urethral stricture requiring dilation (late grade 3 urethral toxicity). Forty-nine percent of men who reported useful erections before treatment experienced erectile dysfunction after treatment.[79]

Toxicity of Brachytherapy Alone

In addition to the acute effects of radiation, acute toxicity secondary to brachytherapy is also due to postimplant bleeding and edema of the prostate. Thus, the acute GU toxicity of brachytherapy alone may be worse than EBRT alone. Brachytherapy may also be associated with higher rates of late urethral stricture. However, brachytherapy appears to be superior with respect to late GI effects and erectile dysfunction. RTOG 9805 prospectively evaluated the toxicity of I-125 brachytherapy alone.[80] This study found that 3% of men experienced acute bleeding requiring a transfusion and 4% experienced acute GU symptoms requiring invasive intervention. With respect to late toxicity, only 2% of men reported late grade 3 bladder toxicity, which is typically manifested as frequent hematuria, with no reports of worse bladder toxicity. There were no cases of rectal bleeding requiring cauterization (late grade 3) or worse bowel toxicity. The rate of urethral stricture was not specifically reported in RTOG 9805; however, a single-institution series from Zelefsky and associates[40] reported a 5-year urethral stricture risk of 10% after I-125 brachytherapy. The rate of moderate to severe impotence after brachytherapy was reported as 10% in RTOG 9805. This is significantly lower than the rate of impotence seen in the series from Zelefsky and associates,[40] which was 29% at 5 years, and it was also lower than many other single-institutional reports. Although it is clear that brachytherapy with I-125 was well tolerated, brachytherapy with Pd-103 may have a superior acute toxicity profile given the shorter half-life of Pd-103.[81]

Evidence suggests that long-term toxicities related to brachytherapy may wane to pretreatment levels several years from the end of treatment. In a prospective evaluation of quality of life after brachytherapy alone, Caffo and colleagues[82] found that urinary function significantly worsened after brachytherapy but returned to pretreatment levels after 3 years. Rectal and sexual functions returned to pretreatment levels sooner and were not significantly different 1 year after treatment.

Toxicity of Combined Brachytherapy and External-Beam Radiation Therapy

In the acute setting, adding supplemental EBRT to brachytherapy does not appear to increase GU or GI toxicity. The acute toxicity of combined brachytherapy and external-beam radiation is mainly a function of the brachytherapy component of the treatment.[83] The late effects of combined treatment appear to be similar to that with IMRT alone, although these treatments have not been prospectively compared.

RTOG P-0019 evaluated the acute and late effects of combined brachytherapy and conventional EBRT in a prospective multi-institutional setting.[84] In this study, patients were initially treated with EBRT to 45 Gy followed by I-125

brachytherapy boost. There were no acute grade 3 or higher rectal toxicities, and 8% of men experienced acute grade 3 GU toxicity. With respect to late toxicity, 2% had severe urinary frequency (grade 3), and less than 1% of men experienced grade 3 GI toxicity or urinary incontinence requiring intervention. Of men who reported no erectile dysfunction at baseline, 45% experienced grade 2 or greater erectile dysfunction 18 months after the initiation of radiation therapy.

Toxicity of Whole Pelvic Radiation

The purpose of whole pelvic radiation is to treat lymph node chains that drain the prostate, primarily the internal and external lymph node chains. To treat these lymph nodes, a greater proportion of a patient's rectum and bladder necessarily receive significant doses of radiation, particularly if conventional radiation techniques are used. As a consequence, whole pelvic radiation has higher rates of acute and late toxicity compared with more limited treatment of the prostate and seminal vesicles.

Patients receiving whole pelvic radiation in RTOG 9413 experienced a 3.9% rate of acute grade 3 or higher GU toxicity (usually hematuria) and a 2.6% rate of acute grade 3 GI toxicity.[85] Late grade 3 GU toxicity was seen in 3.0% of men, and late grade 3 GI toxicity was seen in 4.3% of men. It is important to note that these patients were treated with conventional fields, not IMRT. At our institution, we now perform whole pelvic radiation using IMRT to cover at-risk lymph nodes and to spare the rectum and bladder. This technique may result in a better toxicity profile than that reported in RTOG 9413.

Toxicity of Androgen Suppression

Patients with intermediate- and high-risk prostate cancer are treated with neoadjuvant and concurrent androgen suppression. Patients with high-risk disease continue with androgen suppression for 2 years after completion of radiation treatments. Though an important aspect of definitive management of these patients, androgen suppression is associated with a host of acute and long-term side effects. The earliest side effects of androgen suppression are decreased libido and hot flashes, which are experienced by the majority of men.[86] Side effects that occur after prolonged administration of androgen deprivation include osteoporosis, muscle wasting, changes in fat distribution, anemia, mood disturbance, and cognitive dysfunction.[87-89] A more detailed discussion of the systemic effects of androgen suppression is beyond the scope of this book. The interested reader is directed to an excellent review of these toxicities by MK Brawer.[90]

Toxicity of Adjuvant or Salvage Radiation

The morbidity of adjuvant or salvage radiation can be difficult to discern, given that patients often experience similar side effects from surgery. Nonetheless, we can use data from SWOG 8794 to summarize patients' experiences after both prostatectomy and radiation. With respect to urinary symptoms, patients who received surgery and adjuvant radiation had an 18% rate of urinary stricture and a 7% rate of urinary incontinence. Proctitis was relatively rare at 3%, but erectile dysfunction was common, with 88% of men having some dysfunction 5 years after the end of adjuvant radiation. It is important to note that SWOG 8794 used doses of radiation of 60 to 64 Gy, which are lower than what are currently prescribed in the adjuvant or salvage setting (66 to 70 Gy).[63] This study did not use IMRT, which may decrease the rate of late effects, especially proctitis, by improving conformality of dose around the prostate fossa. The long-term toxicity outcomes of adjuvant and salvage IMRT have not yet been reported.

PSA Follow-up after Radiation Treatment for Localized Disease

The National Comprehensive Cancer Network (NCCN) consensus panel recommends that after definitive radiation treatment for localized prostate cancer, men should have an annual digital rectal exam as well as a PSA drawn every 6 months for 5 years, then annually thereafter.[91] At our institution, we recommend that patients proceed to annual PSA checks after 2 years of follow-up, since clinically important changes in PSA generally occur over long periods of time.

Unlike radical prostatectomy, we do not expect a man's PSA to immediately drop to undetectable levels after radiation to the prostate. In men treated without hormone therapy, the median time to the lowest post-treatment PSA, referred to as *PSA nadir*, is 32 months.[92] Most patients achieve a nadir of less than 1.0 ng/mL.[93]

After the PSA nadir is reached, some patients experience a small rise in PSA followed by a subsequent decline. This phenomenon is called *PSA bounce* and has been observed in anywhere from 17% to 61% of patients treated with various forms of radiation, with the highest rates seen in patients treated with brachytherapy alone and conventional EBRT with concomitant hormone therapy. Benign PSA bounces can occur many months from treatment with the median time to bounce 1.5 to 2.6 years after treatment, depending on the treatment modality.[94-96]

PSA kinetics after radiation treatment provide important prognostic information. Both a lower post-treatment nadir and a longer time to post-treatment nadir have been shown to be correlated with better metastasis-free survival.[97] In addition, shorter post-treatment PSA doubling time has been correlated with increased risk of death from prostate cancer.[98]

If a patient's PSA rises to a level that is greater than 2 ng/mL over the nadir, then he is considered to have experienced a "biochemical failure."[99] Biochemical failure is weakly predictive of subsequent clinical recurrence, and many men with biochemical failure die of other causes.[100] In a study evaluating the effect of biochemical recurrence after EBRT, Kwan and associates[101] found that biochemical recurrence was only associated with worsened overall survival among the subset of patients under age 75 with high-risk cancers. For these reasons, the optimal timing of androgen deprivation following PSA failure remains controversial.[102]

Other Treatment Modalities

High-Dose Rate Brachytherapy

Conformal high-dose rate brachytherapy (HDR) is an alternative means of allowing for dose escalation to the prostate while avoiding the additional toxicity that would be incurred by a biologically equivalent dose delivered via EBRT alone. With this approach, the brachytherapy is delivered in 1 to 3 fractions, separated by 4 to 6 hours, either before, following, or interdigitated with the course of EBRT. Catheters are placed into the prostate under intraoperative transrectal ultrasound guidance. The catheters are then attached to an afterloading unit, which sequentially feeds a high activity (iridium-192) source into predetermined positions within the catheters. The dwell times within each position can be adjusted, thus allowing for development of a treatment plan that optimally conforms to the target volume. The ability to optimize catheter and dwell positions before source deployment is an advantage compared with that of low-dose rate permanent brachytherapy, in which sources cannot be adjusted once placed.

The rationale behind HDR in the treatment of prostate cancer relates to the relative sensitivities of prostate cancer and normal tissues to larger doses of radiation. Recent analyses of clinical and laboratory data suggest that prostate cancer cells are more sensitive to larger doses per fraction than are normal tissues, thus theoretically enhancing the therapeutic ratio.[103,104]

Physicians have started treating prostate cancer using modern HDR brachytherapy only over the past decade, but the preliminary results with technique are encouraging. Deger and colleagues[105] analyzed 411 patients with locally advanced disease treated with HDR and 3D-CRT. Most patients received between 45 and 50.4 Gy via EBRT following two doses of 9 to 10 Gy apiece. The 5-year biochemical progression-free survival rate was 81% for low-risk patients, 65% for intermediate-risk, and 59% for high-risk patients.

Investigators at William Beaumont Hospital have described their experience in a dose escalation trial of HDR with EBRT in 207 patients with poor prognostic factors of PSA higher than 10 ng/mL, Gleason above 7, or clinical stage higher than T2b. At a mean follow-up of 4.7 years, the 5-year actuarial biochemical control rate was 74%. The 5-year biochemical control rate was 85% for one poor prognostic factor, 75% for two, and 50% for all three. Lower HDR dose and higher Gleason score were associated with biochemical failure.[106]

Protons and Neutrons

Particle beams such as those with protons and neutrons have physical advantages over photon or x-ray beams in that they interact more densely with the tissue in the beam path. This results in greater levels of ionization along the length of

the beam and therefore increased radiobiologic effect (RBE). This could theoretically translate into better tumor control.

Proton therapy is not widely available; however, its unique properties of dose distribution have provoked interest in its treatment of prostate cancer. Most of the energy in a proton beam is deposited at the end of its linear track, resulting in what is known as a Bragg peak. Beyond the Bragg peak, the dose falls rapidly to zero. This rapid dose fall-off allows for delivery of high doses of radiation to the target volume with minimal dose to normal surrounding tissues.

Loma Linda University and the Massachusetts General Hospital have been using proton therapy to treat prostate cancer patients for over a decade with good results with respect to cancer control and toxicity.[107,108] Other institutions are in the process of establishing proton therapy programs for prostate cancer.

Neutron-beam therapy for prostate cancer remains investigational in nature at this point. The Neutron Therapy Collaborative Working Group conducted a multi-institutional trial in which 178 men were randomly assigned to conventional radiation therapy with photons to a dose of 70 to 70.2 Gy or 20.4 nGy of neutron therapy. At 5 years, neutron therapy was associated with superior local control and biochemical control, but overall survival was not improved and severe late toxicities were increased.[109] An RTOG study evaluated the use of mixed photon and neutron therapy in 91 patients. The use of neutrons resulted in a superior local control rate and overall survival at 10 years compared with conventional EBRT.[110] More recent reports from Wayne State University cite excellent control rates in patients treated with neutrons alone or in combination with photons, mostly in patients with lower pretreatment PSAs. They also report that a mixture of neutrons and photons of approximately 50% seems to offer the best therapeutic ratio in terms of morbidity and efficacy. Again, increased long-term side effects with neutrons given in this setting were identified.[111]

Summary

Radiation is the most commonly used treatment modality for prostate cancer. Radiation can be delivered externally, most commonly using IMRT, or via brachytherapy at either a low-dose rate or high-dose rate. Radiation plays an important role in the initial management of both early-stage disease and in locally advanced disease, when given in combination with androgen ablation therapy. Furthermore, patients who experience PSA failure following prostatectomy can effectively be salvaged with EBRT, and adjuvant treatment with EBRT has proved effective in patients with high-risk pathologic features. With the tremendous innovations in treatment delivery over the last decade or so, prostate radiation techniques now provide excellent control rates with relatively low morbidity.

References

1. NCDB Hospital comparison Benchmark Reports v7.
2. Kupelian PA, Potters L, Khuntia D, et al: Radical prostatectomy, external beam radiotherapy or ≤ 72 Gy, permanent seed implantation, or combined seeds/external beam radiotherapy for stage T1-T2 prostate cancer. Int J Radiat Oncol Biol Phys 58:25–33, 2004.
3. Lee WR, Moughan J, Owen JB, et al: The 1999 patterns of care study of radiotherapy in localized prostate carcinoma: a comprehensive survey of prostate brachytherapy in the United States. Cancer 98:1987–1994, 2003.
4. Young HH, Frontz WA: Some new methods in the treatment of carcinoma of the lower genito-urinary tract with radium. J Urol 1:505–541, 1917.
5. Barringer BS: Phases of the pathology, diagnosis and treatment of cancer of the prostate. J Urol:407–411, 1928.
6. George FW, Carlton CE, Dykhuizen RF, et al: Cobalt-60 telecurietherapy in the definitive treatment of carcinoma of the prostate: a preliminary report. J Urol 93:102–109, 1965.
7. Kaplan HS, Bagshaw MA: The Stanford Medical Linear Accelerator. III. Application to clinical problems of radiation therapy. Stanford Med Bull 15:141–151, 1957.
8. Bagshaw MA, Kaplan HS, Sagerman RH: Linear accelerator supervoltage radiotherapy. VII. carcinoma of the prostate. Radiology 85:121–129, 1965.
9. Del Regato JA: Radiotherapy in the conservative treatment of operable and locally inoperable carcinoma of the prostate. Radiology 88:761–766, 1967.
10. Leibel SA, Fuks Z, Zelefsky MJ, et al: Technological advances in external-beam radiation therapy for the treatment of localized prostate cancer. Semin Oncol 30:596–615, 2003.
11. Lee WR, DeSilvio M, Lawton C, et al: A phase II study of external beam radiotherapy combined with permanent source brachytherapy for intermediate-risk, clinically localized adenocarcinoma of the prostate: preliminary results of RTOG P-0019. Int J Radiat Oncol Biol Phys 64:804–809, 2006.
12. Blasko JC, Ragde H, Grimm PD: Transperineal ultrasound-guided implantation of the prostate: morbidity and complications. Scand J Urol Nephrol Suppl 137:113–118, 1991.
13. Terk MD, Stock RG, Stone NN: Identification of patients at increased risk for prolonged urinary retention following radioactive seed implantation of the prostate. J Urol 160:1379–1382, 1998.
14. Nag S, Beyer D, Friedland J, et al: American Brachytherapy Society (ABS) recommendations for transperineal permanent brachytherapy of prostate cancer. Int J Radiat Oncol Biol Phys 44:789–799, 1999.
15. D'Amico AV, Whittington R, Kaplan I, et al: Equivalent biochemical failure-free survival after external beam radiation therapy or radical prostatectomy in patients with a pretreatment prostate specific antigen of >4–20 ng/mL. Int J Radiat Oncol Biol Phys 37:1053–1058, 1997.
16. D'Amico AV, Whittington R, Malkowicz SB, et al: Biochemical outcome after radical prostatectomy, external beam radiation therapy, or interstitial radiation therapy for clinically localized prostate cancer. JAMA 280:969–974, 1998.
17. Bastacky SI, Walsh PC, Epstein JI: Relationship between perineural tumor invasion on needle biopsy and radical prostatectomy capsular penetration in clinical stage B adenocarcinoma of the prostate. Am J Surg Pathol 17:336–341, 1993.
18. Bostwick DG, Qian J, Bergstralh E, et al: Prediction of capsular perforation and seminal vesicle invasion in prostate cancer. J Urol 155:1361–1367, 1996.
19. Cheng L, Slezak J, Bergstralh EJ, et al: Preoperative prediction of surgical margin status in patients with prostate cancer treated by radical prostatectomy. J Clin Oncol 18:2862–2868, 2000.
20. de la Taille A, Katz A, Bagiella E, et al: Perineural invasion on prostate needle biopsy: an independent predictor of final pathologic stage. Urology 54:1039–1043, 1999.
21. de la Taille A, Rubin MA, Bagiella E, et al: Can perineural invasion on prostate needle biopsy predict prostate specific antigen recurrence after radical prostatectomy? J Urol 162:103–106, 1999.
22. Rubin MA, Mucci NR, Manley S, et al: Predictors of Gleason pattern 4/5 prostate cancer on prostatectomy specimens: can high grade tumor be predicted preoperatively? J Urol 165:114–118, 2001.
23. Stone NN, Stock RG, Parikh D, et al: Perineural invasion and seminal vesicle involvement predict pelvic lymph node metastasis in men with localized carcinoma of the prostate. J Urol 160:1722–1726, 1998.
24. Villers A, McNeal JE, Redwine EA, et al: The role of perineural space invasion in the local spread of prostatic adenocarcinoma. J Urol 142:763–768, 1989.
25. Bonin SR, Hanlon AL, Lee WR, et al: Evidence of increased failure in the treatment of prostate carcinoma patients who have perineural invasion treated with three-dimensional conformal radiation therapy. Cancer 79:75–80, 1997.
26. Beard C, Schultz D, Loffredo M, et al: Perineural invasion associated with increased cancer-specific mortality after external beam radiation therapy for men with low- and intermediate-risk prostate cancer. Int J Radiat Oncol Biol Phys 66:403–407, 2006.
27. D'Amico AV, Renshaw AA, Cote K, et al: Impact of the percentage of positive prostate cores on prostate cancer-specific mortality for patients with low or favorable intermediate-risk disease. J Clin Oncol 22:3726–3732, 2004.
28. Carter HB, Walsh PC, Landis P, et al: Expectant management of nonpalpable prostate cancer with curative intent: preliminary results. J Urol 167:1231–1234, 2002.
29. D'Amico AV, Chen MH, Roehl KA, et al: Preoperative PSA velocity and the risk of death from prostate cancer after radical prostatectomy. N Engl J Med 351:125–135, 2004.
30. D'Amico AV, Renshaw AA, Sussman B, et al: Pretreatment PSA velocity and risk of death from prostate cancer following external beam radiation therapy. JAMA 294:440–447, 2005.
31. Ali K, Gunnar A, Jan-Erik D, et al: PSA doubling time predicts the outcome after active surveillance in screening-detected prostate cancer: results from the European Randomized Study of Screening for Prostate Cancer, Sweden section. Int J Cancer 120:170–174, 2007.
32. Klotz L: Active surveillance for prostate cancer: for whom? J Clin Oncol 23:8165–8169, 2005.
33. Fowler JE, Jr, Braswell NT, Pandey P, et al: Experience with radical prostatectomy and radiation therapy for localized prostate cancer at a Veterans Affairs Medical Center. J Urol 153(3 Pt 2):1026–1031, 1995.
34. Gibbons RP, Correa RJ, Jr, Brannen GE, et al: Total prostatectomy for localized prostatic cancer. J Urol 131:73–76, 1984.
35. Hanks GE, Asbell S, Krall JM, et al: Outcome for lymph node dissection negative T-1b, T-2 (A-2,B) prostate cancer treated with external beam radiation therapy in RTOG 77-06. Int J Radiat Oncol Biol Phys 21:1099–1103, 1991.
36. Kupelian PA, Elshaikh M, Reddy CA, et al: Comparison of the efficacy of local therapies for localized prostate cancer in the prostate-specific antigen era: a large single-institution experience with radical prostatectomy and external-beam radiotherapy. J Clin Oncol 20:3376–3385, 2002.
37. Grimm PD, Blasko JC, Sylvester JE, et al: 10-year biochemical (prostate-specific antigen) control of prostate cancer with ^{125}I brachytherapy. Int J Radiat Oncol Biol Phys 51:31–40, 2001.
38. Blasko JC, Grimm PD, Sylvester JE, et al: The role of external beam radiotherapy with I-125/Pd-103 brachytherapy for prostate carcinoma. Radiother Oncol 57:273–278, 2000.

39. Blasko JC, Grimm PD, Sylvester JE, et al: Palladium-103 brachytherapy for prostate carcinoma. Int J Radiat Oncol Biol Phys 46:839–850, 2000.
40. Zelefsky MJ, Wallner KE, Ling CC, et al: Comparison of the 5-year outcome and morbidity of three-dimensional conformal radiotherapy versus transperineal permanent iodine-125 implantation for early-stage prostatic cancer. J Clin Oncol 17:517–522, 1999.
41. Crook J, Lukka H, Klotz L, et al: Systematic overview of the evidence for brachytherapy in clinically localized prostate cancer. CMAJ 164:975–981, 2001.
42. Ward JF, Slezak JM, Blute ML, et al: Radical prostatectomy for clinically advanced (cT3) prostate cancer since the advent of prostate-specific antigen testing: 15-year outcome. BJU Int 95:751–756, 2005.
43. Van Poppel H, Goethuys H, Callewaert P, et al: Radical prostatectomy can provide a cure for well-selected clinical stage T3 prostate cancer. Eur Urol 38:372–379, 2000.
44. Pilepich MV, Krall JM, Sause WT, et al: Prognostic factors in carcinoma of the prostate—analysis of RTOG study 75-06. Int J Radiat Oncol Biol Phys 13:339–349, 1987.
45. Pilepich MV, Winter K, John MJ, et al: Phase III Radiation Therapy Oncology Group (RTOG) Trial 86–10 of androgen deprivation adjuvant to definitive radiotherapy in locally advanced carcinoma of the prostate. Int J Radiat Oncol Biol Phys 50:1243–1252, 2001.
46. D'Amico AV, Manola J, Loffredo M, et al: 6-month androgen suppression plus radiation therapy vs radiation therapy alone for patients with clinically localized prostate cancer: a randomized controlled trial. JAMA 292:821–827, 2004.
47. Potters L, Fearn P, Kattan M: The role of external radiotherapy in patients treated with permanent prostate brachytherapy. Prostate Cancer Prostatic Dis 5:47–53, 2002.
48. Sylvester JE, Grimm PD, Blasko JC, et al: 15-year biochemical relapse free survival in clinical stage T1-T3 prostate cancer following combined external beam radiotherapy and brachytherapy: Seattle experience. Int J Radiat Oncol Biol Phys 67:57–64, 2007.
49. Critz FA, Levinson K: 10-year disease-free survival rates after simultaneous irradiation for prostate cancer with a focus on calculation methodology. J Urol 172(6 Pt 1):2232–2238, 2004.
50. Stock RG, Cesaretti JA, Stone NN: Disease-specific survival following the brachytherapy management of prostate cancer. Int J Radiat Oncol Biol Phys 64:810–816, 2006.
51. Dattoli M, Wallner K, True L, et al: Long-term outcomes after treatment with external beam radiation therapy and palladium 103 for patients with higher risk prostate carcinoma: influence of prostatic acid phosphatase. Cancer 97:979–983, 2003.
52. Bolla M, Collette L, Blank L, et al: Long-term results with immediate androgen suppression and external irradiation in patients with locally advanced prostate cancer (an EORTC study): a phase III randomised trial. Lancet 360:103–106, 2002
53. Lawton CA, Winter K, Murray K, et al: Updated results of the phase III Radiation Therapy Oncology Group (RTOG) Trial 85–31 evaluating the potential benefit of androgen suppression following standard radiation therapy for unfavorable prognosis carcinoma of the prostate. Int J Radiat Oncol Biol Phys 49:937–946, 2001.
54. Hanks GE, Pajak TF, Porter A, et al: Phase III trial of long-term adjuvant androgen deprivation after neoadjuvant hormonal cytoreduction and radiotherapy in locally advanced carcinoma of the prostate: the Radiation Therapy Oncology Group Protocol 92-02. J Clin Oncol 21:3972–3978, 2003.
55. Roach M, III, DeSilvio M, Lawton C, et al: Phase III trial comparing whole-pelvic versus prostate-only radiotherapy and neoadjuvant versus adjuvant combined androgen suppression: Radiat Therapy Oncology Group 9413. J Clin Oncol 21:1904–1911, 2003.
56. Thompson IM, Jr, Tangen CM, Paradelo J, et al: Adjuvant radiotherapy for pathologically advanced prostate cancer: a randomized clinical trial. JAMA 296:2329–2335, 2006.
57. Han M, Partin AW, Piantadosi S, et al: Era specific biochemical recurrence-free survival following radical prostatectomy for clinically localized prostate cancer. J Urol 166:416–419, 2001.
58. Vargas C, Kestin LL, Weed DW, et al: Improved biochemical outcome with adjuvant radiotherapy after radical prostatec-
tomy for prostate cancer with poor pathologic features. Int J Radiat Oncol Biol Phys 61:714–724, 2005.
59. Cozzarini C, Bolognesi A, Ceresoli GL, et al: Role of postoperative radiotherapy after pelvic lymphadenectomy and radical retropubic prostatectomy: a single institute experience of 415 patients. Int J Radiat Oncol Biol Phys 59:674–683, 2004.
60. Hagan M, Zlotecki R, Medina C, et al: Comparison of adjuvant versus salvage radiotherapy policies for postprostatectomy radiotherapy. Int J Radiat Oncol Biol Phys 59:329–340, 2004.
61. Anscher MS, Robertson CN, Prosnitz R: Adjuvant radiotherapy for pathologic stage T3/4 adenocarcinoma of the prostate: ten-year update. Int J Radiat Oncol Biol Phys 33:37–43, 1995.
62. Bolla M, Collette L, Blank L, et al: Long-term results with immediate androgen suppression and external irradiation in patients with locally advanced prostate cancer (an EORTC study): a phase III randomised trial. Lancet 360:103–106, 2002.
63. Thompson IM, Jr, Tangen CM, Paradelo J, et al: Adjuvant radiotherapy for pathologically advanced prostate cancer: a randomized clinical trial. JAMA 296:2329–2335, 2006.
64. Swanson GP, Thompson IM, Tangen C, et al: Phase III randomized study of adjuvant radiation therapy versus observation in patients with pathologic T3 prostate cancer (SWOG 8794). International J Radiat Oncol Biol Phys 63(Suppl 1): (Abstract), 2005.
65. Williams MB, Hernandez J, Thompson I: Luteinizing hormone-releasing hormone agonist effects on skeletal muscle: how hormonal therapy in prostate cancer affects muscular strength. J Urol 173:1067–1071, 2005.
66. Higano CS: Management of bone loss in men with prostate cancer. J Urol 170(6 Pt 2):S59–63; discussion S64, 2003.
67. Wiegel T, Bottke D, Willich N, et al: Phase III results of adjuvant radiotherapy (RT) versus wait and see (WS) in patients with pT3 prostate cancer following radical prostatectomy (RP)(ARO 96-02 / AUO AP 09/95). J Clin Oncol 23(Suppl): 4513, 2005.
68. Zincke H, Oesterling JE, Blute ML, et al: Long-term (15 years) results after radical prostatectomy for clinically localized (stage T2c or lower) prostate cancer. J Urol 152(5 Pt 2):1850–1857, 1994.
69. Trapasso JG, deKernion JB, Smith RB, et al: The incidence and significance of detectable levels of serum prostate specific antigen after radical prostatectomy. J Urol 152(5 Pt 2):1821–1825, 1994.
70. Han M, Partin AW, Pound CR, et al: Long-term biochemical disease-free and cancer-specific survival following anatomic radical retropubic prostatectomy. The 15-year Johns Hopkins experience. Urol Clin North Am 28:555–565, 2001.
71. Catalona WJ, Smith DS: 5-year tumor recurrence rates after anatomical radical retropubic prostatectomy for prostate cancer. J Urol 152(5 Pt 2):1837–1842, 1994.
72. Han M, Partin AW, Piantadosi S, et al: Era specific biochemical recurrence-free survival following radical prostatectomy for clinically localized prostate cancer. J Urol 166:416–419, 2001.
73. Pound CR, Partin AW, Eisenberger MA, et al: Natural history of progression after PSA elevation following radical prostatectomy. JAMA 281:1591–1597, 1999.
74. Stephenson AJ, Shariat SF, Zelefsky MJ, et al: Salvage radiotherapy for recurrent prostate cancer after radical prostatectomy. JAMA 291:1325–1332, 2004.
75. Cox JD, Stetz J, Pajak TF: Toxicity criteria of the Radiation Therapy Oncology Group (RTOG) and the European Organization for Research and Treatment of Cancer (EORTC). Int J Radiat Oncol Biol Phys 31:1341–1346, 1995.
76. ctep.cancer.gov/reporting/ctc.html
77. Jani AB, Su A, Correa D, et al: Comparison of late gastrointestinal and genitourinary toxicity of prostate cancer patients undergoing intensity-modulated versus conventional radiotherapy using localized fields. Prostate Cancer Prostatic Dis 10:82–86, 2007.
78. Christodouleas JP, Song DY, DeWeese TL: Treating physician is the most important predictor of acute gastrointestinal and genitourinary toxicities in men with low and intermediate risk prostate cancer treated by IMRT (Abstract). RSNA Annual Meeting, 2006.
79. Zelefsky MJ, Chan H, Hunt M, et al: Long-term outcome of high dose intensity modulated radiation therapy for patients

with clinically localized prostate cancer. J Urol 176(4 Pt 1):1415–1419, 2006.

80. Lawton CA, Desilvio M, Lee WR, et al: Results of a phase II trial of transrectal ultrasound-guided permanent radioactive implantation of the prostate for definitive management of localized adenocarcinoma of the prostate (Radiation Therapy Oncology Group 98-05). Int J Radiat Oncol Biol Phys 67:39–47, 2007.

81. Wallner K, Merrick G, True L, et al: I-125 versus Pd-103 for low-risk prostate cancer: morbidity outcomes from a prospective randomized multicenter trial. Cancer J 8:67–73, 2002.

82. Caffo O, Fellin G, Bolner A, et al: Prospective evaluation of quality of life after interstitial brachytherapy for localized prostate cancer. Int J Radiat Oncol Biol Phys 66:31–37, 2006.

83. Ghaly M, Wallner K, Merrick G, et al: The effect of supplemental beam radiation on prostate brachytherapy-related morbidity: morbidity outcomes from two prospective randomized multicenter trials. Int J Radiat Oncol Biol Phys 55:1288–1293, 2003.

84. Lee WR, DeSilvio M, Lawton C, et al: A phase II study of external beam radiotherapy combined with permanent source brachytherapy for intermediate-risk, clinically localized adenocarcinoma of the prostate: preliminary results of RTOG P-0019. Int J Radiat Oncol Biol Phys 64:804–809, 2006.

85. Roach M, III, DeSilvio M, Valicenti R, et al: Whole-pelvis, "mini-pelvis," or prostate-only external beam radiotherapy after neoadjuvant and concurrent hormonal therapy in patients treated in the Radiation Therapy Oncology Group 9413 Trial. Int J Radiat Oncol Biol Phys 66:647–653, 2006.

86. Potosky AL, Reeve BB, Clegg LX, et al: Quality of life following localized prostate cancer treated initially with androgen deprivation therapy or no therapy. J Natl Cancer Inst 94:430–437, 2002.

87. Radlmaier A, Bormacher K, Neumann F: Hot flushes: mechanism and prevention. Prog Clin Biol Res 359:131–140; discussion 141–153, 1990.

88. Morley JE, Kaiser FE, Sih R, et al: Testosterone and frailty. Clin Geriatr Med 13:685–695, 1997.

89. Daniell HW: Osteoporosis after orchiectomy for prostate cancer. J Urol 157:439–444, 1997.

90. Brawer MK: Hormonal therapy for prostate cancer. Rev Urol 8(Suppl 2):S35–47, 2006.

91. www.nccn.org

92. Hanlon AL, Diratzouian H, Hanks GE: Posttreatment prostate-specific antigen nadir highly predictive of distant failure and death from prostate cancer. Int J Radiat Oncol Biol Phys 53:297–303, 2002.

93. Shipley WU, Thames HD, Sandler HM, et al: Radiation therapy for clinically localized prostate cancer: a multi-institutional pooled analysis. JAMA 281:1598–1604, 1999.

94. Zietman AL, Christodouleas JP, Shipley WU: PSA bounces after neoadjuvant androgen deprivation and external beam radiation: impact on definitions of failure. Int J Radiat Oncol Biol Phys 62:714–718, 2005.

95. Das P, Chen MH, Valentine K, et al: Using the magnitude of PSA bounce after MRI-guided prostate brachytherapy to distinguish recurrence, benign precipitating factors, and idiopathic bounce. Int J Radiat Oncol Biol Phys 54:698–702, 2002.

96. Rosser CJ, Kuban DA, Levy LB, et al: Prostate specific antigen bounce phenomenon after external beam radiation for clinically localized prostate cancer. J Urol 168:2001–2005, 2002.

97. Ray ME, Thames HD, Levy LB, et al: PSA nadir predicts biochemical and distant failures after external beam radiotherapy for prostate cancer: a multi-institutional analysis. Int J Radiat Oncol Biol Phys 64:1140–1150, 2006.

98. Valicenti RK, Desilvio M, Hanks GE, et al: Posttreatment prostatic-specific antigen doubling time as a surrogate endpoint for prostate cancer-specific survival: an analysis of Radiation Therapy Oncology Group Protocol 92-02. Int J Radiat Oncol Biol Phys 66:1064–1071, 2006.

99. Roach M, III, Hanks G, Thames H, Jr, et al: Defining biochemical failure following radiotherapy with or without hormonal therapy in men with clinically localized prostate cancer: recommendations of the RTOG-ASTRO Phoenix Consensus Conference. Int J Radiat Oncol Biol Phys 65:965–974, 2006.

100. Fitch DL, McGrath S, Martinez AA, et al: Unification of a common biochemical failure definition for prostate cancer treated with brachytherapy or external beam radiotherapy with or without androgen deprivation. Int J Radiat Oncol Biol Phys 66:1430–1439, 2006.

101. Kwan W, Pickles T, Duncan G, et al: PSA failure and the risk of death in prostate cancer patients treated with radiotherapy. Int J Radiat Oncol Biol Phys 60:1040–1046, 2004

102. Shipley WU, Desilvio M, Pilepich MV, et al: Early initiation of salvage hormone therapy influences survival in patients who failed initial radiation for locally advanced prostate cancer: a secondary analysis of RTOG protocol 86-10. Int J Radiat Oncol Biol Phys 64:1162–1167, 2006.

103. Fowler J, Chappell R, Ritter M: Is alpha/beta for prostate tumors really low? Int J Radiat Oncol Biol Phys 50:1021–1031, 2001.

104. Duchesne GM, Peters LJ: What is the alpha/beta ratio for prostate cancer? Rationale for hypofractionated high-dose-rate brachytherapy. Int J Radiat Oncol Biol Phys 44:747–748, 1999.

105. Deger S, Boehmer D, Roigas J, et al: High dose rate (HDR) brachytherapy with conformal radiation therapy for localized prostate cancer. Eur Urol 47:441–448, 2005.

106. Martinez A, Gonzalez J, Spencer W, et al: Conformal high dose rate brachytherapy improves biochemical control and cause specific survival in patients with prostate cancer and poor prognostic factors. J Urol 169:974–979; discussion 979–980, 2003.

107. Slater JD, Rossi CJ, Jr, Yonemoto LT, et al: Proton therapy for prostate cancer: the initial Loma Linda University experience. Int J Radiat Oncol Biol Phys 59:348–352, 2004.

108. Zietman AL, DeSilvio ML, Slater JD, et al: Comparison of conventional-dose vs high-dose conformal radiation therapy in clinically localized adenocarcinoma of the prostate: a randomized controlled trial. JAMA 294:1233–1239, 2005.

109. Russell KJ, Caplan RJ, Laramore GE, et al: Photon versus fast neutron external beam radiotherapy in the treatment of locally advanced prostate cancer: results of a randomized prospective trial. Int J Radiat Oncol Biol Phys 28:47–54, 1994.

110. Laramore GE, Krall JM, Thomas FJ, et al: Fast neutron radiotherapy for locally advanced prostate cancer. Final report of Radiation Therapy Oncology Group randomized clinical trial. Am J Clin Oncol 16:164–167, 1993.

111. Forman JD, Porter AT: The experience with neutron irradiation in locally advanced adenocarcinoma of the prostate. Semin Urol Oncol 15:239–243, 1997.

9

High-Intensity Focused Ultrasound for Prostate Cancer

Stefan Thüroff and Christian Chaussy

<table>
<tr><td colspan="2" align="center">K E Y   P O I N T S</td></tr>
<tr><td valign="top">

- The basic principle of transrectal high-intensity focused ultrasound (HIFU) is the precise destruction of prostatic tissue in one session by depositing large amounts of energy into it. The two principal mechanisms of action are based on mechanical and thermal effects. The thermal effect of HIFU is associated with the absorption of ultrasound energy into the tissue, which is converted into heat. Mechanically, damage to cells is due to acoustic cavitation. Both lead to a reduction in prostate volume to 5 mL.
- The use of HIFU in organ-confined prostate cancer was first examined in 1993 and two commercially available devices for HIFU are currently in use: the Ablatherm and the Sonablate. The main differences between the two systems are patient positioning, treatment and planning, ultrasound frequencies, shoot and delay time, intraprostatic treatment mode, and rectal wall control.
- HIFU is generally indicated for patients with localized prostate cancer (stage T1-T2N0M0 Gleason score [GS] 1–3) who are not candidates for surgery because of their age, general health status or a prohibiting comorbidity, or who would prefer not to undergo a radical prostatectomy.
- The indication for HIFU has been expanded based on clinical experience to include partial therapy in unilateral low-volume, low-GS tumors (T1-2aNx/0M0, GS1–2, prostate-specific antigen [PSA] less than 20 ng/mL); salvage therapy in recurrent prostate cancer after radical prostatectomy, radiation therapy, or hormone ablation (all T Nx/0M0, all GS/PSA); and advanced prostate cancer as a debulking process (T3-4Nx/0M0, all GS/PSA).
- Unlike other local treatment options for prostate cancer, such as surgery, radiation therapy, cryotherapy, and brachytherapy, HIFU treatment can be repeated easily in cases of local recurrence and can be used as a salvage therapy.
- In current practice, a pre-HIFU transurethral resection of the prostate (TURP) allows for the removal of any

</td><td valign="top">

calcifications, abscesses, middle lobe, and large adenomas because it optimizes the prostate shape for HIFU application. The generation of a cavity and its subsequent compression by the rectal balloon increase the accessibility of the HIFU.
- A number of studies have reported the outcome with HIFU, including single-center and multicenter European studies.
- Promising 5-year outcome of HIFU for localized prostate cancer in a procedure not involving prior TURP has been reported, with a 93.4% negative biopsy rate in 137 patients studied.
- Data from one study combining TURP with HIFU in 30 patients with localized prostate cancer with a median follow-up of 20 months report a 83.3% negative biopsy rate at 1 year and an overall negative biopsy rate of 86.6% in patients undergoing one or two HIFU sessions.
- HIFU can be considered a treatment option in patients with high-risk prostate cancer, although long-term studies are still needed. In one study involving 30 patients with locally advanced and advanced disease at 6 months follow-up, positive biopsies were reported in 23% of patients. At 1 year, only three (10%) patients had a PSA level higher than 0.3 ng/mL and less than 1.0 ng/mL.
- As salvage treatment, HIFU treatment results in a good outcome in locally recurrent prostate cancer after external-beam radiation therapy. A 30-month actuarial negative biopsy rate of 73% has been reported in one study involving 71 patients.
- Patients treated with HIFU as a primary local therapy combined with TURP generally have low morbidity. Grade 1 (4%–6%) or grade 2 (0%–2%) urinary stress incontinence and secondary intravesical obstruction (5%–10%) are the most commonly reported adverse events. Urinary tract infections are common (5%–13%), but the incidence has been shown to be significantly reduced in patients undergoing the combined TURP/HIFU procedure compared with HIFU alone.

</td></tr>
</table>

Introduction

The first medical application of ultrasonic waves was made by Fry and coworkers[1] in the 1950s and related to the extracorporeal treatment of neurologic disorders such as Parkinson disease. High-intensity focused ultrasound (HIFU) for focal tissue destruction was established in 1955.[2] Through the use of a set of ultrasound transducers focused on the target area, small biological lesions located deep inside the cerebral cortex could be produced. The technique was originally developed as a means of achieving selective destruction of brain tissue but was not put into routine use because it required a large cranial bone flap. Other limitations were a lack of an imaging device with adequate performance and accuracy. The use of HIFU in the treatment of cancer in both human and animal models was examined by Burov[3] in 1956. Irradiation of experimental tumors using HIFU followed in the late 1970s and early 1980s,[4,5] and in 1986, Lizzi and coworkers[6] applied HIFU in the treatment of specific ocular cancers and glaucoma. The first clinical trials using HIFU in the treatment of benign prostatic hyperplasia (BPH) began in 1993[7,8] and at the same time treatment of organ-confined prostate cancer was being carried out by Gelet and coworkers.[9] It should be noted that HIFU can be delivered as a pulsed or a continuous beam. Continuous-beam processes include solar waves, microwaves, and radar technology, whereas medical HIFU and extracorporeal shock wave lithotripsy (ESWL) involve pulsed HIFU.

Mechanism of Action

The basic principle of transrectal HIFU is the precise destruction of prostatic tissue in one session by depositing large amounts of energy into it. Ultrasound waves, generated by the high-frequency vibration (0.5–10 MHz) of a piezoelectric or piezoceramic transducer, are focused into a small discrete region (the focal point) by concave or parabolic arrangement (Fig. 9-1). Coupling and cooling are performed by degassed colored liquid as interface between the source and the patient's rectal wall. Owing to the similar physical properties of water and tissue, as well as the broad flat coupling surface, ultrasound waves penetrate with minimal absorption or reflection. As the converging ultrasound approaches the focal point, the power density increases. The two principal mechanisms of action of HIFU are based on thermal effects and mechanical effects.

The thermal effect of HIFU is associated with the absorption of ultrasound energy into the tissue, which is converted into heat. Tem-

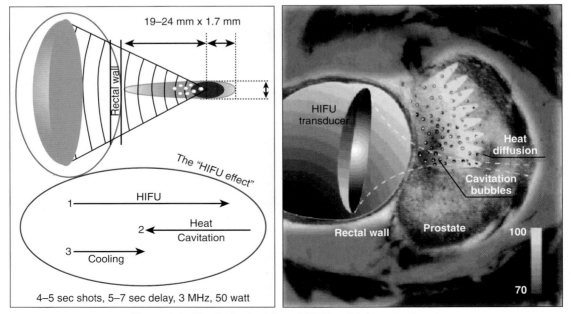

Figure 9-1. Physical principles of HIFU.   Ablatherm treatment.

perature elevation in the tissues depends on the absorption coefficient of the tissue as well as the size, shape, and thermal response. Counterproductive are tissue movement and increased bloodflow in the heated region. The biological changes that are induced by heating depend on the temperature reached and the duration of the exposure (the thermal dose). Above a certain threshold, thermal dose induces irreversible tissue damage in the form of coagulative necrosis. Below the threshold, thermal dose effects depend on the sensitivity of the tissue to heat. A steep temperature gradient exists between the tissue being focused on and the neighboring tissue, as can be seen in the sharp temperature gradient between the necrotic lesion and the normal cells in histologic samples.

From the mechanical perspective, bubbles form inside the cells caused by the negative pressure of the ultrasound wave, and they increase in size to the point at which resonance is achieved. When the bubbles suddenly collapse, high pressure of 20,000 to 30,000 bars develops and damages nearby cells. This acoustic cavitation is complex and must be controlled in its extension. The two activities together lead to a reduction in prostate volume to 5 mL.

Commercially Available Devices

Two commercially available devices for HIFU (Fig. 9-2) are currently in use: the Sonablate (Focus Surgery, Inc., Indianapolis, Indiana) and the Ablatherm (EDAP SA, Lyon, France). Both devices allow transrectal ultrasound-guided imaging with treatment, using a probe (Fig. 9-3) encased within a degassed fluid-filled coupling balloon that cools the rectum. The main differences between the two systems are patient positioning (see Fig. 9-5), treatment and planning ultrasound frequencies, shoot and delay time, intraprostatic treatment mode, and rectal wall control.

Ablatherm has a treatment module that includes the patient's bed, the probe positioning system, the ultrasound power generator, and the cooling system for preservation of the rectal wall (see Fig. 9-2). There is also a treatment and imaging endorectal probe that incorporates both a by-plane imaging probe working at 7.5 MHz and a treatment transducer focused at a maximum of 45 mm and working at 3 MHz. Hence, one size probe fits all prostate sizes and indications (see Fig. 9-3). A variable focusing and rectum distance length of the transducer are shown in Figure 9-4. Real-time rectal wall control is present; automatic applicator adjustment toward the rectal wall and multiple security circuits exclude accidental focusing on the rectal wall, thus avoiding rectal injury. In 2005, modifications were made to the Ablatherm device to incorporate integrated imaging. The advantages of the latest Ablatherm (Integrated Imaging) and the earlier model (Maxis) are

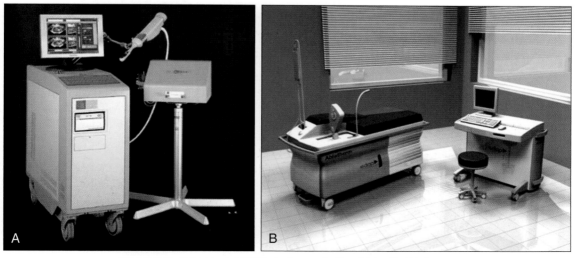

Figure 9-2. Transrectal HIFU devices. A, Sonablate. **B,** Ablatherm.

Sonablate

Ablatherm

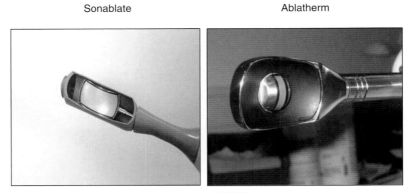

Figure 9-3. Transrectal HIFU applicators.

Sonablate

Ablatherm

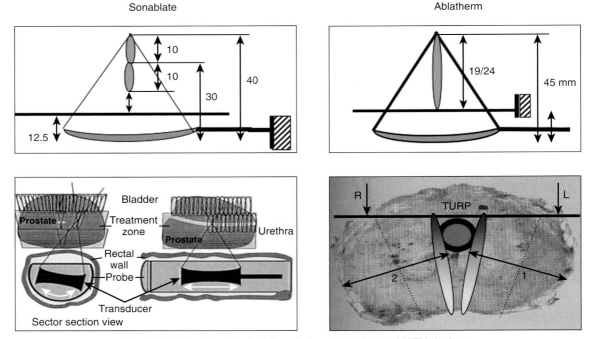

Figure 9-4. Treatment principles of different transrectal HIFU devices.

shown in Table 9-1. Full details of the Ablatherm procedure are described later in this chapter.

Sonablate, unlike the Ablatherm machine, does not have a dedicated bed (see Fig. 9-2). Treatment is performed with the patient in the TURP position under general anesthesia (Fig. 9-5). Several treatment probes are available, and these are selected according to the size of the elementary lesion that is to be generated by the operator. Unlike the Ablatherm device, the Sonablate does not have the dual-frequency probe and operates usually at 4 MHz during the treatment phase and as well at 4 MHz for visualization of the gland. Instead, treatment parameters have to be changed with each parabolic applicator for each treatment layer. For a 25-mm or 45-mm focal length probe, the lesion achieved is 10 mm in length by 2 mm diameter, whereas for a split beam performing with a 30-, 35-, or 40-mm focal length probe, the lesion is 10 mm by 3 mm.[10] In addition, the probe is chosen according to the prostate size, with larger glands requiring longer focal lengths. Treatment is usually conducted in three consecutive coronal layers (see Figs. 9-4 and 9-6)

Sonablate   Ablatherm

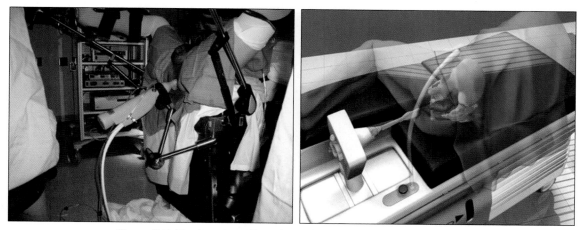

Figure 9-5. Treatment positions for patients in different HIFU devices.

Sonablate   Ablatherm

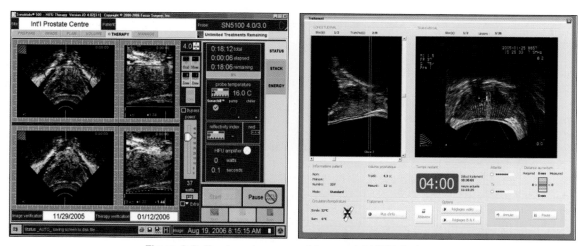

Figure 9-6. Treatment screens of transrectal HIFU devices.

Table 9-1. Features of Different Generations of the Ablatherm High-Intensity Focused Ultrasound Device

Maxis	Integrated Imaging
Electromechanical applicator with inserted 7-MHz alternating TRUS	Electronic applicator with integrated 7.5-MHz real-time TRUS
No real-time control	Excellent TRUS resolution by a new diagnostic ultrasound unit
High TRUS resolution with a standard diagnostic ultrasound unit	Fast and highly precise planning by computerized scanning procedure
Manual therapy planning	Virtual prostate reconstruction
Real-time TRUS control	Real-time TRUS control
Electronic picture and data storage	Electronic picture and data storage
Learning curve: 30 treatments	Ablaview 'blackbox'
	Treatment time reduced by 25%
	Learning curve: 10 treatments (new users); 5 treatments (Ablatherm users)

TRUS, transrectal ultrasound.

starting from the anterior prostate and moving in a progressive manner from the apex to the base. Since one probe integrates two different twistable parabolic piezoapplicators, there is usually at least one change of probe during the process. No real-time rectal wall distance control is present with the Sonablate system, leaving it to the operator to perform manually guided rectal wall–orientated HIFU treatment in the peripheral zone, which is the mostly likely location for a prostate tumor. Sonablate claims restricted indication range for only T1-2 prostate cancer and no use in salvage or palliative HIFU.

Indications and Contraindications

In general, HIFU is indicated for patients with localized prostate cancer (T1-T2N0M0 Gleason score [GS] 1–3) who are not candidates for surgery because of age, general health status, or a prohibiting comorbidity or who prefer not to undergo a radical prostatectomy. However, the indications have been expanded based on clinical experience to include partial therapy in unilateral low-volume, low-GS tumors (T1-2a Nx/0M0, prostate-specific antigen [PSA] less than 20 ng/mL); salvage therapy in recurrent prostate cancer after radical prostatectomy, radiation therapy, or hormone ablation (all TNx/0M0, all GS/PSA); and advanced prostate cancer as an additional neoadjuvant debulking process (T3-4Nx/0M0, all GS/PSA). Of note, other nonsurgical treatment options for localized prostate cancer, such as cryotherapy or brachytherapy, cannot generally be repeated in cases of local recurrence. In comparison, HIFU treatment not only can be repeated but also can be used as a salvage therapy.

Contraindications for the use of Sonablate in prostate cancer patients include a gland size larger than 40 mL due to the focal length of HIFU. For Ablatherm, larger glands can be downsized through transrectal resection of the prostate (TURP) and/or hormonal therapy with a luteinizing hormone-releasing hormone (LHRH) agonist. Contraindications for both devices are a history of rectal fistula since there may be incomplete healing of the fistula, as well as a reduced vascular blood supply to the damaged tissues, making them more prone to injury than normal tissue. Obviously, patients with significant rectal stenosis or rectal amputa-tion are not candidates for HIFU because the probe cannot be placed in the rectum.

HIFU Procedure: Ablatherm TURP

The use of TURP prior to HIFU allows for the removal of any reflecting/deviating calcifications, abscesses, intravesical middle lobes, and large (greater than 40 mL) adenomas. The generation of a cavity and its subsequent compression by the rectal balloon increase the accessibility of the HIFU waves to the remaining gland. TURP should be performed completely in the ventral region but leaving in place a large area of the gland at the bladder neck. This reduces the risk of bladder neck stenosis caused by prostate gland shrinkage during HIFU. The rectal balloon that covers the HIFU probe is then able to squeeze the gland, to stretch and flatten the rectal wall, and to fix it into position.

TURP before HIFU has been used as a standard procedure for most users since 2000. For most (85%) prostates sized, TURP is carried out at the same time as is HIFU. Only for those sized greater than 40 mL (15%) is TURP conducted 1 month before HIFU. In salvage HIFU, TURP use is minimal or only a bladder neck incision is performed. In salvage therapy after radical surgery, HIFU is performed without any additional endoscopic intervention.

Treatment Parameters

Treatment parameters important for effective tissue coagulation include the power setting (watts), the piezoelectric frequency (MHz), shot duration as well as delay between shots, and number of shots per prostate volume (dose). The delay between shots is necessary to prevent overwhelming accumulation of cavitation bubbles in adjacent lesions. The length and diameter of the lesion in the prostate to be generated need to be considered in treatment planning, as well as the possibility of adapting the technology to different tissue types (untreated, preirradiated, or HIFU pretreated). In this regard, three types of software are used involving the application of different levels of energy. Table 9-2 lists the differences between the two Ablatherm devices and shows the settings used for the Maxis system (pre-2005) and the Integrated imaging system (post-2005) and shows that power and shot duration are lower for patients post-radiation than in

Table 9-2. Power Settings for High-Intensity Focused Ultrasound (HIFU) with Ablatherm According to Prostate Tissue Treated

	MHz		Power (%)		Shot Duration (sec)		Delay Duration (sec)	
	M	ii	M	ii	M	ii	M	ii
Standard	3.0		100	100	5	6	5	4
HIFU retreatment	3.0		100	100	4.5	5	5	4
Radiation failure	3.0		90	95	4	5	7	5

M, Maxis; ii, Integrated imaging.

primary HIFU treatment or HIFU retreatment. The rationale is that irradiated prostate tissue has a higher uptake of HIFU energy,[11] and so a lower level is equally efficient and reduces the risk of rectal wall injury to almost zero.

Safety Issues

The safety of Ablatherm was increased with the introduction in 2005 of real-time imaging, made possible through a new electronic probe. Less local movement has also been achieved through fixation of this new probe (see Fig. 9-5), allowing greater accuracy in the delivery of HIFU. Precise control of energy delivery is very important from the safety and efficacy perspective, and this is optimized through the use of the Ablapak transducer fluid. Ablatherm also has inbuilt controls that stop the treatment when the probe is too close or far from the rectal wall. This control compares the three-dimensional position of the applicator to the treatment plan and allows the device to "fire" with a ±1-mm accuracy. In addition, an external motion sensor is in place to detect any patient movement and consequently stop the procedure. The probe itself is held off the rectal wall with a fluid-filled (Ablasonic) balloon. Ablasonic is a blue anticavitation coupling and cooling fluid that prevents cavitation bubbles within the cooling circuit and in front of the applicator. This fluid is cooled to limit the heat damage to the rectal wall tissues by creating a temperature gradient between the rectal mucosa and the prostatic capsule.

Application

Treatment commences with the administration of an enema to cleanse the rectum; prophylactic antibiotics are given and a urethral catheter put into place. Spinal anesthesia with an analgesic sedation is the preferred method for the procedure. The patient is placed in a lateral position and external warming applied to counteract the cooling of the rectum. The transducer is covered with a balloon, which is inserted into the rectum and then filled with 150 mL degassed transmitter fluid (Ablasonic). A roller pump causes the liquid to circulate slowly through the balloon into a cooling unit and back to the rectum at a temperature of 15°C. The prostate is scanned automatically by a 7.5-MHz transrectal ultrasound wave from the base to the apex. A dynamic moveable transrectal ultrasound (TRUS) simulation is created, which allows precise virtual treatment planning, prostate volume calculation, and definition of apex and base to be performed (see Fig. 9-6). Apex definition is one of the most important aspects of treatment planning, involving a balance between preservation of continence and effective treatment. Vertical and lateral borders of the HIFU lesion to be generated are defined at this time. Based on these parameters, generated in just 5 minutes, treatment planning can then be carried out.

Treatment Planning

The TRUS image of the prostate in a longitudinal or transverse view is monitored on the computer screen. Depending on the results of the TRUS-guided biopsies on the localization and volume of the prostate tumor, a complete treatment (in 95% of cases) is performed in one session. Ablatherm treatment typically starts 5 mm cranially from the apex, moving toward the bladder, treating first the left lobe and then the right lobe of the prostate.

The actual plan of how the HIFU will be delivered is then generated by the computer software. The treatment planning divides the prostate into 1.6-mm transverse sections, which are subdivided into single lesions (see Fig. 9-3). The position of slices and lesions is defined by the operator on the control screen and adapted individually; slice by slice, up to 800 lesions may be defined depending on the size of the prostate. Subsections of the prostate (approximately 25% each) are targeted at any one time to integrate the ongoing tissue edema into the consecutive planning process.

Active Treatment

Treatment is carried out by a single operator—making the process highly cost-efficient—who follows the treatment plan and goes through all the predefined regions. For accuracy of the thermal effect, an absolutely stable position of the patient must be maintained. The treatment time is usually 95 (30–150) minutes, and the actual treatment carried out is recorded and can be reviewed after the procedure. Postoperatively, there is minimum pain for the patient, making analgesic medication unnecessary. HIFU perioperative morbidity is low: no significant bleeding, no blood transfusion, no intensive care, and no thrombosis or pulmonary embolism. Antibiotic prophylaxis is usually continued until catheter removal, which usually occurs at 5 (3–10) days postoperatively.

New Treatment Strategies

For optimal efficacy, the entire prostate is normally treated during the HIFU procedure, but in the case of a unilateral tumor and when potency is an important issue for the patient, the contralateral lobe/capsule and neurovascular bundle might be excluded. This is considered only in small-volume, low-GS unilateral cancers. Patients are advised of the risk of tumor recurrence in the untreated area, and selection of patients for this option requires them to have good compliance with follow-up.

Patient Follow-up

PSA measurement is made at 3-month intervals postoperatively, and TRUS-guided sextant biopsies are recommended at between 6 and 12 months after HIFU to identify microscopic residual tumor volumes that may require retreat-ment with HIFU. In this early stage, these microscopic residues would not necessarily be identified through the rising PSA level. The patient is judged as being in complete remission if the biopsy is negative and the PSA level is low and the PSA velocity remains stable below 0.2 ng/mL/year. If the PSA level increases to pathologic levels, then repeat biopsy is performed; depending on the results, the patient is retreated with a second local therapy. If HIFU was used for palliative treatment in local debulking of systemic disease, then retreatment for residual microscopic tumor appears not to be indicated.

Efficacy

A number of studies have reported the outcome of HIFU using Ablatherm, including single-center and multicenter European studies. Most of the studies have focused on localized prostate cancer, but there are also reports on the use of HIFU as salvage therapy after external-beam radiation therapy (EBRT). Reviewed in this section are the key studies with the Ablatherm device reported in the literature.

Localized Disease

Chaussy and Colleagues[12] (1999)

Reported are 3-year data on 184 patients treated with HIFU between 1996 and 1999. Of the patient group, 90 were treated in the period of the learning curve (April 1996 to October 1997) at a frequency of 2.25 MHz and a power of 50 watts. The remaining patients received 3.0-MHz frequency and the same power. Other differences between the two treatment groups were an increased rectum-capsule distance from 3 mm to 6 mm and the treatment started at 5 mm from the anatomic apex. Additional security features in the later patient group included rectal cooling. Patients included in the study had biopsy-proven localized prostate cancer (T1-2 NxM0), a mean age of 72 years, a mean prostate volume of 26 mL, and a mean serum PSA level at the time of treatment of 2.2 ng/mL due to previous hormonal ablation by LHRH agonist in 48% of patients. Mean serum level in patients not pre-treated with hormonal therapy was 12.0 ng/mL. GS was 2–4 in 9.5% of patients, 5–7 in 80%, and 8–10 in 10.5%. Mean follow-up was 193 days, with all patients receiving at least one biopsy post-HIFU. Results showed that 97% of patients reached a PSA nadir of less than 4 ng/mL, and 61% had a nadir of less than 0.5 ng/mL. Of the biopsies taken, 80% were cancer free. There was a distinction in patients treated during the learning curve in that there was a 30% and 23% incidence of residual cancer in the subcapsular and central zones, respectively, compared with incidences of 1% and 17% in the later treatment group. Mean prostate size was reduced by 50%. This study confirmed the local efficacy of HIFU in terms of ablation of prostate cancer tissue and consequently low PSA nadir.

Gelet and Associates[13] (2000)

This study reports outcome in 82 consecutive patients treated from 1996 with a 3.0-MHz frequency, a 5-second treatment pulse, and a 5.0-second shot interval. Patients included in the study had stage T1/T2 cancer, any GS, and a pretreatment PSA level less than 20 ng/mL. Mean (SD) age was 71 (5.7) years; mean (SD) PSA and prostate volume at baseline were 8.11 (4.64) ng/mL and 34.9 (17.4) mL, respectively. Neoadjuvant hormonal therapy was used in seven patients, and four patients had local recurrence after definitive EBRT. On average, 1.8 sessions of HIFU were applied per patient: 34 patients had one session; 32 patients had two sessions; 9 patients had three sessions; 6 patients had four sessions; and 1 patient had six sessions. Mean postoperative catheterization time was 8.5 days. Progression was defined as any positive biopsy result, regardless of PSA level, or three consecutive rises in PSA in patients with a negative biopsy. During the 3-month period after HIFU, negative biopsies were reported in 64 (78%) patients and positive biopsies in 18 (22%). Overall, mean (SD) PSA nadir and prostate volume post-HIFU were 1.02 (1.54) ng/mL and 20.9 (13.1) mL, respectively. Mean follow-up was 17.6 months (range 3–68 months). Magnetic resonance imaging (MRI) indicated that in large prostates (larger than 40 mL) the anterior region of the base was not reached by the ultrasound beam. However, no association with PSA nadir was shown in such patients. Kaplan-Meier estimates of disease-free survival (DFS) at 60 months was 62%. Kaplan-Meier statistical analysis of outcome predictors of DFS was conducted and revealed that pretreatment PSA ($P < .001$)

and GS ($P = .034$) were significantly predictive of DFS rate, whereas prostate volume and number of positive biopsies were not.

Thüroff and Coworkers[14] (2003)

This European multicenter study reported the short-tem results of HIFU in 402 patients with T1-2 N0-xM0 prostate cancer treated from 1995 to 1999 at six centers. Baseline patient characteristics included the following mean (SD) values: age 69.3 (7.1) years; prostate volume 28.0 (12.7) mL; PSA 10.9 (8.7) ng/mL, and GS 6.0 (1.3). Patients were also classified according to the risk groups shown in Table 9-3; 28.4%, 48.0%, and 23.6% of patients were classified as low, intermediate, and high risk, respectively. During the course of the study, several device prototypes were used, and there was a progressive increase in frequency from 2.25 to 3 MHz and in shot duration, from 4 to 5 seconds. Four major treatment protocols (TP) were identified: TP1, frequency 2.25 MHz, shot duration 4.5 seconds, and no cooling system; TP2, frequency less than 3 MH, shot duration 4.5 seconds; TP3, frequency 3 MHz, shot duration 4.5 seconds; and TP4, frequency of 3 MHz, shot duration 5 seconds.

From 1995 to 1998, patients were treated in two sessions (one session/lobe); thereafter a single session was used. A total of 62.4% of patients were treated with a single session and 27.9% with two sessions. Of the 288 patients assessable for sextant biopsy results, a negative biopsy rate of 87.2% was reported (Table 9-4).

Table 9-3. Risk Group Classifications for Patients Treated in the European Multicentre Study on High-Intensity Focused Ultrasound (Ablatherm)

Risk Group	Stage	PSA (ng/mL)	Gleason Score
Low* (n = 114)	T1–2a	≤10	≤6
Intermediate† (n = 193)	T2b	>10 ≤ 20	7
High† (n = 95)	T2c	>20	≥8

*All three parameters required.
†One parameter only required.
PSA, prostate-specific antigen.
Data from Chaussy C, Thüroff S: The status of high-intensity focused ultrasound in the treatment of localized prostate cancer and the impact of a combined resection. Curr Urol Rep 4:248–252, 2003.

Table 9-4. Biopsy and Prostate-Specific Antigen (PSA) Nadir Outcome in the European Multicentre Study on High-Intensity Focused Ultrasound (Ablatherm)

	Negative Biopsy (%)	Mean PSA Nadir (ng/mL)
Overall	87.2	1.8
Prostate volume (mL)		
≤40	88.4	1.5*
>40	85.0	2.9
AP diameter (mm)		
≤25	85.4	1.4
>25	88.1	1.3
Risk		
Low	92.1	1.3
Intermediate	86.4	1.4
High	82.1	3.1
Treatment		
Partial	87.2	1.8†
Complete	91.7	1.4
Protocol		
TP1	44.4‡	5.1§
TP2	82.1	3.3
TP3	91.2	1.3
TP4	94.8	0.9

*$P = 0.0001$.
†$P = 0.016$.
‡$P < 0.0001$.
§$P = 0.0001$ for PSA nadir.
AP, anteroposterior.
Data from Chaussy C, Thüroff S: The status of high-intensity focused ultrasound in the treatment of localized prostate cancer and the impact of a combined resection. Curr Urol Rep 4:248–252, 2003.

Significant differences were observed in negative biopsy rate when patients were stratified according to TP used, but the authors point out that there could be an inherent bias in this because of the time effect, the differences in technical protocols during the course of the study, and the first patients' having a longer time period in which to reveal a recurrent or residual tumor. No significant differences in negative biopsy rates were observed with regard to prostate volume, anteroposterior diameter, risk group, or partial or complete treatment of the prostate gland.

Results of PSA nadir for patients with at least 6-months' follow-up (n = 212) are shown in Table 9-4. Nadir was generally achieved within 3 to 4 months of treatment (mean 163.5 days) A statistically significant difference was observed for PSA nadir with regard to baseline prostate volume of 40 mL and more than 40 mL ($P = .0001$), for complete versus partial treatment of the prostate ($P = .016$) and for TP ($P = .0001$).

The results from this study demonstrate the short-term good local control of prostate cancer achieved with HIFU, despite a high proportion of high-risk patients being treated.

Blana and Coworkers[15] (2004)

Five-year outcome from HIFU conducted between 1997 and 2002 in 146 patients with biopsy proven T1-2N0M0 cancer have been published. Mean (SD) age, PSA level, GS, and prostate volume were: 66.9 (6.7) years, 7.6 (3.4) ng/mL, 5 (1.2), and 23 (7.7) mL, respectively. A total of 63 patients had received neoadjuvant hormonal therapy. The 3.0-MHz frequency was used for HIFU treatment, and the majority of patients received a 5-second treatment pulse. Up to 1000 lesions 1.7 mm in diameter were treated with HIFU during each treatment according to the size of the gland. On average, 1.17 sessions of HIFU were applied per patient: 123 patients had one session, 21 patients had 2 sessions, and 2 patients had 3 sessions. The mean (SD) treated volume was 33.6 (16.3) mL, which when compared with the mean volume of prostates treated meant that 146% of the volume was treated by overlapping the treatment areas. Mean postoperative catheterization time was 12.7 days. A randomized control sextant biopsy was performed at 3, 12, and 24 months or when there was evidence of biochemical failure; PSA was recorded at 3-month intervals. Mean follow-up was 22.5 months (range 4–62). Nine patients were lost to follow-up, seven of whom had no control biopsy data.

The median PSA nadir achieved at 3 months was 0.07 ng/mL (range 0–5.67 ng/mL); the level after 22 months follow-up was 0.15 ng/mL (range 0–12.11 ng/mL). Of the 137 patients, 93.4% had constant negative control biopsies. This study confirms the promising 5-year outcome of HIFU for localized prostate cancer in a procedure not involving prior TURP. Of note, TURP or bladder neck incision was required for infravesical obstruction post-HIFU in 16 (11.7%) patients.

Poissonnier and Coworkers[16] (2007)

Data on 227 consecutive patients treated between 1994 and 2003 are present in the publication from the Lyon group in France. A total of 51 patients were treated before 2000 and 176

Table 9-5. Evolution of the High-Intensity Focus Ultrasound (HIFU) Devices Used During the Study Period 1991–2003

Time Period	Device	Transducer Frequency (MHz)	Shot Duration (sec)	No. of HIFU Sessions
1993–1995	Prototype no 1	2.5	4	2
1996–1998	Prototype no 2	3	4.5	2
1998–1999	Prototype no 3	3	5	1
2000–2003	Ablatherm Maxis	3	5	1

Data from Vallancien G, Prapotnich D, Cathelineau X, et al: Transrectal focused ultrasound combined with transurethral resection of the prostate for the treatment of localized prostate cancer: feasibility study. J Urol 171:2265–2267, 2004.

since 2000. The later group also underwent a TURP at the time of the HIFU procedure. The HIFU devices used during the study as well as the number of treatment sessions are shown in Table 9-5. The mean number of HIFU sessions conducted per patient was 1.4; 10 patients received three sessions or more. On average, 581 shots of HIFU were delivered per patient, and compared with the mean prostate, the mean volume of the gland treated during the first HIFU session was 111% and 156% after the second session, indicating overlapping treatment areas. Catheterization was stopped at a mean of 7 days post-HIFU; duration was considerably lower in patients who had undergone TURP compared with those receiving HIFU alone—5 versus 12 days. Of the patient cohort, 76 had received neoadjuvant hormone therapy (mean duration 4.7 months), primarily for size reduction in prostates larger than 40 mL. Assessment criteria involved PSA nadir, negative biopsy rate and DFS rate, which was defined as any positive biopsy or a PSA greater than 1 ng/mL with three consecutive rises.

Mean (SD) follow-up was 27.5 (20) months. Negative control biopsies were recorded in 86% of patients, and median PSA nadir was 0.10 ng/mL. Actuarial DFS rate at 5 years was 66% based on the combination of pathology and biochemical outcome. Actuarial DFS rates according to initial PSA level, GS, clinical stage, neoadjuvant hormone therapy, and HIFU device used are shown in Table 9-6. The only significant variable identified was pretreatment PSA level ($P = .008$).

HIFU with TURP

The combined procedure of TURP and HIFU in patients with localized prostate cancer has

Table 9-6. Disease-Free Survival (DFS) Rates According to Pretreatment Parameters in Patients Treated with High-Intensity Focused Ultrasound (Ablatherm)

Parameter	DFS (%)	P Value
PSA (ng/mL)		
0–4 ($n = 50$)	90	.008
4.1–10 ($n = 132$)	57	
10.1–15 ($n = 45$)	61	
Gleason score		
2–6 ($n = 152$)	66	.944
7 ($n = 75$)	67	
Clinical stage		
T1 ($n = 122$)	66	.519
T2 ($n = 105$)	67	
Neoadjuvant hormonal therapy		
Yes ($n = 76$)	59	.839
No ($n = 151$)	67	
TURP		
Yes ($n = 175$)	70	.119
No ($n = 52$)	58	

Data from Vallancien G, Prapotnich D, Cathelineau X, et al: Transrectal focused ultrasound combined with transurethral resection of the prostate for the treatment of localized prostate cancer: feasibility study. J Urol 171:2265–2267, 2004.

been reported in two publications, which are reviewed below.

Chaussy and Thüroff[17] (2003)

Outcomes following the combined procedure of TURP and HIFU were reported in 175 patients and compared with outcomes in 96 patients previously treated with HIFU alone. Initial PSA level at diagnosis was 15 ng/mL, and patients with any GS were included. Mean (SD) prostate volume in the HIFU group was 21.7 (6.8) mL and in the combined group 20.5 (9.8) mL. Mean (SD) ages in the HIFU and combined groups were 65.8 (7.6) and 68.4

Table 9-7. Biopsy Results After the First High-Intensity Focused Ultrasound (HIFU) Session and at the Last Follow-Up (Including Retreatments) in Patients Treated with HIFU or Transurethral Resection of the Prostate (TURP) Plus HIFU

	HIFU	TURP + HIFU
Negative biopsy rate after first HIFU	66.3%	70.6%
Retreatment rate	25%	4%
Negative biopsy rate after last follow-up	87.7%	81.6%

All treatments involved the ablatherm device.
Data from Ficarra V, Antoniolli SZ, Novara G, et al: Short-term outcome after high-intensity focused ultrasound in the treatment of patients with high-risk prostate cancer. BJU Int 98:1193–1198, 2006.

(9.6) years, respectively. All HIFU treatments involved a 3-MHz frequency and a 5-second shot duration. PSA was measured at 3-month intervals and considered to be stable according to the 1997 ASTRO definition.[18] Control biopsies were performed at 6 and 12 months and in patients with a rising PSA level.

Mean (SD) follow-up was 18.7 (12.1) months in the HIFU group and 10.9 (6.2) in the combined group. The mean resected weight during TURP was 15.7 g. The mean (SD) PSA nadirs in the HIFU and combined groups were 0.48 (1.10) ng/mL and 0.26 (0.90) ng/mL (NS). PSA stability at last follow-up was 84.2% and 80% in the HIFU and combined groups, respectively (NS). Biopsy results after the first HIFU session and at the last follow-up are shown in Table 9-7. The outcome results showed no significant differences between the two groups, but this should be treated with caution owing to the short follow-up in the combined-treatment group and the lower retreatment rates in the combined-therapy group. This lower retreatment rate is suggestive of the benefits of TURP prior to HIFU in that it allows removal of calcifications of the transitional zone that would prevent HIFU treatment. In addition, it assists the treatment of enlarged prostates and allows the complete treatment of the peripheral zone in a single HIFU session. However, a longer follow-up is needed to confirm the decreased retreatment rate.

Vallancien and Colleagues[19] (2004)

The outcome following the combined treatment of HIFU and TURP or bladder neck incision has been reported in 30 patients treated between 1999 and 2001. All patients were treated under general anesthesia first with TURP (n = 22) or bladder neck incision in those with prostate smaller than 30 mL (n = 8), and then HIFU at a frequency of 3 MHz and a shot duration of 5 seconds. Patients received a single HIFU session. PSA was measured at 3, 6, 12, 18, and 24 months and yearly thereafter, whereas biopsy was carried out at 1 year after treatment and in the case of rising PSA. Mean patient characteristics were as follows: age 72 (range 61–79) years; prostate volume 30 (range 11–45) mL; PSA 7 (range 1–10) ng/mL; and GS 6 (range 4–7).

Median follow-up was 20 (range 3–38) months. At 1 year, 22 (73.3%) patients had a negative biopsy and a mean PSA of 0.9 ng/mL (range 0–2.6 ng/mL). Five (16.7%) patients had a positive biopsy at 1 year and received a repeat HIFU session; negative biopsies were subsequently recorded in four patients 6 months later when the mean PSA was 0.4 ng/mL (range 0.1–0.9 ng/mL). This gave an overall negative biopsy and PSA control rate following one or two HIFU sessions as 86.6%, which is comparable to the results reported by Chaussy and Thüroff.[17]

High-Risk Patients

Ficarra and Associates[20] (2006)

The efficacy of HIFU has been comprehensively reported in a number of studies as evidenced above, but studies are now being extended to patients with locally advanced or advanced prostate cancer as in the report by Ficarra and associates. This series involved 30 patients treated with HIFU in association with an LHRH agonist; TURP was conducted simultaneously. Median patient age was 73.5 (interquartile range 69.75–77.0) years. Median PSA was 18 (range 9–35) ng/mL, and clinical stage assessed at DRE was T2b and T3 in 9 and 21 patients, respectively. GS was 7 (n = 5), 8 (n = 10), 9 (n = 11), or 10 (n = 4). Median prostate volume was 35 (29.4–43.4) mL, and the median weight of resected tissue following TURP was 15 (10–20) g. The most current frequency settings of 3 MHz and shot duration of 5 seconds were used and 100% of the prostate was treated in all cases. The treatment strategy involved dividing the prostate into six areas: apex/medium regions and medium/basal regions of the left and right lobes and the prostatic urethra. The lateral limits of the treatment were widened for these high-risk patients to include one or two HIFU lesions for each area beyond the prostatic capsule. Nerve-sparing procedures were not used in view of the risk status of the patients and their age. PSA was measured at 3, 6, 9, and 12 months after HIFU, and disease recurrence was defined as a PSA level greater than 0.3 ng/mL; sextant biopsies were conducted at 6 months.

After this period, median prostate volume was 4.1 (1.3–6.6) mL, and positive biopsies were reported in seven (23%) patients. In four of these patients, cancer was present in one core, and in the remaining three patients it was present in two cores. At 1 year, only three (10%) patients had a PSA level of more than 0.3 ng/mL and less than 1.0 ng/mL, and each of them had two positive cores at the 6-month biopsy. These findings suggest that HIFU is a feasible treatment option in patients with high-risk prostate cancer and that further studies with a longer follow-up should be conducted.

Salvage Therapy

Gelet and Colleagues[11] (2004)

HIFU treatment can be used as salvage therapy after other local therapies, and Gelet and coworkers have reported good outcome in locally recurrent prostate cancer after EBRT. The study involved 71 patients treated with HIFU between 1995 and 2003 following local recurrence after radiation. Initial cancer stage at diagnosis was T1 ($n = 15$), T2 ($n = 28$), T3 ($n = 15$) and unknown in 13 patients. The pre-EBRT GS was 2 to 6 in 32 patients, seven in 17 patients, 8 to 10 in 7 patients and unknown in 15 patients. The mean PSA level at diagnosis was 20.4 ng/mL (range 3.5–60.0), and after EBRT, the mean PSA nadir was 1.46 ng/mL (range 0–4.3). The mean time of recurrence after EBRT was 38.5 months (range 6–120). Antiandrogen therapy was given to 22 (30%) patients prior to HIFU salvage therapy.

Confirmation of cancer recurrence was demonstrated by biopsy in all patients. Mean PSA prior to HIFU was 7.7 ng/mL (range 0.5–54) ng/mL, and the mean (SD) prostate volume

was 21.4 (11.1) mL. GS was recorded as 2–6 ($n = 24$), 7 ($n = 13$) and 8–10 ($n = 34$). The mean number of HIFU sessions applied per patient was 1.2, and post-HIFU, the mean (SD) prostate volume decreased to 14.4 (10.9) mL. The mean follow-up was 14.8 months (range 6–86) and at last follow-up, 57 (80%) of patients had a negative biopsy, which corresponded to a 30-month actuarial negative biopsy rate of 73%. Mean (SD) PSA nadir was 1.97 (4.58) ng/mL, and a PSA nadir within 3 months of 0.5 ng/mL or less was achieved by 43 (61%) patients. This is in view of the fact that before HIFU salvage therapy, 66.2% of patients had poorly or moderately differentiated prostate tumors (GS = 7). Of the 71 patients undergoing HIFU, 40 patients required additional therapy with hormone ablation ($n = 35$) or hormone ablation plus chemotherapy ($n = 5$) due to a rising PSA or residual cancer foci. Actuarial disease free rate, based on biopsy and PSA response, at 30 months was 38%. These findings indicate that HIFU is a potential treatment option with the possibility of cure in prostate cancer patients with local recurrence following EBRT.

Safety

Patients treated with HIFU as a primary local therapy combined with TURP generally have low morbidity. Grade 1 (4%–6%) or grade 2 (0%–2%) urinary stress incontinence and secondary infravesical obstruction (5%–10%) are the most commonly reported adverse events. Urinary tract infections (UTIs) are common (5%–13%) but the incidence has been shown to be significantly reduced in patients undergoing the combined TURP/HIFU procedure compared with HIFU alone: 11.4% versus 47.9% ($P < .001$).[17] Rare events include grade III incontinence and recto-urethral fistula (0.7%). A study of HIFU dose and its relationship to side effects as well as outcome was conducted in two European centers: Lyon and Munich.[21] Thirty patients with similar baseline characteristics were treated with two different treatment regimens; at Lyon a less aggressive strategy involving nonoverlapping prostate treatment areas was used compared with 30 patients treated with an overlapping strategy and more aggressive treatment at Munich. Results showed that the higher energy dose per treatment resulted in a higher cancer-free rate and lower PSA nadir level. However, this had to be balanced against a longer duration of urinary retention due to the presence of increased necrotic debris if adjuvant TURP was not performed.

Urinary Retention

Studies have been conducted examining the benefits of TURP immediately prior to HIFU as a means of reducing the risk of HIFU-related prolonged urinary retention. Prolonged retention can result from the elimination of necrotic debris in contrast to immediate retention, which occurs following edema induced by tissue coagulation. The study by Chaussy and Thüroff[17] described previously compared HIFU with simultaneous TURP and HIFU in 271 patients. After HIFU alone, the mean (SD) and median suprapubic catheter times were 45.1 (31.4) and 40 days, respectively. This compares with values of 13.7 (16.6) and 7.0 days, respectively, in the combined-therapy group. Vallancien and coworkers[19] reported a transurethral catheter time of 2 days in patients treated with TURP followed immediately by HIFU. Mean post-treatment International Prostate Symptom Score (IPSS) was 6.7 post-treatment compared with 7.5 before treatment.

Stress Incontinence

Stress incontinence can result from treatment of apical tissue, but the condition is usually transient. In the HIFU European Multicentre study, which was an early patient series, Grade 3 stress incontinence was reported in six patients. Resolution of the condition was achieved through implantation of an artificial urinary sphincter in four patients and pelvic floor training or collagen injection in one patient each. To minimize these side effects the first apical lesions are put at 5 mm cranially from the anatomic apex. This treatment strategy has led to a reduction in incidence of mild stress incontinence from around 25% to 3.9%.[22] Another study involving 227 patients has reported similar findings with a rate of 27% during the treatment period 1993 to 1999 (n = 51) and 9% during 2000 to 2003 (n = 176).[16] Reduced rates of incontinence have been recorded with the use of the combined TURP/HIFU treatment in addition to greater improvements in the IPSS (Table 9-8).[17]

Table 9-8. Urinary Complications Following Treatment with High-Intensity Ultrasound (HIFU) or a HIFU/Transurethral Resection of the Prostate (TURP) Combination

	HIFU	HIFU + TURP	P Value
Incontinence			
Grade 1	9.1%	4.6%	<.05*
Grade 2	6.3%	2.3%	
Grade 3	0%	0%	
IPSS (mean [SD])			
Before	6.47 (6.92)	6.69 (7.29)	<.05
After	8.91 (10.89)	3.37 (3.21)	

All treatments involved the ablatherm device.
*For grades 1 and 2 comparisons.
Data from Ficarra V, Antoniolli SZ, Novara G, et al: Short-term outcome after high-intensity focused ultrasound in the treatment of patients with high-risk prostate cancer. BJU Int 98:1193–1198, 2006.

Rectourethral Fistula

Rectourethral fistulas are extremely rare, occurring in less than 0.1% of T1-2 cases. In radiation failures, since the adoption of new software the fistula rate has decreased from 2.0% to 0.1%.[11] Patients experiencing such a complication are usually treated with prolonged catheterization or fibrin glue, but stoma diversion of urine and feces may be necessary, for example in salvage radiation therapy cases. More recently, the incidence of rectourethral fistula has been reduced to almost zero as a result of specific software, rectal safety margins, and the introduction of rectal cooling. The rate has also been reduced by observing contraindications for treatment, for example, patients with a rectal-wall thickness of over 6 mm due to local infection and those with abnormal rectal anatomy (e.g., after rectal surgery). This reduction is exemplified in one study that reported an incidence of rectourethral fistula of 3.5% prior to 1997 compared with 0.5% after this time when safety features were introduced.[22]

Erectile Dysfunction

Erectile dysfunction (ED), as with other treatments for localized prostate cancer, is common with rates of 55% to 66%. A nerve-sparing protocol can be instituted for men with positive biopsy results on one side of the prostate. This involves leaving a 5-mm lateral margin on the contralateral side. Poissonier and coworkers[16] report potency rates in 67 patients treated with

HIFU, 26 of whom received a nerve-sparing procedure and 41 who did not. ED was observed in 6 (31%) patients who had the nerve-sparing procedure compared with 16 (39%) patients in whom the nerves were not spared. This conservative approach has to be balanced against a higher retreatment rate.[22,30-32]

Future Directions

MRI is the gold-standard technique for assessing the efficacy of HIFU treatment. The extent of necrosis can be clearly visualized on gadolinium-enhanced T1-weighted images, as hyposignal zones.[23] MRI has also been used to guide HIFU treatments, since it is possible to monitor the temperature changes within tissues with MRI during HIFU.[23,24] Magnetic resonance elastography (MRE) has also been proposed as a method for assessing the effects of thermal tissue ablation by measuring the mechanical properties of the lesion.[25] HIFU-induced lesions are visible using standard ultrasound as hyperechoic regions,[26] but the extent of lesions is not always accurate. Other ultrasound-based techniques have been proposed to assess the extent of HIFU-induced lesions, such as MRE,[27] the use of contrast-enhanced power Doppler,[28] or different techniques for characterizing the acoustic properties of tissues.[29]

Conclusions

HIFU is a highly effective standard treatment with a large indication range over all tumor stages. In localized prostate cancer treatment, HIFU is associated with high-efficacy, low-operative morbidity and no systemic side effects. As a palliative therapy, an effective local tumor reduction decreases local morbidity and even kills cells insensitive to hormone therapy or radiation therapy. Unlike certain other localized therapies, HIFU is effective in salvage therapy and can result in acceptable side effects. The use of HIFU does not preclude other therapeutic options, such as hormonal therapy. and unlike such therapies, HIFU does not provoke a negative cell selection.

References

1. Fry WJ, Mosberg WH, Barnard JW, et al: Production of focal tissue destructive lesions in the central nervous system with ultrasound. J Neurosurg 11:471–478, 1954.
2. Fry WJ, Barnard JW, Fry FV, et al: Ultrasonic lesions in mammalian central nervous system. Science 122;517–518, 1955.
3. Burov AK: High-intensity ultrasonic vibrations for action on animal and human malignant tumours. Dokl Akad Nauk SSSR 106:239–241, 1956.
4. Fry FJ, Johnson LK: Tumor irradiation with intense ultrasound. Ultrasound Med Biol 4:337–341, 1978.
5. Goss SA, Fry FJ: The effects of high-intensity ultrasonic irradiation on tumour growth. IEEE Trans Sonics Ultrasonics SU-31:491–496, 1984.
6. Lizzi FL, Coleman DJ, Driller J, et al: A therapeutic ultrasound system incorporating real time ultrasonics scanning. In MacAvoy BR (ed): Proceedings of the 1986 Ultrasonics Symposium Institute of Electrical and Electronic Engineers. New York, 1987, pp 981–984.
7. Bihrle R, Foster RS, Sanghvi NT, et al: High intensity focused ultrasound for the treatment of benign prostatic hyperplasia: early United States clinical experience. J Urol 151:1271–1275, 1994.
8. Vallancien G, Chartier-Kastler E, Chopin D, et al: Focused extracorporeal pyrotherapy: experimental results. Eur Urol 20:211–219, 1991.
9. Gelet A, Chapelon JY, Bouvier R, et al: Treatment of prostate cancer with transrectal focused ultrasound: early clinical experience. Eur Urol 29:174–183, 1996.
10. Uchida T, Sanghvi NT, Gardner TA, et al: Transrectal high-intensity focused ultrasound for treatment of patients with stage T1b-2N0M localized prostate cancer: a preliminary report. Urology 59:394–398, 2002.
11. Gelet A, Chapelon JY, Poissonnier L, et al: Local recurrence of prostate cancer after external beam radiotherapy: early experience of salvage therapy using high-intensity focused ultrasonography. Urology 63:625–629, 2004.
12. Chaussy C, Thüroff S: High-intensity focused ultrasound in prostate cancer: results after 3 years. Mol Urol 4:179–182, 2000.
13. Gelet A, Chapelon JY, Bouvier R, et al: Transrectal high-intensity focused ultrasound: minimally invasive therapy of localized prostate cancer. J Endourol 14:519–528, 2000.
14. Thüroff S, Chaussy C, Vallancien G, et al. High-intensity focused ultrasound and localized prostate cancer: efficacy results from the European multicentric study. J Endourol 17:673–677, 2003.
15. Blana A, Walter B, Rogenhofer S, Wieland WF: High-intensity focused ultrasound for the treatment of localized prostate cancer: 5-year experience. Urology 63:297–300, 2004.
16. Poissonnier L, Chapelon JY, Rouviere O, et al: Control of prostate cancer by transrectal HIFU in 227 patients. Eur Urol 51:381–387, 2007.
17. Chaussy C, Thüroff S: The status of high-intensity focused ultrasound in the treatment of localized prostate cancer and the impact of a combined resection. Curr Urol Rep 4:248–252, 2003.
18. Consensus statement: Guidelines for PSA following radiation therapy. Int J Radiat Oncol Biol Phys 37:1035–1041, 1997.
19. Vallancien G, Prapotnich D, Cathelineau X, et al: Transrectal focused ultrasound combined with transurethral resection of the prostate for the treatment of localized prostate cancer: feasibility study. J Urol 171:2265–2267, 2004.
20. Ficarra V, Antoniolli SZ, Novara G, et al: Short-term outcome after high-intensity focused ultrasound in the treatment of patients with high-risk prostate cancer. BJU Int 98:1193–1198, 2006.
21. Thüroff S, Chaussy C, Gelet A: Focused ultrasound (HIFU) in the treatment of prostate cancer: energy/efficacy correlation. WCE Congress, 2001. J Endourol 15(Suppl 1): 32, abstract A3-P10, 2001.
22. Chaussy C, Thüroff S: Results and side effects of high-intensity focused ultrasound in localized prostate cancer. J Endourol 15:437–440, 2001.
23. Hynynen K, Freund WR, Cline HE, et al: A clinical, noninvasive, MR imaging-monitored ultrasound surgery method. Radiographics 16:185–195, 1996.
24. Damianou C, Pavlou M, Velev O, et al: High intensity focused ultrasound ablation of kidney guided by MRI. Ultrasound Med Biol 30:397–404, 2004.
25. Wu T, Felmlee JP, Greenleaf JF, et al: Assessment of thermal tissue ablation with MR elastography. Magn Reson Med 45:80–87, 2001.

26. Vaezy S, Shi X, Martin RW, et al: Real-time visualization of high-intensity focused ultrasound treatment using ultrasound imaging. Ultrasound Med Biol 27:33–42, 2001.

27. Souchon R, Rouviere O, Gelet A, et al: Visualisation of HIFU lesions using elastography of the human prostate in vivo: preliminary results. Ultrasound Med Biol 29:1007–1015, 2003.

28. Sedelaar JP, Aarnink RG, van Leenders GJ, et al: The application of three-dimensional contrast-enhanced ultrasound to measure volume of affected tissue after HIFU treatment for localized prostate cancer. Eur Urol 37:559–568, 2000.

29. Lu J, Ying H, Sun Z, et al: In vitro measurement of speed of sound during coagulate tissue heating. Ultrasonics Symp Proc IEEE 2:1299–1302, 1996.

30. Thüroff S, Chaussy C: Status of high intensity focused ultrasound (HIFU) in Urology in 2005. In Chaussy C et al (eds): Therapeutic Energy Applications in Urology. Stuttgart: Thieme Verlag 2005, pp 92–102.

31. Chaussy C, Thüroff S: High intensity focused ultrasound for the treatment of prostate cancer. In Moore RG, Bishoff JT (eds): Minimally Invasive Uro-oncologic Surgery. London: Taylor & Francis, 2005, pp 327–335.

32. Chaussy C, Thüroff S, Rebillard X, et al: Technology insight: high intensity focused ultrasound for urologic cancers. Nature Clin Pract Urol 2:191–198, 2005.

10 Prostate Cryoablation: Successful Therapy for Clinically Localized Prostate Cancer

Daniel B. Rukstalis and Mary Ann Kenneson

KEY POINTS

- Prostate cryoablation represents an effective image-guided percutaneous treatment for clinically localized prostate cancer.
- Metal cryoprobes were first developed in the 1960s for delivering liquid nitrogen and have evolved to 1.4 mm needles that carry argon gas as the cryogen.
- Modern prostate cryoablation was developed with the application of transrectal ultrasound guidance in the 1980s.
- Tissue temperatures below −40°C cause cell death through vascular injury, stimulation of apoptosis, and creation of intracellular ice crystals.
- Salvage prostate cryoablation for persistent prostate cancer following radiation therapy eradicates the cancer in 86% to 95% of cases.
- Primary prostatic cryoablation is associated with a positive postprocedure biopsy rate of 1% to 5% with a low risk of incontinence.
- Primary prostatic cryoablation is the least costly treatment alternative for clinically localized prostate cancer.
- The technique of prostate cryoablation provides flexibility in treatment planning that allows for a whole gland or subtotal gland destruction.
- A significant minority of men diagnosed with localized prostate cancer harbor small-volume and unilateral cancers that can be destroyed with an individualized subtotal cryoablation, further reducing treatment intensity and cost.

Introduction

Adventurers and physicians alike have long understood the lethal effects of cold temperatures on human tissues. The deleterious results of frostbite were obvious to early explorers and during military campaigns. In particular, the cycle of freezing followed by thawing and reperfusion produced visible injury to the fingers and toes of people exposed to cold temperatures. Physicians have also attempted to harness these destructive effects for treatment of surface lesions of the skin and cervix. Technologic advances in the 1960s enabled physicians to deliver lethal cold temperatures to deeper anatomic structures such as the retina, brain, kidney, and prostate. Metal needles called *cryoprobes* (demonstrated in Fig. 10-1) were cooled to temperatures below −150°C with liquid nitrogen and positioned into structures such as the prostate using transurethral or open exposure.[1,2] Clinical reports demonstrated the efficacy of these approaches but also emphasized the challenges of limiting the tissue damage to the targeted organ or tissue site.

In particular, open prostate cryoablation was attempted for the treatment of both benign and malignant prostatic diseases with acceptable efficacy.[3,4] Furthermore, both animal models and clinical experience in men with prostate cancer suggested an advantageous immunologic effect of the cryoprostatectomy.[5,6] However, clinical trials also demonstrated persistence of cancer on follow-up biopsy and associated injury to the nearby bladder and rectum. In addition, concomitant injury of the urethra resulted in bladder outlet obstruction from sloughing of necrotic tissue and the development of fibrotic strictures. Therefore, further innovation was required to improve the placement of the cryoprobes, improve the control of the iceball created within the prostate, and avoid injury to adjacent structures.

The remainder of this chapter details the process of innovation in prostatic cryosurgery, examines the basic and translational science behind this technique, and reviews the clinical

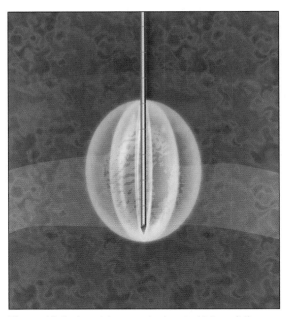

Figure 10-1. A metal cryoprobe inserted into soft tissue is depicted with a surrounding iceball. (Courtesy of Endocare, Inc.)

reports that have established prostate cryoablation as an effective treatment alternative for clinically localized prostatic adenocarcinoma.

History of Cryosurgical Innovation

Physicians became interested in cryoablation of the prostate before robots, biomedical engineering programs, and quality-of-life instruments. However, the principles of engineering and outcomes research lie at the center of the series of innovations that together have resulted in modern cryosurgery. Once a metal probe that could be cooled by liquid nitrogen became available in the 1960s, Soanes and coworkers[7] inserted the blunt-ended probe transurethrally into the prostatic adenoma to treat bladder outlet obstruction. The size of the iceball was monitored by digital examination. The subsequent need for improved patient safety resulted in the procedural modification of open placement of the cryoprobes through a perineal incision that could protect the rectum. Although apparently efficacious, the unattractive outcome of urethral sloughing and further obstruction inhibited further innovation for cryosurgery in the treatment of benign prostatic hyperplasia.

Treatment for prostatic cancer, on the other hand, provided an opportunity for technical application of cryoablation in an attempt to reduce therapy-related adverse events. Flocks and coworkers used a flat cryoprobe that was placed against the prostate through a perineal incision designed to avoid both urethral and sphincteric injury.[8] This experience reinforced the tissue destructive effects of cold temperatures and demonstrated the requirement for more precise methods of application. Subsequently, Megalli and coworkers[9] reported in 1974 on the percutaneous placement of a 6.3-mm cryoprobe into the prostate through a small skin incision. Digital examination was used to guide the freezing process while the cryoprobes were repositioned to ensure complete destruction of the prostate. Again, this approach demonstrated effective tissue destruction but was associated with unacceptable rates of urethral and rectal injury.

Prostate cryoablation remained only a potential therapeutic option until the development and application of transrectal ultrasound (TRUS) in the late 1980s. TRUS provided a minimally invasive mechanism for guiding the percutaneous placement of the cooling probes while identifying the extent of the freezing process. Onik and coworkers[10] first described the ultrasound characteristics of the advancing ice front as a hyperechoic rim. Subsequently, this same group demonstrated the appearance of the frozen prostate again as a hyperechoic rim with posterior shadowing.[11] Furthermore, TRUS also proved useful for the real-time monitoring of the percutaneous placement of the echogenic cryoprobes into the prostate. This advance in imaging established the platform for what has become modern cryoablation of the prostate.

Although improvements in ultrasound imaging provided the opportunity for improved probe placement and the ability to monitor the anatomic location of the ice front, challenges remained with the actual process of freezing the prostate. The percutaneous technique appeared highly effective in animal models.[12] However, the challenges became clear once men were treated with the new TRUS-guided percutaneous prostate cryoablation procedure in 1990.[13] Translational research experiments had established the requirement for cold temperatures to reach below $-20°C$ to reliably eradicate prostatic cancer cells.[14] Therefore, initial cryoablation systems were designed to achieve those temperatures as rapidly as possible. These early units were based on the application of liquid nitrogen as the cryogen with the ability to independently power five individual cryoprobes. The iceball created by the vacuum insulated cryoprobes reached −209°C at the center with an elongated ellipsoid shape that engulfed the prostate and a margin of surrounding tissue.[13] Preliminary clinical series confirmed the efficacy of the procedure but also identified significant associated toxicities of urethral sloughing, urinary obstruction and rectal injury resulting in rectourethral fistula. The associated adverse events were due primarily to the inherent limitations of controlling the delivery of liquid nitrogen. Despite the ability of TRUS to visualize the advancing ice front and the ability of thermocouples to measure the temperature of the tissue at critical points, the iceball often advanced into nearby structures such as the rectum with deleterious consequences. It is important to note that clinical evidence of oncologic efficacy from pooled patient series was sufficient to convince the Centers for Medicare and Medicaid Services (CMS) to approve prostate cryoablation for reimbursement.[15] However, the procedure was quickly relegated to the periphery of medical practice until further technologic advancements were completed.

Cryosurgical innovators and their engineering counterparts focused on three critical aspects of the prostate cryoablation procedure. Oncologic efficacy required the ability to rapidly and accurately shape the lethal iceball to fit the desired volume of tissue to be destroyed. Furthermore, such destruction threatened the urethra and the rectum with injury and therefore limited the ability to effectively treat the prostate cancer. Although the use of liquid nitrogen as the cryogenic agent resulted in sufficiently cold temperatures for tissue destruction, the inability to rapidly alter the freezing process stimulated innovative solutions. The solution was to develop argon gas–based units that took advantage of the Joule-Thompson effect to cool the cryoprobes. This effect occurs when a gas under high pressure expands through a narrow orifice into a lower pressure chamber. The expanding argon gas rapidly cooled to approximately −186°C at the probe tip, resulting in lethal cold temperatures that could be switched on and off very easily to more safely shape the ice to fit the treatment volume of tissue. In addition, the argon gas system can power many more probes,

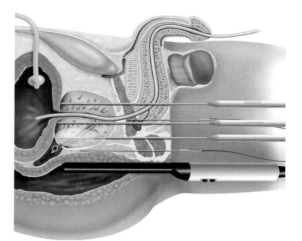

Figure 10-2. The position of the endorectal ultrasound probe with percutaneous placement of several cryoprobes and thermosensors.   A warming catheter is present in the urethra. A suprapubic tube has been placed, as was common with the initial technique. (Courtesy of Endocare, Inc.)

again facilitating a more accurate shape of the lethal ice to fit the desired treatment plan. These cryoprobes were designed to facilitate percutaneous placement through the perineum under ultrasound guidance, as demonstrated in Figure 10-2.

Another seminal advance involved the development of a urethral warming catheter designed to maintain the urethral wall at a warm temperature. Previous prostate cryoablation techniques resulted in injury to the urethral wall with secondary necrosis, obstruction, and stricture formation. The urethral warming catheter comprises a pump and fluid warmer that circulates a saline solution through a balloon catheter designed to preserve a thin layer of urethral mucosa and approximately 3 mm of underlying tissue.[16] The routine application of this catheter, which is considered an integral aspect of modern prostate cryoablation, has been associated with a reduction in the incidence of both urethral sloughing and rectal injury.

The third important quality improvement in the technique of prostate cryoablation focused on the technique rather than technology. The rapid expansion of the lethal iceball toward the rectum with the liquid nitrogen units was associated with an unacceptably high incidence of rectal injury and secondary rectourethral fistula. The development of argon gas–based equipment facilitated the use of multiple small cryoprobes that allowed the development of a new template for probe placement. The initial template with the liquid nitrogen machines involved the placement of five cryoprobes, with one of the probes placed anterior to the rectum beneath the urethra. This template often resulted in growth of ice into the anterior rectal wall before the remainder of the posterior prostatic capsule was completely engulfed in lethal ice. The development of smaller cryoprobes (1.4 to 2.4 mm) cooled with the Joule-Thompson effect provided the opportunity for cryosurgeons to establish a new probe orientation. The modern orientation involves placement of six to eight cryoprobes with no cryoprobe placed anterior to the rectum. The placement of cryoprobes into the prostate in an array designed to cover the entire prostate with ice is depicted in Figure 10-3. This approach has successfully reduced the incidence or rectal injury and rectourethral fistula while improving the ability to completely ablate the prostatic tissue.[17]

The overall outcome of these quality improvements in the equipment and technique of prostatic cryoablation has been the development of a minimally invasive outpatient procedure for the management of clinically localized prostatic adenocarcinoma. This treatment approach is potentially the optimal approach for several of the most vexing clinical problems urologists face with prostate cancer. These problems include salvage therapy for clinically persistent prostate cancer within the prostate gland following primary radiation therapy and locally advanced prostate cancer that is difficult to manage with radical prostatectomy or external-beam radiation therapy.[18–21]

Basic Science of Prostate Cryoablation

Clinical investigators have long recognized the sensitivity of human tissue to cold-induced injury. Cold ice-salt mixtures were used in the 19th century to treat breast and cervical cancer. The use of metallic probes to deliver cold temperatures more precisely were first reported in the 1960s. In 1965, Cooper[22] first reported that temperatures of −20°C for 1 minute would induce necrosis and cell death. Subsequently, both basic science and clinical physician-scientists began an effort to understand and optimize the treatment of human disease with cold temperatures.

Cryosurgery involves the freezing and thawing of tissue by means of cryoprobes inserted into a targeted tissue area. Isotherms are created around each probe and extend radially until a normothermic temperature is reached. The temperatures can be as low as −190°C at the cryoprobe and warm to 0°C at the ice ball periphery.[23] The margin of the cold zone appears hyperechoic on ultrasound examination providing a definable freeze margin. Beyond this margin, tissues gradually transition to a normothermic temperature. As a result, cells in different regions experience varying thermal histories. The cells near the probe are cooled rapidly and to a lower temperature than those farther from the probe. The mechanisms of cellular injury from cold temperatures are related to the thermal conditions experienced by the cells. Cellular death can result from direct cell injury from mechanical destruction with ice formation, vascular injury with ischemia due to endovascular cell death, and apoptosis resulting from cellular biochemical injury.

There are two proposed mechanisms for direct cellular injury. The first mechanism results from rapid cooling of cells nearest the cryoprobe with the formation of intracellular ice crystals. During rapid cooling, the water in the cell fails to equilibrate with the extracellular environment such that the intracellular solution becomes supercooled, leading to the formation of intracellular ice. The ice crystals form on a nucleation site and result in mechanical disruption of the

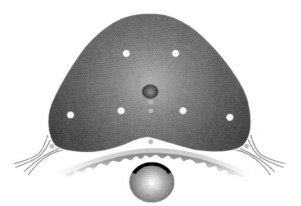

Figure 10-3. A transverse depiction of the prostate with an endorectal ultrasound probe in rectum and an array of six cryoprobes positioned in the prostate. The central smaller dots represent positions for thermal monitoring probes. (Courtesy of Endocare, Inc.)

cell membrane.[24] All living cells exposed to the effect of intracellular ice formation are destroyed. Several investigators working with both cell and tissue culture experiments have determined that the critical temperature for complete cell destruction is −40°C.[14,25] The region nearest the cryoprobe where intracellular ice develops is called the *zone of direct cell destruction* and has been located 10 to 17 mm from the leading edge of the ice ball.

The second proposed mechanism for cellular injury and secondary cell death involves slow cooling with a resultant solution effect. During slow cooling, which occurs farther from the cryoprobe near the periphery of the visible ice ball, ice forms preferentially in the extracellular space. The development of ice crystals incorporates only pure water, thereby causing an increase in extracellular osmolality. Water shifts from the intracellular compartment to the extracellular space with secondary dehydration of the cells.[24] Both the intracellular osmolality and the intracellular pH are altered leading to protein denaturation. The process appears to be cumulative, time dependent, and most damaging during the thaw phase. These biochemical effects damage the cell membrane, increasing the permeability to ion flow, and weaken the cytoskeleton, thus leading to increased sensitivity to mechanical injury. Figure 10-4 demonstrates the cellular effects of both rapid and slow cooling.

The ability of cold temperatures to damage cells can also invoke other pathways that result in cell death and tissue necrosis. In particular, vascular endothelial cells are highly sensitive to cold-related injury. The damaged endothelial cells become more permeable, which leads to platelet aggregation and microthrombus formation.[26] The specific temperature required to cause irreversible vascular injury is uncertain. However, experiments suggest that the temperature range between −10°C and −20°C is likely to be sufficiently cold.[27,28]

Finally, cold temperatures in the range of −5°C to −15°C have been shown to induce mitochondrial-mediated apoptosis through the upregulation of BCL-2-related proteins.[29,30] Tissue freezing activates apoptotic cascades through modulation of the opposing members of the BCL-2 protein family. Clarke and coworkers[31,32] demonstrated the synergistic effect of cold-induced cellular injury and pro-apoptotic chemotherapeutic agents in a cell culture model, suggesting that the addition of systemic pharmacologic agents may be helpful in the clinical applications of cryoablation.

Clinical Applications of Prostate Cryoablation

Salvage Cryoablation for Persistent Clinically Localized Prostate Cancer Following Radiation Therapy

The delivery of ionizing radiation to the prostate has long been an acceptable treatment option for men with prostatic adenocarcinoma. The potential for a curative treatment with minimal morbidity is attractive to many men and their physicians. In addition, other men with multiple medical comorbid conditions elect radiation therapy for prostate cancer in an effort to avoid the actual and perceived risks of radical prostatectomy. Ultimately, a total of approximately 60,000 men each year receive radiation therapy by one of several modalities to try to eradicate their putatively clinically localized disease.

Several prospective and retrospective clinical investigations have demonstrated that between 11% and 71% of men managed with definitive radiation therapy harbor persistent adenocarcinoma within the prostate gland on prostate biopsy after treatment with the various forms of prostatic radiation therapy.[33–39] Salvage radical prostatectomy specimens further demonstrate that the persistent cancer is located at the site of the primary cancer within the prostate. This suggests that improved targeting of salvage therapy will eradicate the remaining cancer

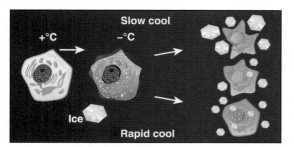

Figure 10-4. The development of ice in tissue as the temperature is reduced.   Ice crystals form in the extracellular compartment initially. During a rapid cool process, intracellular ice crystals form, mechanically disrupting the cell membrane. During a slow cool process, ice continues to form extracellularly, resulting in solute effects on the cell. (Courtesy of Endocare, Inc.)

volume.[40] Also, clinical evidence suggests that locally persistent prostate cancer after radiation therapy is a likely cause of subsequent metastatic disease.[41] Therefore, as many as 20,000 men will be identified each year with nonmetastatic and clinically localized prostate cancer and may be candidates for curative salvage therapy. Although the treatment options available to these men at this new juncture may mirror the options initially presented to them, the implications of the prostate cancer do not.

Persistent adenocarcinoma within the prostate after definitive radiation therapy represents a more aggressive disease state compared with the situation before therapy. These cancers demonstrate a 24% increase in Gleason score of 8–10 cancers and a 31% increase in aneuploid tumors when compared with pretreatment characteristics.[38] Salvage radical prostatectomy series further reveal that these cancers are often large in volume and associated with extracapsular extension with positive margins in 40% to 60% and with lymph node metastases in 14% to 34%.[42] Furthermore, only 30% to 62% of the radical prostatectomy specimens contain organ-confined cancer with the majority (51%) exhibiting a cancer volume of greater than 5 cm^3.[43] Clearly, recurrent prostatic adenocarcinoma following curative radiation therapy represents a serious health risk to these patients. Although some patient subgroups such as men older than 70 years of age may manifest a lower risk of cancer related adverse events from recurrent clinically localized cancer, most men likely require additional salvage treatment.[44]

Radiation therapy of all forms damages both benign and malignant glandular epithelium, which is subsequently removed from the prostate through the process of apoptosis. This process can be delayed and may require many months following the completion of therapy. Therefore, it is difficult to develop an effective pathway for the timely diagnosis of residual cancer. In particular, serum PSA levels decline slowly over 6 to 18 months after radiation, sometimes requiring 33 months to reach the nadir value.[37,45] Serum PSA levels can actually rise after brachytherapy and often fluctuate during post-treatment surveillance due to benign disease. The optimal PSA value for the diagnosis of residual disease and treatment failure following radiation therapy is uncertain with multiple criteria under consideration.[46,47]

Note that several salvage radical prostatectomy patient series have emphasized that early diagnosis and treatment of persistent clinically localized disease, prior to a PSA higher than 10 ng/mL, result in improved cancer-specific survival rates.[43,48] Because the timely diagnosis of persistent prostatic cancer confined to the prostate is critical for a second chance at curative therapy, a decision must be made for post-radiation prostate biopsy. A potentially clinically useful PSA parameter would be a PSA nadir lower than 0.5 ng/mL. Approximately 90% of men who achieve such a level within 2 years remain free of recurrent disease.[49] It can be proposed that a treatment algorithm that includes a prostatic biopsy at 12 to 24 months after definitive radiation therapy—for either an elevation in the serum PSA or failure to reach an acceptable nadir value—is likely to identify clinically significant residual cancer in a large minority of men. The timing of this diagnosis is consistent with the expectation of clinically localized cancer amenable to salvage curative treatment.

Current clinical practice often results in the delayed diagnosis of persistent prostatic cancer following radiation therapy. This general approach is likely a result of the community understanding of the overall toxicity of a salvage radical prostatectomy and the inability of systemic hormonal therapy to eradicate the cancer. Therefore, an early diagnosis of persistent cancer is unattractive for most patients and their physicians. This hypothesis is supported by the finding that most physicians treat radiation-recurrent prostate cancer with testosterone ablation therapy and believe that only 2% to 5% of men are candidates for curative salvage therapy.[50] However, modern salvage radical prostatectomy series have demonstrated an improved toxicity profile, whereas new modalities such as prostate cryoablation offer a minimally invasive option with fewer adverse consequences.[51–54]

The remainder of this section focuses on the clinical evidence supporting the application of ultrasound-guided percutaneous prostate cryoablation for the treatment of prostatic adenocarcinoma following definitive radiation therapy.

One of the earliest publications regarding salvage prostate cryoablation demonstrated an 86% negative biopsy rate at 3 months after the procedure but was associated with an almost universal incidence of aderse events.[55] This report suggested that salvage cryoablation—at least with the liquid nitrogen–based equipment available at the time—was associated with excessive morbidity. However, other investigators continued to report attractive negative biopsy rates of salvage cryoablation as high as 93%, which served to maintain a modest interest in this modality.[56] The advent of gas-based cryoablation equipment in the late 1990s created the clinical platform to readdress the application of cryoablation in the salvage setting. Katz and coworkers demonstrated in 2000 that the new technology could maintain the high negative biopsy rate while reducing the incidence of adverse events such as incontinence and rectourethral fistula.[57] Since that time, several single-institution patient series have been published that firmly established salvage prostate cryoablation as an effective and minimally morbid second-chance curative treatment for prostate cancer.[18,58–60] These publications consistently demonstrate a negative prostate biopsy rate of 86% to 95%. This is associated with a 5- to 7-year biochemical disease-free survival rate of 40% to 68% for a PSA cutoff of less than 0.5 ng/mL. This rate increases to 71% to 92% when using the ASTRO definition for PSA failure following radiation therapy.[61] Furthermore, the incidence of rectourethral fistula has been reduced to 0% to 3% and that of urinary incontinence to 0% to 13%.[18,62]

In summation, ultrasound-guided percutaneous cryoablation of the prostate with argon gas–based equipment represents an attractive treatment option for men diagnosed with persistent clinically localized prostate cancer following radiation therapy. The efficacy of cryoablation, as with all salvage options, is enhanced with early detection efforts that identify the residual cancer with a serum PSA lower than 4 to 10 ng/mL. Since any therapy in the salvage setting is associated with an unavoidable incidence of adverse events, these men must receive a complete staging evaluation before an attempt at curative treatment. This evaluation should include a bone scan, pelvic nodal imaging, and possibly a pelvic lymph node dissection.[60,63] Properly selected men should expect disease-specific survival rates as high as 92% at 8 years. A comparison of clinical outcomes of salvage radical prostatectomy and salvage cryoablation patient series is presented in Table 10-1.

Table 10-1. Clinical Outcomes of Salvage Therapy

Author	Type	No.	% Incont	Rectal Injury	BR (%)
Pontes, 1993[52]	RP	43	30	9	60
Rogers, 1995[53]	RP	40	58	15	75
Amling, 1999[51]	RP	108	23	6	74
Lee, 1997	Cryo	46	9	9	53
Bahn, 2003[59]	Cryo	59		0	31
Katz, 2006*	Cryo	161	8.8	0	31

BR, biochemical recurrence; Cryo, cryoablation; RP, radical prostatectomy.
*Treatment outcomes from Katz 2006 were published in Rukstalis DB, Katz A (eds): Handbook of Urologic Cryoablation. Informa UK, Ltd. London: 2007.

Cryoablation as Primary Therapy for Clinically Localized Prostate Cancer

Sometimes it may seem to men with newly diagnosed prostate cancer that there are as many treatment options as there are physicians who treat the disease. The bewildering variety of treatments and modifications of those treatments make selecting therapy a challenge for patients and physicians alike. However, despite the apparently disparate collection of options, there are several unifying concepts for all validated treatment approaches for clinically localized prostate cancer. Each treatment has been developed to eradicate the entire cancer while minimizing the treatment-associated side effects and cost. This conceptual framework has resulted in the development of nerve-sparing radical prostatectomy approaches, which now include robotic and laparoscopic techniques. Radiation therapy pathways have grown to include brachytherapy and targeted approaches such as intensity-modulated radiation therapy. Both the surgical and radiation categories of treatments have successfully improved oncologic efficacy and reduced, but not eliminated, treatment-related side effects. Therefore, it should come as no surprise that alternative options continue to be pursued by physician-scientists and patients alike. Ultrasound-guided percutaneous cryoablation of the prostate represents such an alternative option. This technique is capable of treating the entire prostate gland including the investing periprostatic fascia with a low rate of adverse events and the least cost of all validated treatment approaches. Figure 10-5 demonstrates such a procedure with the echogenic iceball clearly visible in the prostate.

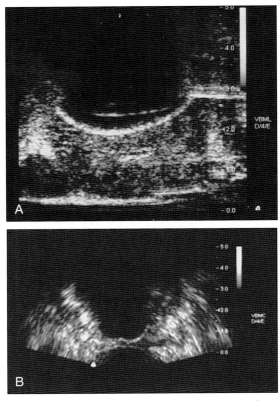

Figure 10-5. These ultrasound images demonstrate the hyperechoic iceball rim in the sagittal (**A**) and transverse (**B**) planes.

The application of a cryogen for the treatment of benign and malignant diseases of the prostate was first described in 1964 through an open surgical incision.[64] However, the addition of TRUS guidance in 1988 was required to establish the technique as a viable clinical alternative for men with prostate cancer.[11] The initial patient series, published in 1993, demonstrated that the percutaneous placement of five 3-mm cryoprobes into the prostate under ultrasound guidance resulted in an 82% negative postprocedure prostate biopsy.[13] These preliminary results involved liquid nitrogen as the cryogen delivered to the prostate percutaneously through the perineal skin. Despite the promising oncologic efficacy, the procedure was associated with many adverse effects including freezing of the rectal wall, the development of rectourethral fistula, urethral sloughing with secondary obstruction, perineal ecchymosis, and erectile dysfunction. Also important, stress urinary incontinence was an infrequent effect and remains rare in all subsequent published clinical series. The finding of

urethral sloughing emphasized the need for clinical innovation designed to protect the prostatic urethral lumen while destroying the surrounding prostatic parenchyma. Therefore, a urethral catheter was designed that served to circulate warm fluid through the urethral lumen during the cryoablation process.[65] Ultimately, the placement of the urethral warming device has become an established component of the prostate cryoablation technique.

In 1996, Cohen and coworkers[66] published an updated patient series that included 383 patients most of whom were followed up for over 21 months using a prostate biopsy. A total of 60% of men were found to have a negative biopsy after one cryoablation and 82% after a second cryoablation was performed. Serum PSA information was available for 163 subjects after 21 months of evaluation, with 60% exhibiting a PSA below 0.4 ng/mL and 77% below 1.0 ng/mL. It is noteworthy that the incidence of adverse events had greatly decreased with urethral sloughing—now occurring in 10% of cases with the urethral warming device. These initial reports confirmed the oncologic efficacy of the new ultrasound-guided procedure. Moreover, a subsequent multi-institutional pooled analysis was published by Long and co-investigators in 2001 that resulted in approval for reimbursement of the procedure from CMS.[15] This report analyzed the outcomes of prostate cryoablation as primary therapy in 975 men with clinically localized prostate cancer. The surgical approach was designed to destroy the entire prostate and incorporated some form of the urethral warming catheter. It is interesting that this pooled analysis also demonstrated that 82% of the men were without persistent cancer on follow-up prostate biopsy. The information regarding adverse outcomes included erectile dysfunction in 93%, incontinence in 7.5%, and rectourethral fistula in 0.5%. This analysis established the oncologic efficacy of prostate cryoablation with liquid nitrogen–based equipment and further documented a stable reduction in adverse consequences of the treatment.

As with most technical aspects of modern medicine, the drive for process and technologic improvement has been relentless in the field of cryoablation. The liquid nitrogen–based machines provided the initial platform for the in situ destruction of the prostate with an energy source other than radiation. However, these machines possessed inherent limitations, such as a limit of five cryoprobes per procedure, the inability to terminate the freeze process once a desired endpoint was reached, and the lack of a method for warming tissue that could reduce operative times. These limitations stimulated clinical innovation and resulted in the development of argon gas–based units that were capable of delivering cold temperatures with 8 to 20 probes. These units incorporated thermosensors for monitoring the temperature of the treated tissues and the use of helium gas to warm the probes. In 1999, Lee and coworkers[17] reported a comparison of the new gas-based equipment with six to eight cryoprobes per each prostate with the liquid nitrogen technique using five cryoprobes. The new equipment resulted in an improved ability to ablate the entire prostatic parenchyma with a reduction in the median postprocedure serum PSA level (0.07 ng/mL versus 0.1 ng/mL). Subsequently, additional authors have provided patient series that confirm, and further extend, the oncologic and toxicity data from this initial report.[61,67–69] Perhaps most important, the rate of persistent cancer within the prostate gland after an initial cryoablation has fallen from the early reports of 18% positive biopsy rates to 1% to 5%.[70,71]

The modern conceptual framework for process and technologic innovation in prostatic cancer treatment incorporates patient-reported quality-of-life outcomes. Specific health services research uses validated instruments such as questionnaires to extend the traditional toxicity data produced from retrospective chart reviews and physician-based reports. Several investigators have published such patient-focused data for primary prostatic cryoablation. Smith and co-investigators[72] performed a retrospective analysis of 2234 men diagnosed with prostate cancer in a longitudinal prostate cancer screening program using a mailed quality-of-life questionnaire. A total of 2% of the men received treatment with cryoablation. This study found that only 9% of men treated with any modality complained of significant urinary incontinence at 12 months after therapy. It is interesting that only 45% of men treated with cryoablation described significant bother from erectile dysfunction with only observation performing better in this domain. Despite the small number of men treated with cryoablation, this study demonstrated that this technique compares very

favorably with the other established treatment approaches. This finding was echoed by Ball and coworkers[73] with a prospective quality-of-life analysis of 719 men treated with each of the established modalities. This group discovered that 498 men adequately completed 12 months of follow-up with completion of the UCLA Prostate Cancer Index and that 18% of those men treated with cryoablation returned to baseline in the sexual function domain by 12 months. Moreover, cryoablation appeared equivalent to brachytherapy at 6 months regarding urinary function except for a poorer outcome of brachytherapy for irritative urinary symptoms.

Several publications have provided more focused information regarding the experiences of men treated with cryoablation. In 1999, Robinson and colleagues[74] reported the results of a 12-month prospective analysis using the Functional Assessment of Cancer Treatment-Prostate questionnaire (FACT-P), which demonstrated that men had returned to baseline quality of life in all domains except for sexual functioning by 12 months. This group updated the results at 3 years after cryoablation, which demonstrated stable quality of life without new complications. A total of 13% of men had returned to baseline sexual function, and an additional 34% resumed sexual activity with therapy.[75] Badalament and coworkers[76] reported on 223 men managed with primary cryoablation who were evaluated with a questionnaire mailed retrospectively following treatment. These men described a 4.3% incidence of incontinence that required one absorbent pad each day; erectile dysfunction was a complaint in 85%, and 10% required a subsequent procedure to manage urethral sloughing. Overall, 96% of men reported a high degree of satisfaction with the treatment.

The final tenet for a successful prostate cancer treatment modality involves the cost of treatment. Several investigators have examined the cost of cryoablation relative to the other established management techniques. One comparison of open radical prostatectomy to cryoablation demonstrated a 27% lower cost for cryoablation, which was predominantly related to operative room costs and length of hospital stay.[77] A second report evaluated costs of treatment for 452 men treated with an open retropubic prostatectomy, a radical perineal prostatectomy, a laparoscopic prostatectomy, or cryoablation.[78] Again, prostate cryoablation was the least costly strategy despite an elevated equipment cost in the operating room. The cost reduction was due primarily to a reduction in pathology charges and hospital length-of-stay differences. Taken together, these patient-focused investigations with the financial cost analysis support prostate cryoablation for the management of clinically localized prostatic adenocarcinoma and emphasize the low risk of serious adverse outcomes for treatment.

Patient-Specific Modifications of Prostate Cryoablation for Primary Treatment of Low-Risk Prostate Cancer

The surgical approach to prostate cryoablation has been established as a whole gland treatment designed to destroy the entire prostate and periprostatic tissue. This technique is consistent with the therapeutic intentions of all other treatment options such as radical prostatectomy and radiation therapy. The core scientific principle underlying the desire to treat the entire prostate, with the obligatory risks of collateral damage to adjacent structures, states that prostatic adenocarcinoma is a multifocal disease that is often peppered throughout a palpably normal prostate.[79] The analysis of prostatic specimens from radical prostatectomy series consistently demonstrates an incidence of multifocal prostatic cancer of 70% to 85%.[80-82] Therefore, it has long been assumed that total prostate gland ablation is absolutely required to ensure long-term survival for men diagnosed with localized prostate cancer.

This assumption should be reexamined since clinical research into the natural history of prostatic cancer in men has suggested that the disease commonly exhibits a protracted course. In 1994, Chodak and coworkers published a pooled analysis of 828 men managed with observation for the diagnosis of localized prostatic cancer.[83] The 10-year disease-specific survival for well and moderately well differentiated cancers was 87%. This finding has been extended further by Carter and others[84] into the concept of active surveillance with curative therapy delivered if evidence of progression is identified. In a report examining a total of 407 men, the majority (59%) remained on observation at a median follow-up of 3.4 years.[84] Increasingly, extended prostate biopsy protocols appear to identify men with clinically insignificant prostate cancer volume.[85]

Certainly, many men harbor cancers that are unlikely to result in their death but still present a challenging therapeutic dilemma.

Although the pathologic analysis of radical prostatectomy specimens consistently demonstrates multifocal prostate cancer, serum PSA-based early detection programs appear to have resulted in a reduction in the number of individual cancers and an overall reduction in the tumor volume at the time of diagnosis and treatment. One early analysis of multifocal cancer discovered 500 individual cancers in the prostate specimens from 234 men.[86] It is interesting that 117 of the glands contained only a single cancer considered to be the palpably manifest cancer. These investigators also demonstrated that most prostates contained cancer volumes greater than $4 \, cm^3$ and that only 10% were below $0.5 \, cm^3$. Despite the larger total cancer volume and the identification of multiple cancers in 50% of specimens, the authors concluded from this analysis that prostate cancer was never diffusely distributed within the prostate but rather an expansion of cancer from a single region of the prostate. In addition, the total volume of all cancer foci within the prostate is rarely larger than the volume of the known or index cancer. These same investigators examined a cohort of 139 prostate glands from men treated with cystoprostatectomy for bladder cancer.[87] A total of 55 of the 139 samples contained at least one focus of prostatic adenocarcinoma, with 92% demonstrating a total cancer volume of less than $0.5 \, cm^3$. Taken together, these two reports provided the data that established the cancer volume of $0.5 \, cm^3$ as the threshold for clinically significant prostate cancer.

In 2001, Noguchi and coworkers[88] evaluated the histologic features of cancer in 222 radical prostatectomy specimens. The mean volume of the index cancer was $1.86 \, cm^3$, and it appeared that the overall cancer volume was now below $4 \, cm^3$. It is noteworthy that 73% of the men were found to have unilateral prostate cancer on prostate biopsy before the radical prostatectomy. In addition, approximately 19% to 35% of men with a single positive prostate biopsy or no evidence of Gleason pattern 4/5 cancer on biopsy had less than $0.5 \, cm^3$ cancer volume in the radical prostatectomy specimen. Despite the finding that no single parameter on biopsy was found to be predictive of the tumor volume, it did appear that a growing percentage of men treated with radical prostatectomy possess small volume and potentially regionally localized prostate cancer. Chan and associates[89] further demonstrated in 2001 that 25% of 297 men treated with radical prostatectomy manifested cancer volumes less than 0.5 cm^3 and that the mean tumor volume of the study population was 1.6 cm^3. Again, these results suggest that early detection programs identify men with a reduced overall tumor volume associated with fewer ancillary lesions. Epstein and coworkers[90] completed this analysis with a report in 2005 examining the prostates of 103 men treated with radical prostatectomy with the expectation of low volume prostate cancer on the preoperative saturation prostate biopsy. The biopsy parameters that appeared to correlate with low-volume cancer included no single prostate core with more than 50% involvement, Gleason score less than 7, and fewer than three cores involved. If these characteristics were present in the biopsy, a total of 71% of the prostates contained less than 0.5 cm^3 total cancer volume. Table 10-2 provides further information regarding the results of reported prostate biopsy series demonstrating that a large minority of men present with putative low-volume prostate cancer. These publications analyzed the results of prostate biopsy paradigms relative to the pathologic findings on radical prostatectomy to understand the predictive ability of the biopsy.

Against this backdrop of a significant minority of men with low-volume prostate cancer, the toxicity profile of whole gland destructive strategies must be evaluated. Certainly, a strong argument can be made for noncurative therapy such as active surveillance for men in this clinical situation, because the cancer would be unlikely to progress to systemic disease within 10 years of diagnosis. However, the finding of clinical local progression in up to 31.5% of men with putatively low-volume and low-risk cancer by 3 years supports the risk-based strategy of curative therapy even in this circumstance.[90] It is likely that many patients and their physicians would find a minimally invasive and targeted ablative approach to the destruction of the cancer-containing region of the prostate as attractive. Ultrasound-guided percutaneous prostate cryoablation has demonstrated the flexibility to achieve this individualized treatment outcome. As a result, many patients have received such a focal therapy with the understanding that the toxicity is low and that the procedure can be repeated if necessary.

The initial report of focal cryoablation appeared in 2002 and contained the experience of nine men treated with a focal nerve-sparing cryoablation.[92] The men were followed up for a mean of 36 months with six men receiving a negative postcryoablation prostate biopsy. None of the patients developed urinary incontinence, and 70% maintained normal potency. This potentially transformative publication has been followed subsequently by reports from other investigators that suggest similar outcomes. Bahn and associates[93] described a series of 31 men treated with focal cryoablation for low-volume prostate cancer with a 96% negative follow-up biopsy rate, 88% preservation of potency, and no evidence of urinary incontinence. Lambert and coworkers[94] published their series of 25 men treated with focal therapy in 2007 and demonstrated that 17 of the men maintained normal potency without evidence of incontinence or urethral toxicity. Note that with a mean follow-up of 28 months, three of seven men exhibited persistent microscopic prostate cancer on postcryoablation biopsy. These reports support the hypothesis that a less than total individualized prostate cryoablation technique

Table 10-2. Results of Prostate Needle Biopsy Patient Series

Author	No. of Men	No. of Cores	No. of Cores Positive	Unilateral/Unifocal Insignificant
Terris, 1992[91]	124	6	NA	21.7% Unifocal
Chan, 2001[89]	107	≤8	2.1	22.6% Insignificant
	190	≥9	2.8	25.4% Insignificant
Noguchi, 2001[88]	222	6.4 (6–13)	2.1 (1–7)	73%/35.1%
Epstein, 2005[90]	56	44 (24–54)	3 (1–21)	73% Insignificant
Haas, 2007[85]	164	18	NA	50% Insignificant

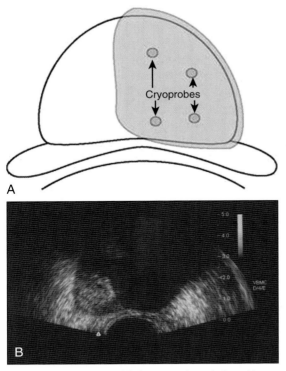

A

B

Figure 10-6. A, A cryoablation procedure designed to ablate the left side of the gland with the placement of four cryoprobes. (Courtesy of Endocare, Inc.) **B,** The ultrasound appearance of the iceball as it develops within the prostate.

can eradicate small-volume prostate cancer in the majority of men with minimal treatment-related toxicity. However, enthusiasm for this exciting new strategy must be tempered by the real likelihood of persistent prostatic cancer in 10% to 20% of men and the potential requirement for a second therapeutic procedure. The images in Figure 10-6 demonstrate the capability of an individualized prostate cryoablation to treat selected regions of the prostatic gland.

Summary

Ultrasound-guided percutaneous prostate cryo-ablation represents an attractive treatment modality for men with clinically localized prostatic adenocarcinoma. The scientific foundation of the destructive effect of cold temperatures suggests that even high-grade cancers can be eradicated with a local in situ-based approach. Clinical innovation has resulted in an improvement in the cryoablation equipment available to urologists and their patients over the past 15

years with an associated reduction in the adverse events associated with the therapy.

The generalized adoption of PSA-based early detection programs for prostate cancer has resulted in a shift to earlier-stage cancers with lower cancer volumes at the time of diagnosis. Therefore, more men are likely to be attracted to the minimally invasive nature of cryoablation for eradication of this lower-risk cancer. The technique is highly flexible and can be provided to men following radiation therapy as a salvage treatment. In addition, prostate cryoablation has been demonstrated to be an effective option for the primary treatment of localized prostate cancer with the capacity for further reduction in cost and toxicity by individualizing the treatment to focus on the cancer-containing region of the prostate gland.

References

1. Cooper IS, Lee AS: Cryostatic congelation: a system for producing a limited, controlled region of cooling or freezing of biologic tissues. J Nerv Ment Dis 133:259, 1961.
2. Gonder MJ, Soanes WA, Shulman S: Cryosurgical treatment of the prostate. Invest Urol 3:372, 1966.
3. Haschek H: Cryosurgery of prostate adenoma: evaluation of the method. Prog Clin Biol Res 6:73, 1976.
4. Petersen DS, Milleman LA, Rose EF, et al: Biopsy and clinical course after cryosurgery for prostatic cancer. J Urol 120:308, 1978.
5. Lubaroff DM, Reynolds CW, Culp DA: Immunologic studies of prostatic cancer using the R3327 rat model. Trans Am Assoc Genitourin Surg 70:60, 1978.
6. Guinan P, Ray P, Shaw M: Immunotherapy of prostate cancer: a review. Prostate 5:221, 1984.
7. Soanes WA, Gonder MJ, Shulman S: Apparatus and technique for cryosurgery of the prostate. J Urol 96:508, 1966.
8. Flocks RH, Nelson CM, Boatman DL: Perineal cryosurgery for prostatic carcinoma. J Urol 108:933, 1972.
9. Megalli MR, Gursel EO, Veenema RJ: Closed perineal cryosurgery in prostatic cancer. New probe and technique. Urology 4:220, 1974.
10. Onik G, Cooper C, Goldberg HI, et al: Ultrasonic characteristics of frozen liver. Cryobiology 21:321, 1984.
11. Onik G, Cobb C, Cohen J, et al: US characteristics of frozen prostate. Radiology 168:629, 1988.
12. Onik G, Porterfield B, Rubinsky B, et al: Percutaneous transperineal prostate cryosurgery using transrectal ultrasound guidance: animal model. Urology 37:277, 1991.
13. Onik GM, Cohen JK, Reyes GD, et al: Transrectal ultrasound-guided percutaneous radical cryosurgical ablation of the prostate. Cancer 72:1291, 1993.
14. Tatsutani K, Rubinsky B, Onik G, et al: Effect of thermal variables on frozen human primary prostatic adenocarcinoma cells. Urology 48:441, 1996.
15. Long JP, Bahn D, Lee F, et al: Five-year retrospective, multi-institutional pooled analysis of cancer-related outcomes after cryosurgical ablation of the prostate. Urology 57:518, 2001.
16. Cohen JK, Miller RJ, Shuman BA: Urethral warming catheter for use during cryoablation of the prostate. Urology 45:861, 1995.
17. Lee F, Bahn DK, Badalament RA, et al: Cryosurgery for prostate cancer: improved glandular ablation by use of 6 to 8 cryoprobes. Urology 54:135, 1999.
18. Anastasiadis AG, Sachdev R, Salomon L, et al: Comparison of health-related quality of life and prostate-associated symptoms after primary and salvage cryotherapy for prostate cancer. J Cancer Res Clin Oncol 129:676, 2003.

19. Galosi AB, Lugnani F, Muzzonigro G: Salvage cryosurgery for recurrent prostate carcinoma after radiotherapy. J Endourol 21:1, 2007.
20. Chin JL, Ng CK, Touma NJ, et al: Randomized trial comparing cryoablation and external beam radiotherapy for T2C-T3B prostate cancer. Prostate Cancer Prostatic Dis 11:40–45, 2008.
21. Mouraviev V, Polascik TJ: Update on cryotherapy for prostate cancer in 2006. Curr Opin Urol 16:152, 2006.
22. Cooper IS: Cryogenic surgery for cancer. Fed Proc 24:S237, 1965.
23. Baust J, Gage AA, Ma H, et al: Minimally invasive cryosurgery—technological advances. Cryobiology 34:373, 1997.
24. Mazur P: Cryobiology: the freezing of biological systems. Science 168:939, 1970.
25. Bischof JC, Smith D, Pazhayannur PV, et al: Cryosurgery of dunning AT-1 rat prostate tumor: thermal, biophysical, and viability response at the cellular and tissue level. Cryobiology 34:42, 1997.
26. Rubinsky B: Cryosurgery. Annu Rev Biomed Eng 2:157, 2000.
27. Hoffmann NE, Bischof JC: The cryobiology of cryosurgical injury. Urology 60:40, 2002.
28. Hoffmann NE, Bischof JC: Cryosurgery of normal and tumor tissue in the dorsal skin flap chamber: part I—thermal response. J Biomech Eng 123:301, 2001.
29. Baust JG, Gage AA, Clarke D, et al: Cryosurgery—a putative approach to molecular-based optimization. Cryobiology 48:190, 2004.
30. Clarke DM, Baust JM, Van Buskirk RG, et al: Addition of anticancer agents enhances freezing-induced prostate cancer cell death: implications of mitochondrial involvement. Cryobiology 49:45, 2004.
31. Clarke DM, Baust JM, Van Buskirk RG, et al: Chemo-cryo combination therapy: an adjunctive model for the treatment of prostate cancer. Cryobiology 42:274, 2001.
32. Clarke DM, Robilotto AT, Van Buskirk RG, et al: Targeted induction of apoptosis via TRAIL and cryoablation: a novel strategy for the treatment of prostate cancer. Prostate Cancer Prostatic Dis 10:175–184, 2007.
33. Morgan PB, Hanlon AL, Horwitz EM, et al: Timing of biochemical failure and distant metastatic disease for low-, intermediate-, and high-risk prostate cancer after radiotherapy. Cancer 110:68, 2007.
34. Deger S, Boehmer D, Roigas J, et al: High dose rate (HDR) brachytherapy with conformal radiation therapy for localized prostate cancer. Eur Urol 47:441, 2005.
35. Horwitz EM, Uzzo RG, Hanlon AL, et al: Modifying the American Society for Therapeutic Radiology and Oncology definition of biochemical failure to minimize the influence of backdating in patients with prostate cancer treated with 3-dimensional conformal radiation therapy alone. J Urol 169:2153, 2003.
36. Aygun C, Blum J, Stark L: Long-term clinical and prostate-specific antigen follow-up in 500 patients treated with radiation therapy for localized prostate cancer. Md Med J 44:363, 1995.
37. Crook JM, Choan E, Perry GA, et al: Serum prostate-specific antigen profile following radiotherapy for prostate cancer: implications for patterns of failure and definition of cure. Urology 51:566, 1998.
38. Siders DB, Lee F: Histologic changes of irradiated prostatic carcinoma diagnosed by transrectal ultrasound. Hum Pathol 23:344, 1992.
39. Stone NN, Stock RG, Unger P, et al: Biopsy results after real-time ultrasound-guided transperineal implants for stage T1-T2 prostate cancer. J Endourol 14:375, 2000.
40. Pucar D, Hricak H, Shukla-Dave A, et al: Clinically significant prostate cancer local recurrence after radiation therapy occurs at the site of primary tumor: magnetic resonance imaging and step-section pathology evidence. Int J Radiat Oncol Biol Phys 69:62, 2007.
41. Coen JJ, Zietman AL, Thakral H, et al: Radical radiation for localized prostate cancer: local persistence of disease results in a late wave of metastases. J Clin Oncol 20:3199, 2002.
42. Lerner SE, Blute ML, Zincke H: Critical evaluation of salvage surgery for radio-recurrent/resistant prostate cancer. J Urol 154:1103, 1995.
43. Cheng L, Sebo TJ, Slezak J, et al: Predictors of survival for prostate carcinoma patients treated with salvage radical prostatectomy after radiation therapy. Cancer 83:2164, 1998.
44. Petit JH, Chen MH, Loffredo M, et al: Prostate-specific antigen recurrence and mortality after conventional dose radiation

45. Critz FA, Levinson AK, Williams WH, et al: The PSA nadir that indicates potential cure after radiotherapy for prostate cancer. Urology 49:322, 1997.
46. Shipley WU, Thames HD, Sandler HM, et al: Radiation therapy for clinically localized prostate cancer: a multi-institutional pooled analysis. JAMA 281:1598, 1999.
47. Roach M III, Hanks G, Thames H, Jr, et al: Defining biochemical failure following radiotherapy with or without hormonal therapy in men with clinically localized prostate cancer: recommendations of the RTOG-ASTRO Phoenix Consensus Conference. Int J Radiat Oncol Biol Phys 65:965, 2006.
48. Stephenson AJ, Eastham JA: Role of salvage radical prostatectomy for recurrent prostate cancer after radiation therapy. J Clin Oncol 23:8198, 2005.
49. Zietman AL, Tibbs MK, Dallow KC, et al: Use of PSA nadir to predict subsequent biochemical outcome following external beam radiation therapy for T1–2 adenocarcinoma of the prostate. Radiother Oncol 40:159, 1996.
50. Schellhammer PF, Kuban DA, el-Mahdi AM: Treatment of clinical local failure after radiation therapy for prostate carcinoma. J Urol 150:1851, 1993.
51. Amling CL, Lerner SE, Martin SK, et al: Deoxyribonucleic acid ploidy and serum prostate specific antigen predict outcome following salvage prostatectomy for radiation refractory prostate cancer. J Urol 161:857, 1999.
52. Pontes JE, Montie J, Klein E, et al: Salvage surgery for radiation failure in prostate cancer. Cancer 71:976, 1993.
53. Rogers E, Ohori M, Kassabian VS, et al: Salvage radical prostatectomy: outcome measured by serum prostate specific antigen levels. J Urol 153:104, 1995.
54. Sanderson KM, Penson DF, Cai J, et al: Salvage radical prostatectomy: quality of life outcomes and long-term oncological control of radiorecurrent prostate cancer. J Urol 176:2025, 2006.
55. Bales GT, Williams MJ, Sinner M, et al: Short-term outcomes after cryosurgical ablation of the prostate in men with recurrent prostate carcinoma following radiation therapy. Urology 46:676, 1995.
56. Pisters LL, von Eschenbach AC, Scott SM, et al: The efficacy and complications of salvage cryotherapy of the prostate. J Urol 157:921, 1997.
57. de la Taille A, Hayek O, Benson MC, et al: Salvage cryotherapy for recurrent prostate cancer after radiation therapy: the Columbia experience. Urology 55:79, 2000.
58. Chin JL, Pautler SE, Mouraviev V, et al: Results of salvage cryoablation of the prostate after radiation: identifying predictors of treatment failure and complications. J Urol 165:1937, 2001.
59. Bahn DK, Lee F, Silverman P, et al: Salvage cryosurgery for recurrent prostate cancer after radiation therapy: a seven-year follow-up. Clin Prostate Cancer 2:111, 2003.
60. Ng CK, Moussa M, Downey DB, et al: Salvage cryoablation of the prostate: follow-up and analysis of predictive factors for outcome. J Urol 178:1253, 2007.
61. Bahn DK, Lee F, Badalament R, et al: Targeted cryoablation of the prostate: 7-year outcomes in the primary treatment of prostate cancer. Urology 60:3, 2002.
62. Ismail M, Ahmed S, Kastner C, et al: Salvage cryotherapy for recurrent prostate cancer after radiation failure: a prospective case series of the first 100 patients. BJU Int 100:760, 2007.
63. Chin JL, Lim D, Abdelhady M: Review of primary and salvage cryoablation for prostate cancer. Cancer Control 14:231, 2007.
64. Gonder MJ, Soanes WA, Smith V: Experimental prostate cryosurgery. Invest Urol 1:610, 1964.
65. Cohen JK, Miller RJ: Thermal protection of urethra during cryosurgery of prostate. Cryobiology 31:313, 1994.
66. Cohen JK, Miller RJ, Rooker GM, et al: Cryosurgical ablation of the prostate: two-year prostate-specific antigen and biopsy results. Urology 47:395, 1996.
67. Bahn DK, Silverman P, Lee F, Sr, et al: In treating localized prostate cancer the efficacy of cryoablation is independent of DNA ploidy type. Technol Cancer Res Treat 3:253, 2004.
68. Ellis DS: Cryosurgery as primary treatment for localized prostate cancer: a community hospital experience. Urology 60:34, 2002.
69. Zisman A, Pantuck AJ, Cohen JK, et al: Prostate cryoablation using direct transperineal placement of ultrathin probes through

therapy in select men with low-risk prostate cancer. Cancer 107:2180, 2006.

a 17-gauge brachytherapy template-technique and preliminary results. Urology 58:988, 2001.

70. Polascik TJ, Nosnik I, Mayes JM, et al: Short-term cancer control after primary cryosurgical ablation for clinically localized prostate cancer using third-generation cryotechnology. Urology 70:117, 2007.

71. Ellis DS, Manny TB, Jr, Rewcastle JC: Cryoablation as primary treatment for localized prostate cancer followed by penile rehabilitation. Urology 69:306, 2007.

72. Smith DS, Carvalhal GF, Schneider K, et al: Quality-of-life outcomes for men with prostate carcinoma detected by screening. Cancer 88:1454, 2000.

73. Ball AJ, Gambill B, Fabrizio MD, et al: Prospective longitudinal comparative study of early health-related quality-of-life outcomes in patients undergoing surgical treatment for localized prostate cancer: a short-term evaluation of five approaches from a single institution. J Endourol 20:723, 2006.

74. Robinson JW, Saliken JC, Donnelly BJ, et al: Quality-of-life outcomes for men treated with cryosurgery for localized prostate carcinoma. Cancer 86:1793, 1999.

75. Robinson JW, Donnelly BJ, Saliken JC, et al: Quality of life and sexuality of men with prostate cancer 3 years after cryosurgery. Urology 60:12, 2002.

76. Badalament RA, Bahn DK, Kim H, et al: Patient-reported complications after cryoablation therapy for prostate cancer. Arch Ital Urol Androl 72:305, 2000.

77. Benoit RM, Cohen JK, Miller RJ, Jr: Comparison of the hospital costs for radical prostatectomy and cryosurgical ablation of the prostate. Urology 52:820, 1998.

78. Mouraviev V, Nosnik I, Sun L, et al: Financial comparative analysis of minimally invasive surgery to open surgery for localized prostate cancer: a single-institution experience. Urology 69:311, 2007.

79. Stamey TA, Donaldson AN, Yemoto CE, et al: Histological and clinical findings in 896 consecutive prostates treated only with radical retropubic prostatectomy: epidemiologic significance of annual changes. J Urol 160:2412, 1998.

80. Rukstalis DB, Goldknopf JL, Crowley EM, et al: Prostate cryoablation: a scientific rationale for future modifications. Urology 60:19, 2002.

81. Mouraviev V, Mayes JM, Madden JF, et al: Analysis of laterality and percentage of tumor involvement in 1386 prostatectomized specimens for selection of unilateral focal cryotherapy. Technol Cancer Res Treat 6:91, 2007.

82. Epstein JI, Lecksell K, Carter HB: Prostate cancer sampled on sextant needle biopsy: significance of cancer on multiple cores from different areas of the prostate. Urology 54:291, 1999.

83. Chodak GW, Thisted RA, Gerber GS, et al: Results of conservative management of clinically localized prostate cancer. N Engl J Med 330:242–248, 1994.

84. Carter HB, Kettermann A, Warlick C, et al: Expectant management of prostate cancer with curative intent: an update of The Johns Hopkins Experience. J Urol 178:2359–2364, 2007.

85. Haas GP, Delongchamps NB, Jones RF, et al: Needle biopsies on autopsy prostates: sensitivity of cancer detection based on true prevalence. J Natl Cancer Inst 99:1484, 2007.

86. Villers A, McNeal JE, Freiha FS, et al: Multiple cancers in the prostate. Morphologic features of clinically recognized versus incidental tumors. Cancer 70:2313, 1992.

87. Stamey TA, Freiha FS, McNeal JE, et al: Localized prostate cancer. Relationship of tumor volume to clinical significance for treatment of prostate cancer. Cancer 71:933, 1993.

88. Noguchi M, Stamey TA, McNeal JE, et al: Relationship between systematic biopsies and histological features of 222 radical prostatectomy specimens: lack of prediction of tumor significance for men with nonpalpable prostate cancer. J Urol 166:104, 2001.

89. Chan TY, Chan DY, Stutzman KL, et al: Does increased needle biopsy sampling of the prostate detect a higher number of potentially insignificant tumors? J Urol 166:2181, 2001.

90. Epstein JI, Sanderson H, Carter HB, et al: Utility of saturation biopsy to predict insignificant cancer at radical prostatectomy. Urology 66:356, 2005.

91. Terris MK, McNeal JE, Stamey TA: Detection of clinically significant prostate cancer by transrectal ultrasound guided systematic biopsies. J Urol 148:829–832, 1992.

92. Onik G, Narayan P, Vaughan D, et al: Focal "nerve-sparing" cryosurgery for treatment of primary prostate cancer: a new approach to preserving potency. Urology 60:109, 2002.

93. Bahn DK, Silverman P, Lee F, Sr, et al: Focal prostate cryoablation: initial results show cancer control and potency preservation. J Endourol 20:688, 2006.

94. Lambert EH, Bolte K, Masson P, et al: Focal cryosurgery: encouraging health outcomes for unifocal prostate cancer. Urology 69:1117, 2007.

11 Alternative Medicine for Prostate Cancer: Diet, Vitamins, Minerals, and Supplements

Aaron Katz

KEY POINTS

- Prostate cancer is an excellent candidate for chemoprevention with nutrition because of its long latency, high incidence, and strong correlation with specific dietary factors.
- The highest likelihood of chemoprevention of prostate cancer is in the very earliest stages of the disease, that is, prostatic intraepithelial neoplasia (PIN).
- Current evidence supports a chemopreventive approach that incorporates reduction of inflammation (using omega-3 fatty acids and anti-inflammatory herbal supplements) and protection against oxidant damage (using antioxidant nutrients and herbs).
- Research into nutritional chemoprevention of prostate cancer is ongoing and highly promising, and it can be applied now with patients in the early stages of prostate cancer.
- Nutritional chemopreventive agents have no negative impact on potency or continence.

Introduction

Prostate cancer foci are believed to occur in 30% of men over age 50 and in 75% of men over 80.[1] Most of these foci remain latent and do not end up growing or spreading to any significant extent, and the occurrence of such foci is fairly consistent worldwide. Much evidence from epidemiologic surveys, as well as from laboratory, intervention, and case-control studies, suggests that diet may be a crucial factor in the transformation of a latent or slow-growing focus into a more aggressive form that requires invasive treatment. Western men have a much greater risk for developing advanced, invasive prostate cancer and prostate cancer death. Migration studies find that risk rises substantially within a single generation in lower-risk men who relocate to the United States.[2,3]

These factors—high incidence, long latency, and strong environmental influence—make prostate cancer an ideal target for chemopreventive approaches. In this context, the term *chemoprevention* is used to describe nutritional interventions, that is, changes in diet and the use of specific nutritional supplements to slow or reverse the progression of early prostate cancer or PIN. Chemoprevention can also be used in a more proactive fashion to help prevent prostate cancer from ever occurring in the first place.

In research performed at the Preventive Medicine Research Institute at the University of California, San Francisco, Ornish and associates[4] demonstrated the power of diet and lifestyle changes in 87 men with prostate cancer (PSA 4 to 10 ng/mL; Gleason score less than 7) who chose not to undergo conventional treatments. The study period was 1 year. Subjects were enrolled either in a program of extensive, comprehensive lifestyle changes, including a low-fat, vegetarian, soy-rich diet and nutritional supplements, exercise, psychosocial support, and stress reduction, or in a usual care control group. None of the men in the experimental group required conventional treatment during the study period, whereas six of the control subjects required such treatment (Table 11-1).

This and other research studies—many of which will be discussed in detail in this chapter—strongly suggest that if men who would otherwise be told to watchfully wait were offered the information and motivation they need to enter into a focused chemoprevention program, we could have significant impact on disease progression, as well as on other important aspects of men's overall health.

Table 11-1. Effect of Intensive Lifestyle Changes on PSA and Serum-Stimulated LNCaP Cell Growth

PSA		
Time from Study Initiation	Experimental Group	Control Group
3 months	PSA ↓ 1%	PSA ↑ 5%
1 year	PSA ↓ 3%	PSA ↑ 7%
LNCaP		
Experimental group	67% growth inhibition	
Control group	12% growth inhibition	

LNCaP, lymph node carcinoma of the prostate; PSA, prostate-specific antigen.
Data from Ornish D, Weidner G, Fair WR, et al: Intensive lifestyle changes may affect the progression of prostate cancer. J Urol 174:1065–1070, 2005.

The research community is well on its way to deducing which dietary factors can be applied in the earliest stages of prostate carcinogenesis to reduce the risk of morbidity and mortality from this disease. As tools for early detection improve, applying these chemopreventive factors will be an increasingly practical, inexpensive, and effective path to decreasing prostate cancer incidence. Most nutritional chemoprevention agents have the added benefit of being good for the cardiovascular system and for the prevention of other cancers (Fig. 11-1).

A sizable body of research suggests that nutritional interventions can be valuable for patients with early-stage prostate cancers. This is particularly true in patients with prostatic intraepithelial neoplasia (PIN), which we have found to be responsive to herbal and dietary therapies in our research at the New York-Presbyterian Hospital/Columbia Center for Holistic Urology. Reversing PIN with chemopreventive agents could turn out to be our best primary defense against prostate cancer.

This chapter addresses the research evidence that supports a role for dietary factors in the initiation and progression of prostate cancer; and, by association, the promise of manipulation of those factors in prostate cancer chemoprevention. First, there is a brief discussion of the putative influence of macronutrient elements of the diet, including the controversial role of total fat intake and the less disputed role of subtypes of fat, particularly the role of omega-3 to omega-6 balance and its effects on inflammation, a factor now strongly suspected in the etiology of prostate cancer.

Next, a discussion of the micronutrients, specifically lycopene, vitamin E, and selenium, and

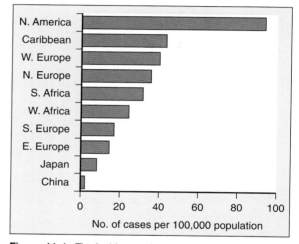

Figure 11-1. The incidence of prostate cancer (PCa) worldwide has been strongly associated with differences in diet and lifestyle. (Figure created by Ronald Morton, MD, based on data from Willett WC: Goals for nutrition for the year 2000. CA Cancer J Clin 49:331–352, 1999.)

of specific nutrient-dense foods, plant chemicals, and herbs that have shown promise as prostate cancer chemopreventives is offered. I also share the nutritional protocol that has shown the most promise in my own research—still preliminary at this writing—for slowing the progression of and even reversing PIN (Table 11-2).

Diet and Prostate Cancer Risk

Fat content of the diet, overall caloric intake, the ratio of omega-6 to omega-3 fatty acids in the diet, and consumption (or lack thereof) of meat, antioxidants, and soy foods are the major factors that appear to correlate most closely

Table 11-2. Dietary Factors, Foods, Nutrients, Plant Chemicals, and Herbs with Putative Effects on Prostate Cancer Growth

Macronutrients	Specific Foods/Herbs	Micronutrients/Phytochemicals
Dietary fat	Pomegranate	Antioxidants, especially
Dietary fiber	Tomato	selenium/vitamin E
Meat	Soy	Phytoestrogens, especially
Dietary balance of	Green tea	genistein from soy
individual classes	Ginger	Lycopene
of fatty acids	Ginseng	Omega-3 fats from fish oil
(omega-3,	Holy basil	Indole-3-carbinol
omega-6,	Medicinal mushrooms	Inositol hexaphosphate (IP-6)
saturated,	Zyflamend (an herbal combination that includes curcumin,	
trans fats)	ginger, holy basil, Baikal scullcap, green tea, and *hu zhang*)	
	Prostabel (an herbal combination that includes *Pao pereira*	
	and *Rauwolfia vomitoria*)	
	Saw palmetto	

with risk of prostate cancer and risk of death from this disease. These dietary factors may act as late-stage promoters rather than initiators, transforming a relatively harmless, latent prostatic neoplasia into a more aggressive form.

Fat Content of the Diet

In a 31-country study, investigators found a close correlation between fat intake and prostate cancer mortality.[5,6] On the other hand, the Netherlands Cohort Study found no association between prostate cancer and total fat intake.[7] Other population surveys have found moderate correlations. Within populations with low risk of prostate cancer, such as Chinese men, the percentage of fat in the diet is strongly predictive of whether they ultimately develop the disease.[8] Another case-control study, performed in Utah, found that men with high fat intake had the highest risk of aggressive prostate tumors.[9]

Laboratory results conflict in this regard as well: Some animal models find increased tumor growth with higher-fat diets, whereas others find no relation between these variables. Reducing dietary fat in LAPC-4 xenografted severe combined immunodeficient mice was found to delay the progression of prostate cancer to androgen insensitivity and to prolong survival,[10] but other preclinical investigations find no relation among fat intake, androgen sensitivity, and survival.[11-13] In a comprehensive review article, Sonn and associates point out that "most clinical evidence on the role of fat is from observa-

tional, not interventional studies."[1] Case-control studies on this subject often find a positive correlation between fat in the diet and prostate cancer risk, but most of these studies "differ with selection of controls and method of dietary assessment."[1]

Possible explanations for a correlation between total fat intake and prostate cancer incidence include effects of dietary fat on serum androgen levels, oxidative stress, or increases in insulin-like growth factor 1 (IGF-1). On the other hand, more fat in the diet may boost conversion of testosterone to estrogens, which may have protective effects. It is also important to consider the potential role of xenoestrogenic, persistent pollutants found in high concentrations in animal fat.

Caloric Intake

Caloric restriction has been found consistently and independently to reduce prostate tumor growth in animal models. As long as intake of vitamins, minerals, and accessory nutrients is adequate, caloric restriction reduces inflammation, free radical stress, high insulin levels, and body weight—all factors that can accelerate cancer growth. Caloric restriction reduces DNA damage and enhances DNA repair. Results from animal studies of caloric restriction are among the most impressive in the small but growing realm of chemoprevention research (Tables 11-3 and 11-4).

Unfortunately, dramatic effect like this requires drastic reduction in caloric intake—one

Table 11-3. Caloric Restriction and Tumor Growth in Mice

Mouse Strain	Carcinogen	Site	Number of Tumors Fed	Number of Tumors Underfed
DBA	Spontaneous	Breast	13	3
DBA	Spontaneous	Breast	20	1
ABC	Benzo(a)pyrene	Skin	22	7
Swiss	Benzo(a)pyrene	Skin	24	6
C57	Benzo(a)pyrene	Subcutaneous	36	22

From Kritschevsky D: Caloric restriction and experimental carcinogenesis. Toxicol Sci 52(Suppl):13–16, 1999, Table 1. Copyright © 1999 by the Society of Toxicology.

Table 11-4. Influence of 40% Energy Restriction and Fat on DMBA-Induced Mammary Tumors in Rats

Fat Type	Amount (%)	Regimen	Tumor Incidence (%)
Coconut oil	4.0	*Ad libitum*	14/24 (58%)
Coconut oil	7.9	Restricted	0/23 (0%)
Corn oil	4.0	*Ad libitum*	16/20 (80%)
Corn oil	7.9	Restricted	4/20 (20%)

DMBA, dimethylbenzanthracene.
From Kritschevsky D: Caloric restriction and experimental carcinogenesis. Toxicol Sci 52(Suppl):13–16, 1999, Table 3. Copyright © 1999 by the Society of Toxicology.

third or 40% below what an animal would eat if given unlimited access to food. Most patients (and, no doubt, physicians) would balk at this regimen, which entails being hungry most of the time. However, the potency of this very simple intervention should not be disregarded just because patients may have difficulty adhering to a physician's advice to eat fewer calories. Although the most potent effect is seen with greater restriction, even moderate caloric restriction has been found to reduce gastrointestinal cancer risk in mice by 60%.[14] Prostate and breast cancers have shown similar vulnerability to caloric restriction. A study by investigators at the University of California–Berkeley found that restricting caloric intake through every-other-day fasts in mice reduced cell proliferation in several organ systems.[15]

Some nutritional interventions (i.e., supplements) show promise as substitutes for caloric restriction, mimicking the effect of a low-calorie diet at the cellular level. However, such research is still in its earliest stages. A nutrient-dense diet extremely rich in vegetables and fruits and with reduced consumption of meats and sugars has been found to have cancer-preventive effects

similar to the calorically restricted diet, although not to the same extent.

Obesity

Obesity may in some cases be correlated to high fat intake—although the more likely culprit is high caloric intake—and obesity has been strongly implicated as an independent risk factor for high-grade prostate cancer and prostate cancer mortality.[16,17]

Excess body fat alters estrogen and testosterone activity. Lower testosterone is associated with lower prostate-specific antigen (PSA) at diagnosis. Tymchuk and coworkers[18] found that when 27 obese men were put on very low-fat (less than 10% of calories from fat), high-fiber diet, and exercise programs, all the men who had high PSA levels (over 2.5 ng/mL) saw these values fall. Sex hormone-binding globulin (SHBG) rose and free testosterone levels dropped, possibly decreasing growth-promoting effects on the prostate. It is interesting that diabetes appears to independently *reduce* the risk of prostate cancer.[19]

Ratio and Types of Dietary Fatty Acids

Today we know that singling out dietary fat for blame in heart disease and obesity is to oversimplify a complex picture, and in oversimplifying in this manner, we may be missing a factor that is at the crux of the chemoprevention issue. The various classes of dietary fatty acids have very different physiologic effects, and the expansion of our knowledge in this area has revealed a similar picture in terms of prostate cancer risk: Overall fat content in the diet appears to be less influential than the ratio of the various fatty acids.

High intake of saturated fatty acids (SFA), trans-fatty acids (from processed, hydrogenated vegetable oils), and omega-6 polyunsaturated fatty acids (PUFAs)—particularly arachidonic acid (AA) and linoleic acid (LA)—have all been associated with both increased prostate cancer incidence and mortality or no effect on these variables. On the other hand, higher intake of the omega-3 fatty acids docosahexaenoic acid (DHA), eicosapentaenoic acid (EPA) and alpha-linolenic acid (ALA) is associated with reduced risk and a protective effect. A Western high-fat diet is likely to be high in omega-6 PUFAs and trans fats. This could explain the connection between total fat and prostate cancer risk that has continued to come up in the research.

Olive oil in the diet, a source of neutral omega-9 fatty acids, has been found to be protective against many cancers, including cancer of the prostate. Unrefined vegetable oils rich in phytosterols, including B-sitosterol and campesterol, are believed to reduce the risk of prostate cancer. Asian and Mediterranean diets, both rich in phytosterols, confer reduced risk compared with the standard American diet with its abundance of cholesterol, refined oils, and saturated fats. Animal and cell culture studies have found that olive oil phytosterols directly inhibit prostate cancer cell growth and migration, as well as their binding to membrane proteins of normal cells.

The balance of omega-3 (n-3) and omega-6 (n-6) fats in the diet affects hormone levels and activity and eicosanoid balance. Eicosanoids are potently bioactive lipids and autocrine and paracrine mediators that are involved in the initiation of the inflammatory response, fever production, regulation of blood pressure, blood clotting, control of reproductive processes and tissue growth, and regulation of the sleep/wake cycle. AA and LA are altered by lipoxygenase (LO) and cyclooxygenase (COX) enzymes to produce leukotrienes and prostaglandins; these eicosanoids and enzymes are implied, in current research, in tumor development, progression, and metastasis. This cascade appears to be of particular importance in the earliest stages of prostate cancer (Figs. 11-2 and 11-3).

ALA, EPA, and DHA, when altered by COX and LO enzymes, form anti-inflammatory prostaglandins, leukotrienes, and thromboxanes. Because these various types of fatty acids compete for the same enzymes, the balance of n-3 and n-6 fats in the diet strongly influences the balance of pro- and anti-inflammatory eicosanoids in the body.

Laboratory research offers robust support for the role of n-3/n-6 imbalance in prostate cancer etiology. So far, this has been difficult to demonstrate in vivo in humans, but a recent study by Kelavkar and coworkers[20] at the University of Baroda, India, provides some support for dietary manipulation of the balance of these fatty acids, either through dietary changes or supplements. These investigators compared the

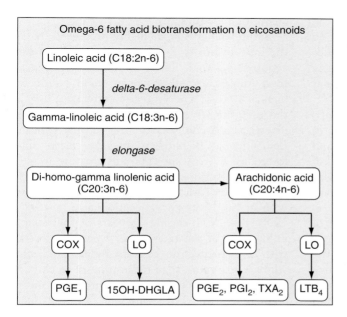

Figure 11-2. Linoleic acid (omega-6) biotransformation into eicosanoids.
Those derived from arachidonic acid have pro-inflammatory effects and may be associated with prostatic intraepithelial neoplasia and prostate cancer. Dietary manipulation of eicosanoids appears to be an important chemopreventive tool.

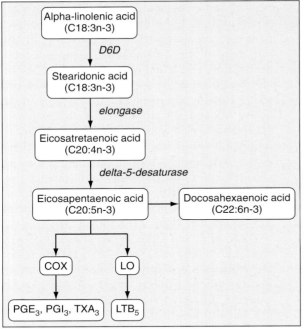

Figure 11-3. Omega-3 fatty acid biotransformation to eicosanoids. Omega-3 fats such as DHA and EPA compete for the same enzymes, reducing the production of pro-inflammatory eicosanoids and enhancing production of anti-inflammatory versions. Manipulation of eicosanoid production through diet and herbal therapies may be a keystone of prostate cancer chemoprevention.

expression of cyclooxygenases and lipoxygenases in 18 normal donor prostates with that of 60 prostate tumors, as well as activity of desaturase enzymes that help to transform AA into pro-inflammatory eicosanoids. They found that normal prostate had lower 15-LO-1 expression and higher elongase, delta-6-desaturase, delta-5-desaturase, and 15-LO-2 expression, whereas cancerous prostate had the opposite profile: higher 15-LO-1 and lower 15-LO-2, delta-6 and delta-5-desaturase expression. In conclusion, the authors state: "[o]ur study underscores the importance of promising dietary intervention agents such as the omega-3 fatty acids as substrate competitors of LA/AA, aimed primarily at high 15-LO-1 and COX-2 as the molecular targets in PCa initiation and/or progression."[20]

COX enzymes are the target of most anti-inflammatory drugs. The two main isoforms of cyclooxygenase are COX-1 and COX-2, and these enzymes are responsible for production of the eicosanoid class known as the prostaglandins. The COX-1 isoform has many important housekeeping functions in the cell and is produced throughout the body as a matter of course. COX-2 is produced in response to pro-inflammatory stimuli and is implicated in the progression of many disease states, including cancer. Elevated COX-2 levels have been detected in lung, colon, pancreatic, head and

neck, and prostate cancers. COX-2 (and, to some extent, COX-1) elevation has been found in numerous studies of prostate tumor samples; benign prostatic tissues from the same patients had significantly lower concentrations of COX-2. Elevations in COX-2 activity and its attendant prostaglandins are implicated in angiogenesis; COX-2 inhibition has been observed to induce apoptosis in prostate cancer cells. Many researchers are considering these enzymes as useful targets for development of novel chemotherapeutics.

Before the advent of highly processed diets, the ratio of n-6 to n-3 fats in typical diets was about 2 or 3 to 1. Today's standard processed-food American diets, however, yield a ratio as high as 40 to 1. The protective effects of fish in the diet further support this hypothesis. One investigation, published in the journal *Cancer Epidemiology, Biomarkers and Prevention*, followed up 47,882 subjects participating in the Health Professionals' Follow-Up Study. Dietary intake of individuals in Sweden was assessed with a food frequency questionnaire in 1986, 1990, and 1994; during 12 years of follow-up, 2482 cases of prostate cancer were diagnosed, with 278 metastatic cancers found. Subjects who ate fish more than three times a week had almost half the risk of metastatic prostate cancer compared with those who ate fish less than twice a month. Each additional daily intake of 0.5 grams of marine fatty acid from food was associated with a 24% decreased risk of metastatic cancer.[21]

Fish oil supplements rich in DHA and EPA are promising chemopreventive agents. Herbal supplements have also been studied for their potential to push the balance of COX and LO enzymes and eicosanoid balance in an anti-inflammatory direction. In our investigations, we have found that doing so can stall or even reverse PIN. Both fish oil supplements and herbal anti-inflammatory supplements are discussed in greater detail later in this chapter.

Meat in the Diet

Colli and Colli,[22,23] in two retrospective population studies published in *Urologic Oncology* in 2005 and 2006, found strong correlations between prostate cancer mortality and intake of total meat, added fats and oils, ice cream, vegetable shortening, margarine, and salad and cooking oils. In their international survey of prostate cancer mortality in 71 countries, they found increased risk in those who ate more animal calories, more animal fat calories, more meat, more sugar, and more alcoholic beverages. These results lend further epidemiologic credence to the theory that overconsumption of n-6 fats and trans-fatty acids, with the lack of n-3 fats, vegetables, whole grains, and fruit characteristic of diets abundant in meat, sugar, and processed oils and margarines, is an important point to address in a chemoprevention program.

A link between meat intake and prostate cancer makes sense on several fronts. Fats from nonorganic animal sources contain more organochlorines and other xenoestrogens (environmental estrogens) than vegetable fats. These chemicals are known carcinogens that can damage the prostate, and evidence from animal studies indicate that this damage to prostate cellular function and microstructure can begin during the fetal stage of life.[24-26] Prostate and breast tissues are particularly good at concentrating these ubiquitous, fat-soluble xenoestrogens. To ignore the potential influence of these chemicals because we cannot control their presence in the environment or in the body is to leave out what is probably a crucial piece of the puzzle as we consider the design of a chemoprevention program.

Meat (including red meat, chicken, and fish) cooked at high temperatures contains high concentrations of polyaromatic hydrocarbons (HCAs), which are known prostate carcinogens. A meat-rich diet can crowd out vegetables and fruits, which leaves the body with an excess of carcinogens to deal with and few of the naturally occurring carcinogen-detoxification enzyme inducers and antioxidants that are abundant in plant foods and that are effective at reducing cancer risk.

Phytoestrogens

Differences in the level of consumption of traditionally prepared soy foods (miso, tofu, tempeh, natto) are believed to contribute to the large difference in prostate cancer incidence and mortality between Asian and Western males. A large-scale epidemiologic study by Hebert and associates[27] of 59 countries found that soy-derived products offered highly significant protection against prostate cancer. Animal studies reveal that soy isoflavones, particularly genistein, inhibit prostate cancer growth in cell cultures.[28] In rat models, genistein has been found to offer significant chemopreventive activity against advanced prostate cancer. Possible mechanisms include estrogenic properties and inhibition of 5-α reductase. Soy foods contain protease inhibitors, saponins, and phytates, all of which have putative anticarcinogenic effects.

Fiber/Lignan Intake

Lignans are found in seeds, whole grains, vegetables, fruit, and legumes, but the richest dietary source is flax seed. Diets rich in this and other fibers have consistently been correlated with reduced prostate cancer risk.[29] Lignans are fermented in the bowel, yielding the phytoestrogenic metabolites enterodiol and enterolactone. These metabolites influence sex hormone metabolism in ways that are believed to reduce the risk of hormonally influenced cancers; they reduce the action of growth factors, malignant cell proliferation and differentiation, and angiogenesis.[30] An investigation by Swedish researchers found that the lowest blood levels of enterolactone correlated with higher prostate cancer risk.[31] Duke University investigators

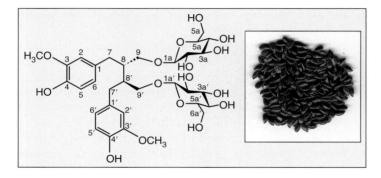

Figure 11-4. Lignan and flax seeds.
Lignan, a type of fiber, is transformed in the colon to phytoestrogenic enterolactone, which may aid in prostate cancer prevention. Flax seeds, the best source of lignans, should be a part of the chemoprevention diet.

added 30 grams of ground flax seed per day for an average of 34 days (21–77 days) to the diets of 25 patients scheduled for prostatectomy. (The men were also placed on a 20% fat diet for the study's duration.) Testosterone and free androgen levels fell; proliferation rate fell and apoptosis was enhanced[32] (Fig. 11-4).

Laboratory studies find that lignans and enterodiol/enterolactone enhance apoptosis, downregulate sex steroid receptor activity, and inhibit the growth of prostate cancer cell lines (both androgen-dependent and androgen-independent).[33] Lignans inhibit estrogen binding to alpha-fetoprotein.

The Ideal Prostate Cancer Chemoprevention Diet

Slowing the growth of latent foci is best achieved with a combination of diet and nutritional supplementation. Current evidence supports a diet rich in vegetables, fruits, and whole grains. Red meat should be a small part of the diet, if consumed at all, and grass-fed, organic beef, free-range poultry, game, eggs, and wild-caught ocean fish are the best options for flesh foods. Encourage patients to try tempeh, tofu, and miso as alternate protein sources. Nuts and seeds are good additions to the chemopreventive diet; unrefined extra-virgin olive oil should be the oil of choice; and ground flax seeds can be added to the diet, stirred into organic, low-fat, live-culture yogurt (the best choice of dairy product) or oatmeal. Have patients minimize refined flour and sugar intake, as well as the consumption of trans fats and other highly refined vegetable oils, all of which promote the pro-inflammatory eicosanoid cascade.

A vegetable or fruit serving is equivalent to ½ cup fresh or ¼ cup dried; a cup of leafy greens; or six fluid ounces of fruit or vegetable juice. Advise patients to aim for at least 5, but preferably 8 to 10, servings of these foods per day (Fig. 11-5).

To enhance lignan intake, patients may be advised to supplement their diets with 3 tablespoons of flax seed daily; the seed meal can be added to yogurt, hot cereals, soups, stews, or nut butters. The seeds can be ground in a coffee grinder or purchased already ground. Advise patients to keep ground seeds in the freezer.

Superfoods for Prostate Cancer Chemoprevention

The popular media frequently use the term "superfood" to describe foods discerned to contain high concentrations of health-promoting nutrients; foods that have been found in epidemiologic studies to increase lifespan and healthy lifespan in various parts of the world; and foods that appear to support the smooth function of multiple organ systems. Spinach, wild-caught salmon, blueberries, soy foods, oats, broccoli, and green tea all have been defined as superfoods. Although all of these foods have value in men's health and cancer prevention, investigations specific to prostate health suggest that a few additional foods qualify for a list of superfoods with specific value for prostate health. Where relevant, concentrated versions of these foods available as nutritional supplements are addressed.

Pomegranate

Pomegranate, which is actually a very large berry, contains a wide range of antioxidant polyphenolic flavonoids, anti-inflammatory phytochemicals, lignans, and plant estrogens, all of which may aid in efforts toward prostate and

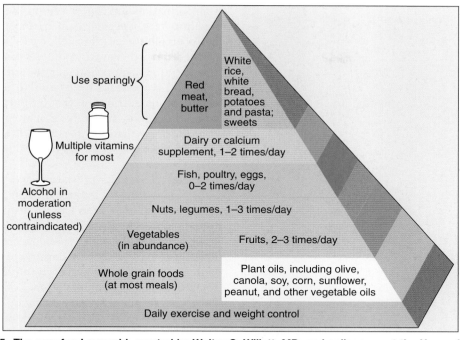

Figure 11-5. The new food pyramid, created by Walter C. Willett, MD, and colleagues at the Harvard School of Public Health. This pyramid reflects a diet ideal for prostate cancer chemoprevention and is easy for patients to understand. (From *EAT, DRINK, AND BE HEALTHY* by Walter C. Willett, MD. Copyright © 2001, 2005 by the President and Fellows of Harvard College.)

breast cancer chemoprevention and as an adjunct nutritional therapy (Fig. 11-6).

The pomegranate has been used medicinally for thousands of years. This fruit is anti-inflammatory, cardioprotective, and protective against diabetic complications. Its components protect against platelet aggregation, low-density lipoprotein (LDL) oxidation, and general oxidative stress.[34] Pomegranate also has antibiotic and neuroprotective effects.[35]

In their investigations at the University of Wisconsin Department of Dermatology, Malik and associates[36] first discovered that pomegranate fruit extract (PFE) had notable antitumor effects in mouse skin. The team then used human prostate cancer cells to assess the antiproliferative, proapoptotic activities of PFE, and found a dose-dependent inhibition of highly aggressive PC3 prostate cancer cells. Cell growth and viability fell and apoptosis was induced in this experiment. In a follow-up investigation, they administered PFE orally to athymic nude mice implanted with androgen-sensitive prostate cancer cells; the result was a significant inhibition of tumor growth and a fall in PSA. Albrecht and coworkers,[37] in a multicenter study based at Philipps University in

Marburg, Germany, had similar results in an investigation of cold-pressed pomegranate seed oil, fermented juice polyphenols, and pericarp (the whitish, bitter "cuticle" of the fruit) polyphenols. They found that all of these components of the pomegranate had significant antitumor activity. Human prostate cancer cell xenograft growth in vivo was inhibited. Measurements of proliferation, cell cycle distribution, apoptosis, gene expression, and invasiveness all supported this conclusion. Normal prostatic cells were unaffected by the treatments. At this writing, the Center for Holistic Urology at Columbia University Medical Center is an active site for a clinical trial of pomegranate in 250 patients. The study is a randomized, placebo-controlled clinical trial of pomegranate juice, pomegranate liquid extract, and placebo supplementation in men with rising PSA levels after treatment for localized prostate cancer.

Advise patients to add pomegranate to their diets as juice or as a whole fruit. Concentrated supplements of whole pomegranate fruit are available. These appear to be safe for use as a dietary supplement, with benefits to multiple body systems.

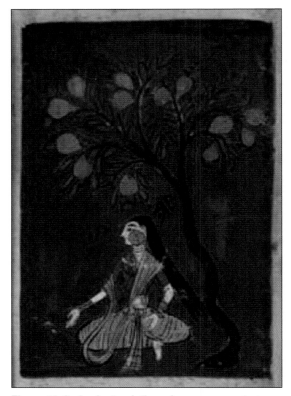

Figure 11-6. Ancient painting of a pomegranate tree. This painting, dating back to 1570, depicts a woman sitting under a pomegranate tree. The tree's fruits symbolize fertility and abundance and have been important medicinal plants for most of recorded history. Modern research suggests that pomegranate is an important source of prostate cancer chemopreventive substances.

Tomato

Lycopene, the red carotenoid pigment abundant in tomatoes, has garnered a good deal of attention in recent years as a preventive against cancer, prostate disease, and cardiovascular disease. Epidemiologic studies find that greater consumption of foods rich in lycopene correlate with reduced risk of prostate cancer and cardiovascular disease. Giovannucci's[38] 1999 review found that 57 of 72 studies revealed inverse associations between cancer risk at various sites and blood lycopene level, and further investigations found protective effects of lycopene against prostate cancer specifically.[39]

Lycopene is not an essential nutrient, but is a major operator in the body's antioxidant network, protecting lipids, proteins, and DNA in circulating blood against free radical damage—particularly from singlet oxygen. Laboratory studies find that lycopene inhibits malignant

transformation and cancer cell proliferation in a highly potent, specific manner, and that it is a better inhibitor of the cell cycle than beta-carotene. It is believed to do so by modulating transcription factors integral to cell proliferation.[40,41] Lycopene has been found to help restore cell membrane structures that enable cell-to-cell communication—structures that are more abundant in nonmalignant than malignant cells. It also enhances the activity of phase II liver detoxification enzymes.

Lycopene inhibits prostate cancer growth in vitro,[42] and in a rat model, Boileau and associates[43] found that both caloric restriction and tomato powder, but not pure lycopene, protected against prostate carcinogenesis. In an investigation by Chen and coworkers,[44] 32 men with prostate cancer were given dishes with tomato sauce containing 30 mg of lycopene every day for the 3 weeks leading up to prostatectomy. Serum PSA and markers of oxidative DNA damage fell in prostatic tissues in men on the tomato sauce regimen than in controls ($P = .0003$). In the removed prostates, tumor areas of men who had eaten the lycopene-rich diet had 3.3-fold the number of apoptotic cells compared with control subjects.

Lycopene may be a beneficial nutrient to supplement, but so far it appears that isolated lycopene is a source inferior to a whole-food tomato concentrate that contains complementary nutrients. Advise patients to consume tomatoes and tomato products often—daily, if possible. Tomato cooked with oil is the most bioavailable form in which to get this nutrient into the body. Men who wish to supplement this nutrient may benefit more from a whole-food tomato concentrate than from isolated lycopene.

Soy Foods

The epidemiologic link between soy food consumption and reduced risk of prostate and breast cancers is well established. Asian men with soy-rich diets have far less cancer of the prostate than do Western men. One often-cited study found a 70% reduction of prostate cancer risk in American Seventh-Day Adventist men who consumed soy milk at least once per day. This strong link has led many researchers to investigate soy foods and individual components of soy as cancer preventives and as complementary cancer therapies. Genistein is an isoflavone plant pigment that has weak estrogenic properties. Its best known source is soy. Because of its mild hormone-modulating effects, genistein has been studied as a potential chemopreventive agent in prostate cancer.

Data from investigations into isoflavones support their usefulness in a chemoprevention program, but more research is needed to determine effective dosage in supplement form. Advise patients to consume soy foods once per day, particularly fermented soy foods such as miso and tempeh. Patients interested in trying genistein-combined polysaccharide (see next section) at the recommended dose of 5 grams per day should be informed that the cost of this supplement may be prohibitive. At this writing, a month's supply can cost up to $600.

Medicinal Mushrooms

Medicinal mushrooms, another aspect that the US diet does not share with the Asian diet, have a variety of physiologic effects valuable for a chemoprevention program. Medicinal mushrooms such as shiitake, maitake, and reishi have been found to have antitumor and immunostimulant properties. Men will probably reap health benefits simply from adding shiitake, maitake, and reishi mushrooms—good sources of B vitamins, fiber, and antioxidants—to the diet.

Genistein-combined polysaccharide (GCP) is a supplement that is a combination of medicinal mushroom polysaccharides and genistein (Amino Up, Sapporo, Japan), which has been found to have potent anticancer effects in vitro. Naturally occurring isoflavones are poorly absorbed; they exist in soy foods predominantly in glycosylated form. GCP, a fermented extract of soy and basidiomycetes mycillae, contains highly bioavailable isoflavones, and in vivo and in vitro studies have found GCP to have potent anticancer activity.[45]

In a case study, which was documented at the College of Physicians and Surgeons of Columbia University, a male patient with biopsy-proven prostate cancer took GCP for 44 days before radical prostatectomy. His PSA fell from 19.7 to 4.2, and no cancer could be observed in his radical prostatectomy specimen.[46] Further research is needed to determine what role GCP might have in the prevention and early treatment of prostate cancer.

Active hexose-correlated compound (AHCC), another mushroom polysaccharide preparation, has been used in conjunction with GCP as a complementary therapy for prostate cancer, particularly in Japan. AHCC has been found to stimulate natural killer cell and macrophage activity. Anecdotal reports suggest that it and other medicinal mushroom preparations help to relieve chemotherapy-related nausea, pain, liver damage, and immunosuppression.

Various supplements containing medicinal mushroom fractions are available, and may be valuable for overall health and immunomodulation. Further research is needed to determine the role of isolated mushroom polysaccharides in the treatment of early-stage prostate cancer, but no harmful effects are likely to come with their use by patients who wish to try them. Their promise of benefit appears to outweigh any risk.

Cruciferous Vegetables

Consumption of cruciferous vegetables, including broccoli, cauliflower, and cabbage, is inversely related to the incidence of prostate cancer. Sulfur-containing glucosinolate breakdown products indole-3-carbinol (I3C) and sulforaphane are phytochemicals found in crucifers, and both have been demonstrated to reduce the proliferation of prostate cancer in vivo in a dose-dependent manner. I3C causes growth arrest and increases apoptosis; some investigations have found that supplemental doses of this nutrient chemosensitize chemoresistant prostate cancer cells, aiding in the treatment of hormone-resistant cancers.[47]

Inhibition of Akt and NF-kappaB are putative mechanisms for this effect; beneficial effects of cruciferous vegetables on liver detoxification enzymes, theoretically improving the body's ability to rid itself of carcinogens, are also suspected to play a role in the chemopreventive effects of these foods. Much evidence also points to I3C's effects on estrogen binding and metabolism.[48,49] A tumor-promoting effect of I3C has been found in a few models of chemical carcinogenesis, but the general thrust of the research suggests broad chemopreventive effects in breast and prostate cancers.

Advise patients to consume broccoli, cabbage, cauliflower, kale, mustard greens, bok choy, watercress, horseradish, and brussels sprouts, all good sources of this nutrient. Broccoli sprouts, which are widely available in supermarkets, are an excellent source of I3C. Supplements of I3C and sulforaphane are available, but more research is needed to determine whether these supplements are more useful chemopreventives than the foods from which they are derived.

Fish and Fish Oils

The long-chain omega-3 fats DHA and EPA, which are abundant only in fish, crustaceans, and some forms of algae, have been found to suppress cancer initiation, induce apoptosis, and counter the enhancing effects of AA on risk of atherosclerosis and several cancers, including cancer of the prostate. This appears especially true when the overall diet is altered to reduce intake of red meat, dairy products, hydrogenated oil, and highly unsaturated vegetable and seed oils—staples of the standard American processed-food diet and sources of saturated fats, omega-6 polyunsaturated fats, and trans fats.[50,51] These three classes of fat all have been linked with increasing incidence of cancer in the prostate and breast.

The short-chain omega-3 found in plant foods such as flax seeds and ALA has not matched DHA and EPA in its chemopreventive effects; to act as a substrate for the production of anti-inflammatory eicosanoids, ALA must first be converted to long-chain omega-3 PUFAs, an inefficient process. Flax seeds, walnuts, and soybeans, the most important dietary sources of ALA, are still good foods to include in the chemoprevention diet, but they should not be relied on as sole sources of omega-3 fats.

Numerous investigations have found that consumption of fish three to four times per week confers a significant reduction in prostate cancer occurrence (a two- to threefold reduction in one study and a 40% to 44% reduction in risk in two others).[52–54]

One interesting investigation by Narayanan and coworkers[55] found that low-dose celecoxib plus DHA had a significant anticancer effect on prostate cancer cell lines, including enhanced apoptosis, favorable effects on NF-kB (the number of NK-kBp65-positive cells in nucleus versus cytoplasm fell in prostate cancer cells treated with omega-3 plus celecoxib [Celebrex] in comparison with controls), and inhibitory effects on cell growth that lead to apoptosis and improved differentiation. Several transcription factors were modulated in a beneficial fashion by this intervention. This study provides support for an approach involving fish oil plus herbal COX inhibitors—a topic covered in a later section of this chapter.

A 2006 review by the Southern California Evidence-Based Practice Center (RAND Health) in Santa Monica, California, published in the *Journal of the American Medical Association*, found equivocal evidence in favor of a chemopreventive role for omega-3 fatty acids in 38 human studies published between 1966 and 2005. On the other hand, in vitro and animal studies continue to demonstrate significant potential for long-chain omega-3 fats in chemoprevention.[56]

Although the chemopreventive value of fish oil rich in EPA and DHA is strongly supported by epidemiologic and experimental studies, the mechanism of fish oil chemoprotection is not yet well understood. The long-chain PUFAs EPA and DHA elicit a decrease in prostaglandin E_2 (PGE_2), which in turn has been found to retard the growth of tumor cells. Increased lipid peroxidation can be measured with long-chain PUFA supplementation; it has been postulated that this could enhance tumor cell lipid peroxidation enough to enhance apoptosis.[57]

Advise patients that consumption of fatty fish, such as salmon, sardines, and anchovies, two to three times weekly may help to prevent or slow the progression of prostate cancer. Instruct patients with concerns over media reports of mercury and other industrial toxins in fish that wild-caught salmon, Pacific flounder, Pacific sole, herring, king crab, sardines, scallops, clams, and anchovies are good choices, and that albacore tuna, tuna steaks, mackerel, shark, Gulf coast oysters, and swordfish should be avoided. For further up-to-date information on safe fish to eat, refer patients to the Web page of Oceans Alive, www.oceansalive.org.

Evidence in favor of fish oil supplementation is adequate to make general recommendations for patients to take one supplement daily. Advise patients to use a fish oil supplement that has been purified (pharmaceutical grade or molecularly distilled), that contains an antioxidant such as vitamin E or rosemary oil to prevent rancidity, and that comes from small, oily cold-water fish such as anchovies or sardines. Current guidelines indicate that patients may benefit from 1000 to 3000 mg per day of combined EPA and DHA, with higher EPA than DHA content.

Anti-Inflammatory Chemoprevention: A Role for Herbs

COX-2 is overexpressed in many cancers, including prostate cancer, and is a well-established and significant target for efforts to forestall cancer growth. Benign prostate tissue in cancerous prostates has been found to have low COX-2, suggesting increased activity of the enzyme with disease progression. COX-2 over-expression is a predictor of worse prostate cancer outcome.[58]

Other studies have suggested that angiogenesis is orchestrated in part by increased COX-2 activity and ensuing prostaglandin production, a hypothesis supported by the effects of some COX-2 inhibitor drugs on the biochemical measures of apoptosis. COX-2 inhibitor drug celecoxib (Celebrex) has been found to be a promising chemotherapy. Inhibition of COX-2 in animals suppresses angiogenesis and prostate cancer growth and enhances sensitivity to radiation therapy.

Lipoxygenase enzymes are also implicated in prostate carcinogenesis. 12-Lipoxygenase and 15-lipoxygenase are pro-inflammatory and are upregulated during prostate cancer progression. Pharmaceutical inhibitors of 5-LO and 12-LO have, as with inhibitors of COX-2, been found to reduce angiogenesis, tumor cell growth, and tumor cell motility and invasiveness.[59]

Thus, the anti-inflammatory aspect of chemoprevention appears to be a pivotal one, particularly in cases of PIN. PIN, which can appear up to 10 years before diagnosable cancer and which coexists with cancer in more than 85% of cases, offers investigators the opportunity to apply chemopreventive measures when dysplasia is present—the point at which prostate carcinogenesis may be at its earliest stages.

Manipulation of pro-inflammatory eicosanoids can be achieved through two approaches: (1) with manipulation of fatty acid intake, providing the body with increased substrate for the production of anti-inflammatory eicosanoids, which then competitively inhibits formation of pro-inflammatory eicosanoids; and (2) with

manipulation of COX and LO enzyme isoforms, inhibiting those that promote the inflammation found to encourage prostate carcinogenesis. So far, it appears that fatty acid intake is a safe and effective intervention in this regard. Manipulating COX and LO with pharmaceutical agents, however, has proved to be a less promising avenue for chemoprevention. Recent case-control studies have found significant risks with long-term COX-2 inhibitor therapy, with increases in mortality and risk of heart failure and gastrointestinal bleeding.

Highly specific COX-2 inhibition leaves other enzymes, such as 5-lipoxygenase, available to maintain those inflammatory "fires" ignited with arachidonic acid, an inflammation that appears to promote cancer and cardiovascular disease. For example, a series of studies by Myers and Ghosh and colleagues[60,61] at the University of Virginia reveal that 5-HETE, a metabolite of 5-LO, is found in 2.2-fold greater concentration in malignant prostate tumor tissue than in benign tissue. Blocking 5-HETE formation was found to trigger apoptosis in prostate cancer cells; re-introducing 5-HETE rescued cancerous cells from apoptosis. The same research team found that inhibition of 5-LO "triggers massive apoptosis in human prostate cancer cells."[60,61]

Schroeder and colleagues at the MD Anderson Cancer Center have demonstrated that "inhibition of the COX pathway by celecoxib resulted in a time-dependent activation of the LO pathway. Specifically, the production of multiple LO-metabolites . . . e.g. 5-HETE, 12-HETE, and 15-HETE, increased as the PGE$_2$ level declined . . . with celecoxib at one microgram, a concentration that is easily achieved in patients."[62] It appears that selective inhibition of a single pro-inflammatory enzyme shifts rather than decreases inflammation. Herbal anti-inflammatory agents have a broader, less specific effect (Table 11-5).

Before there were pharmaceuticals, there were medicinal herbs. Many modern pharmaceuticals are derived from plant medicines that have therapeutic value—value that has, in the current climate of highly refined pharmaceutical agents, been underappreciated. However, traditional Eastern medicinal practices have used these unrefined plant medicines to control inflammation for far longer than any modern drug has existed. Since herbs are increasingly

Table 11-5. Herbal Combination Zyflamend Inhibits Cyclooxygenase Activity

| | Percent Inhibition | |
	COX-1	COX-2
Zyflamend (0.90 µL/mL)	73.8 ± 1.83	85.7 ± 5.60
Zyflamend (0.45 µL/mL)	36.5 ± 10.46	80.9 ± 12.00
NS-398 (0.15 µM)	ND	52.5 ± 21.26
Indomethacin (6 µM)	45.0 ± 23.32	58.0 ± 13.18

Zyflamend inhibits COX-1 and COX-2 enzyme activity, as determined using purified ovine COX-1 and COX-2 colorimetric screening assay (Cayman Chemical, Michigan).
Findings are reported as means and SEM; n = 3 for all data points.
NS-398, specific COX-2 inhibitor; indomethacin, nonspecific COX-2 inhibitor; ND, not determined.

subjected to the rigors of modern studies, the research community is beginning to recognize their therapeutic value.

Many researchers have explored a variety of natural plant extracts and other natural products to elucidate their specific and nonspecific effects on COX and LO. Curcumin (turmeric), ginger, holy basil, resveratrol (concentrated in grape skins), and berberine (from barberry and Chinese goldthread) are among the most promising candidates in the burgeoning field of herbal anti-inflammatories.

New Chapter, Inc. (Brattleboro, Vermont) is a small company that has created a promising mixture, Zyflamend, which is composed of these and a few other herbs, most of which have nonselective COX-inhibitory effect. Each of the mixture's components has been found to have anti-inflammatory, antioxidant, and/or antiproliferative effects. Some are anti-angiogenic.

In 2005, Bemis and associates[63] published the results of an analysis of Zyflamend's effects on LNCaP (lymph node carcinoma of the prostate) cells. The supplement brought about a dramatic drop in both COX-1 and COX-2 activity; increased p21 expression; attenuated cell growth; and induced apoptosis. It is interesting that the effect of the supplement on LNCaP cells appeared to be due to COX-independent mechanisms, including enhanced expression of p21 and reduced expression of androgen receptor (AR), pStat3, and PKC alpha and beta.

At this writing, a phase I clinical trial is being performed at Columbia in men with PIN to determine whether Zyflamend can influence the progression of biopsy-proven high-grade PIN to prostate cancer.[64] Patients are between ages 40 and 75 years (median age: 65.1), with high-grade PIN without prostate cancer on biopsy within 6 months before enrollment. They have been assigned to one of eight treatment groups, with successive dose escalation in each group. They are evaluated every 3 months for 18 months and monitored for toxicity, PSA and testosterone fluctuations, and inflammatory markers in serum. Twelve-core transrectal ultrasound-guided prostate biopsies are performed at 6, 12, and 18 months, and cores are evaluated for PIN and prostate cancer, then stained for inflammatory markers. The protocol being used for this study includes Zyflamend, DHA, and additional supplements including holy basil, turmeric, Baikal skullcap, green and white tea extracts, a probiotic supplement, and a male-specific multivitamin. All supplements are manufactured and supplied by New Chapter, Inc., Brattleboro, VT.

Preliminary results are promising.[63] At the end of 2006, 26 patients had had at least two follow-up visits; 13 had decrease in PSA, with 46% of those patients having more than a 10% decrease and 27% having more than a 50% decrease. Thirty-five biopsies had been performed on 21 patients at that juncture, and 31 of these showed no cancer development; 21 of the 35 biopsies showed neither PIN nor cancer, suggesting a reversal of PIN. The four patients who had developed cancer, according to this preliminary data, had very small tumors with Gleason scores of 6 or less and good prognosis. One 66-year-old patient had multiple areas of PIN on entering the study, with a starting PSA of 12.2; 1 year later, his PSA had descended to 10, and all three biopsies showed no cancer and no PIN. At this time complete biopsy results are not yet available.

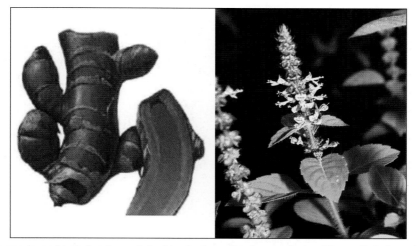

Figure 11-7. Turmeric and holy basil, medicinal herbs from the Ayurvedic tradition.   Both these herbs have anti-inflammatory and antioxidant effects that may aid in prostate cancer chemoprevention.

The individual components of Zyflamend include:

Turmeric (**Curcuma longa**). India has one of the world's lowest rates of prostate, colorectal, and lung cancers, and dietary factors are believed to play a role in this reduced risk (Fig. 11-7). Indian cuisine incorporates a great deal of turmeric, a bright yellow spice rich in curcumin (diferuloylmethane). Curcumin has COX-2 inhibitory activity and has been determined to have chemopreventive and anti-inflammatory activities in multiple prostate cancer cell lines. Turmeric has also been shown to decrease proliferative potential and induce apoptosis in both androgen-dependent and androgen-independent prostate cancer cells in vitro.[65]

Curcumin has been determined to have chemopreventive and growth-inhibitory activity against multiple tumor cell lines. Stanford researchers have elucidated one possible mechanism for these effects: an upregulation of MAP kinase phosphatase-5 (MKP5), which in turn reduces cytokine-induced NF-kB, COX-2, IL-6, and IL-8 in normal and cancerous prostate cells. Resveratrol and [6]-gingerol—both of which are discussed later in this chapter—were found to have the same effect.[66]

Curcumin has also been found to be a potent radiosensitizer that enhances radiation-induced clonogenic inhibition in tumor cells.[67] At Columbia, Dorai and colleagues[68] found that curcumin modulates proteins that suppress apoptosis and interferes with growth factors that promote cancer progression.

Resveratrol from Hu Zhang (**Polygonum cuspidatum**). Resveratrol is a phenolic antioxidant abundant in grape skins and the putative reason for the cardiovascular health benefits of moderate red wine consumption. *Hu zhang* is the Chinese (pinyin) name for the herb *Polygonum cuspidatum*, which contains significant amounts of resveratrol. Anticancer effects of resveratrol are supported by epidemiologic, experimental, and clinical investigations. Effects specific to the prostate include alteration of the activity of p53 and activation of a cascade of genes involved in cell cycle arrest and apoptosis.[69] At nutritionally relevant concentrations, resveratrol inhibits NF-kappaB, which in turn attenuates tumor necrosis factor (TNF)-alpha–induced inflammation.[70]

Green Tea. In cultures where green tea is consumed often, incidence of and mortality from prostate cancer is significantly lower. A *Journal of Nutrition* report observed that the equivalent of six cups of green tea daily "significantly inhibits [prostate cancer] development and metastasis."[71] The antioxidant content of green tea is remarkable, and some 51 compounds with anti-inflammatory activity have been identified in this centuries-old beverage. Several targets for green tea compounds have been elucidated with regard to prostate cancer prevention:

- Green tea polyphenols downregulate ornithine carboxylase, which is overexpressed in prostate cancer patients.
- Green tea phytochemicals reduce concentrations of angiogenic vascular endothelial growth factor (VEGF) and reduce metastasis-related gene expression (matrix metalloproteinases MMP-2 and MMP-9).[71]
- Epigallocatechin-3-gallate (EGCG) from green tea inhibits the growth of both androgen-sensitive and androgen-insensitive prostate cancer in animal studies.[72]
- EGCG induces apoptosis and alters expression of regulatory proteins that are critical for cell survival in ways that indicate promise for this compound as an adjunct therapy for prostate and breast cancers.[73]

One recent study by Hussain and coworkers[74] from the University of Wisconsin, which was published in the *International Journal of Cancer*, found that EGCG selectively inhibits COX-2 in both hormone-sensitive and hormone-refractory human prostate cancer cells.

Most men will not drink six cups per day of green tea; therefore, supplementation with a concentrated extract appears to be an important aspect of herbal chemoprevention.

Chinese Goldthread and Barberry. This herbal combination is rich in berberine, an antibiotic, anti-inflammatory, antidiabetic isoquinoline alkaloid.[75] Berberine has demonstrated antitumor properties in some in vitro systems, inducing cell cycle arrest and apoptosis and inhibiting DNA synthesis in human prostate cancer cells.[76]

Golden Root (Scutellaria baicalensis). This traditional Chinese herbal medicine has been investigated by modern scientists for its anti-inflammatory and free radical-scavenging properties. It has anti-androgenic and growth-inhibitory effects in prostate cancer models.[77,78] Golden root contains several unique flavonoids, including baicalin, baicalein, oroxylin A, scullcapflavone, and wogonin; several of these fractions have inhibitory effects on prostate carcinogenesis and prostate cancer growth. Baicalin has been found to interfere with the inflammatory cascade by binding to chemokines.[79]

Holy Basil (Ocimum sanctum). This traditional Ayurvedic herb has antidiabetic, wound-healing, antioxidant, and cardioprotective properties. It contains ursolic acid, a known inhibitor of COX-2.[80]

Ginger. This root flavors many cuisines and has been an herbal medicine since antiquity. It is used to treat nausea, motion sickness, upper respiratory infection, and intestinal parasites. Modern investigators have discovered in this rhizome more than 20 phytochemicals that inhibit COX-2 and 5-LO. Ginger constituents have potent antioxidant and anti-inflammatory activities; some, such as shogaols and vallinoids [6]-gingerol and [6]-paradol, exhibit cancer-preventive activity in experimental carcinogenesis. This herb's chemopreventive effects have been illustrated in a variety of experimental models.[81]

Zyflamend is a potent but gentle herbal combination that may have significant effect on the progression of PIN to prostate cancer and on the recurrence of prostate cancer (Table 11-6). In studies performed at Columbia, the supplement is being used as part of a larger protocol.

Saw palmetto, usually used as a natural therapy for BPH, appears also to have prostate-

Table 11-6. Zyflamend Prevention Protocol for Prostatic Introepithelial Neoplasia

Supplement	Dosage
Zyflamend	1 capsule with each meal (3 total)
Supercritical DHA 100	1 capsule with lunch
Supercritical Holy Basil	1 capsule with lunch
Turmericforce	1 capsule with lunch
Baikal skullcap	1 capsule with lunch
Green and white tea extract	1 capsule with lunch
Anti-aging formula probiotic with a purpose	1 capsule with breakfast
Every Man one daily multivitamin	1 tablet with breakfast

All supplements supplied by New Chapter, Brattleboro, Vermont.

chemopreventive potential. This herb has been found to inhibit the conversion of testosterone into DHT; it also has been found to lower prostate levels of epidermal growth factor as it enhances men's levels of free testosterone.[82]

Prostabel, an herbal combination containing extracts of *Pao pereira* (an Amazonian tree) and *Rauwolfia vomitoria* (from the bark of a sub-Saharan plant), was created by the late molecular biologist Mirko Beljanski. These plants have been used in indigenous medical traditions for hundreds of years; Beljanski found that they had anticancer activities in various cancer cell lines, including prostate cancer. Investigations at Columbia have revealed that both *Rauwolfia* and *Pao* extracts suppress prostate tumor cell growth in culture and in vivo. At this writing, Katz and colleagues[83] of Columbia are enrolling patients with elevated PSA and negative biopsy results for a phase I study of Prostabel; seven regimens of prostabel are being used, with subjects taking from two to eight capsules daily.

The herbs listed here are relatively free of interactions with prescription drugs. Turmeric may potentiate antiplatelet activity in patients on antiplatelet agents; ginger and turmeric may potentiate the effects of blood thinners. Patients should be advised that herbs and drugs can interact in harmful ways and that they should reveal the use of all medications and supplements to their medical team so that these kinds of interactions can be avoided.

Individual Micronutrients as Chemopreventives

According to a survey by the American Institute of Cancer Research (AICR), roughly half of adults over age 45 take multivitamins specifically to lower their risk of developing cancer. In this same survey, 23% to 36% of subjects reported using other supplements for the same purpose.[84]

With the ever-increasing popularity of nutritional supplementation, patients are likely to ask their medical team about which might benefit their prostate condition. Many advertisements and pseudo-news articles offer consumers vague, exaggerated, or even patently false information about these products. Nutritional products and product claims are not as closely monitored by regulatory agencies, and patients can waste time and resources trying to find something that helps

them get well. A physician who can give sound, research-based advice on nutritional supplements is a valuable ally to patients.

No single nutrient has been found to stand alone as a chemopreventive agent. Current evidence in favor of individual nutrients from animal and in vitro models notwithstanding, the synergistic action and interaction of a wide spectrum of micronutrients constitute the most likely reason for the health benefits of disease-preventive foods—not the isolated action of any one or two nutrients therein.

Nevertheless, the evidence does point strongly to the supplemental use of a handful of nutrients, in addition to a diet composed of beneficial and nutrient-dense foods. Vitamin E, selenium, vitamin D, and calcium all appear to play roles in prostate health. Supplementation of some of these vitamins and minerals may be appropriate as part of a chemopreventive program.

Vitamin E

In the Alpha-Tocopherol, Beta-Carotene (ATBC) Study, 29,133 male smokers received daily doses of 50 mg alpha-tocopherol, 20 mg beta carotene, both, or a placebo for 5 to 8 years. Although beta carotene had no effect on prostate cancer risk—and it increased risk of lung cancer and total mortality in this cohort—alpha-tocopherol supplementation reduced risk of prostate cancer by 32%.[85] Other research by the same Finnish investigators found that higher circulating concentrations of alpha-tocopherol and gamma-tocopherol, the major vitamin E fractions, correlated with reduced risk of prostate cancer. The odds ratio with alpha-tocopherol in this study was 0.49, and for gamma-tocopherol, 0.57.[86] A role for alpha- and gamma-tocopherol in prostate cancer chemoprevention is further supported by the results of serum case-control studies.

Inhibitory effects of vitamin E on prostate carcinogenesis are probably attributable to its antioxidant effect in membrane phospholipids; animal and preclinical studies find that vitamin E also has direct antiproliferative effects unrelated to its antioxidant capacity.[87]

Follow-up analysis of the cohort involved in the ATBC studies found that the risk ratio for prostate cancer rose again to 0.94 in the 6 years following the end of the supplementation protocol, suggesting that continual supplementation with vitamin E is necessary for chemopreventive effects in the prostate.

Vitamin E is a general term referring to a class of related compounds, including alpha-, beta-, gamma-, and delta-tocopherol and alpha-, beta-, delta-, and gamma-tocotrienols. Alpha-tocopherol has the highest biologic activity of all of these compounds. In foods, vitamin E exists as a mixture of these various compounds, each of which ongoing study finds to have unique and interactive effects.

Men should take a minimum of 240 international units (IU) of vitamin E daily as mixed tocopherols (alpha and gamma in particular). A recent analysis found that more than 400 IU per day increased all-cause mortality and heart failure incidence; it seems prudent to limit the dose in light of this finding.

Selenium

This essential trace mineral lends redox potential to vitamin E. The amount obtained in the diet can vary widely due to variations in selenium content of soil in different parts of the world where food is grown. Population studies consistently show that men with higher intake of selenium have lower risk of cancer of the prostate and that men with prostate cancer have lower selenium levels than men who do not have the disease.

In 1996, the Nutritional Prevention of Skin Cancer study found that although daily selenium supplements did not protect against nonmelanoma skin cancer, it reduced prostate cancer risk substantially. Supplementation for 6.5 years correlated with a 60% reduction in the number of new cases of cancer of the prostate in comparison with placebo, and 7.5 years of supplementation yielded 52% fewer cases compared with placebo. These investigators used a form of selenium that had been fermented with *Saccharomyces cerevisisae* yeast, a process that increases the nutrient's bioavailability.[88] These results, and the overall reduction in the risk of other cancers, were so promising that the control arm of the trial was stopped early. Further investigations into selenium for chemoprevention are ongoing.[89,90]

Other studies demonstrate that selenium supplementation alone may slow prostate cancer growth or aid in prevention of recurrence. In one study, 974 men with a history of

prostate cancer received 200 mcg of selenium a day or placebo. With about 4½ years of treatment and a 6½-year follow-up, the authors concluded that selenium treatment was associated with a 63% reduction in prostate cancer recurrence.

Laboratory studies have determined that selenium inhibits the growth of prostate cancer cells[91] and that selenium potentiates vitamin E-induced inhibition of prostate cancer cell growth.[92] Vitamin E plus selenium has been found to induce cellular arrest in abnormal cells. Five of six biomarker-based studies found an association between selenium intake and either reduced risk of prostate cancer or a nonsignificant trend toward lower risk of the disease.[93–97]

The Selenium and Vitamin E Chemoprevention Trial (SELECT), slated to yield results beginning in 2008 or 2009, closed enrollment in 2004. SELECT, the largest prevention trial ever undertaken using a drug or nutrient, involves 32,400 men age 55 and older (50 and older for African Americans) at 435 research centers in the United States, Puerto Rico, and Canada. Subjects receive 200 µg selenium daily, 400 IU of vitamin E, both nutrients, or two placebo capsules.

Men should take 200 µg of selenium with their vitamin E daily.

Calcium and Vitamin D

Current guidelines for calcium intake for osteoporosis prevention recommend that men over 50 take 1200 mg of this mineral daily. However, in epidemiologic studies of calcium intake from diet and supplements, men with the highest intake of calcium have significantly elevated risk of prostate cancer.[98,99] The interplay between vitamin D and calcium is probably the reason behind this association. High calcium intake reduces the production of $1.25(OH)_2$ vitamin D, which has antiproliferative, differentiating, and antimetastatic effects.

The intake of calcium found to raise the risk of prostate cancer was well above 1200 mg; intake of over 2000 mg calcium per day from food and supplements elevated men's risk of this disease to varying extents, with risk ratios for prostate cancer ranging from 1.2 in the 86,404 men enrolled in the CPS-II Nutritional Cohort to 1.71 in the Physicians' Health Study. The risk ratio for metastatic disease was found to be 2.97 in the latter investigation. A very small proportion of men—1% of study subjects—consumes enough calcium to raise risk of prostate cancer, but the link does exist, and it is consistent.

Ensure that patients recognize the upper limit for calcium intake. If the patient consumes a great deal of dairy along with a calcium supplement, it may be prudent to evaluate that patient's diet and work with him to reduce calcium intake.

Inositol Hexaphosphate (IP$_6$) Plus Inositol

IP$_6$ is a derivative of the B vitamin inositol. It is abundant in cereals, legumes, soy, and other fiber-rich foods. In vitro and in vivo studies have found that IP$_6$ has remarkable anticancer effects and no toxicity and that it enhances the differentiation of prostate, colon, breast, and rhabdomyosarcoma cells.

In their excellent review on the subject, Vucenik and Shamsuddin[100] point out that IP$_6$ has been observed to interfere with carcinogenesis and proliferation in mouse, human, and rat prostate cancer cell lines and that this nutrient appears most effective when paired with inositol. They exhaustively list the potential mechanisms by which IP$_6$ plus inositol appear to work to prevent prostate cancer progression: targeting of molecular events associated with prostate carcinogenesis, including mitogenic and survival signaling and cell cycle progression and chelation of iron, which suppresses formation of hydroxyl radicals.[101] Shamsuddin and colleagues[102] have found a strong effect of inositol hexaphosphate on PC-3 cells in vitro, affecting growth inhibition and differentiation. A significant dose- and time-dependent growth inhibition was observed.

IP$_6$ enhances natural killer cell activity. Baten and coworkers[103] illustrated this by depressing natural killer cell activity with colon carcinogen DMH (1,2-dimethylhydrazine) and then treating the culture with IP$_6$. The treatment reversed natural killer cell depression and enhanced the potency of natural killer cells in a dose-dependent fashion.

Dosages of IP$_6$ range between 2 grams and 8 grams daily. IP$_6$ should be taken separately from multivitamins or minerals due to its tendency to bind to minerals in the GI tract, reducing their bioavailability.

Conclusion

Nutritional and herbal interventions in early prostate cancer and PIN enjoy strong support in the published research. The interventions described in this chapter are beneficial for multiple body systems, including the endocrine, cardiovascular, immune, and nervous systems.

In a series of studies, Demark-Wahnefried and associates[103] of the Duke University Program of Cancer Preventive, Detection and Control Research have pointed out the growing role of oncologists as advisors and supporters of cancer patients who will greatly benefit from long-term diet and lifestyle changes. According to their review article on the subject, cancer survivors frequently initiate diet, exercise, and other lifestyle changes after the "wakeup call" of diagnosis, but that older men and less educated men are less likely to do so. They found, in reviewing relevant studies from 1966 to the present, that only 25% to 42% of cancer survivors consume adequate fruits and vegetables and that some 70% of prostate and breast cancer survivors are obese or overweight. They write, "Oncologists can play a pivotal role in health promotion, yet only 20% provide such guidance."[104]

With the number of cancer survivors continually rising thanks to early detection and improved treatments, and with our increasing understanding of the benefits of dietary changes and nutritional interventions in early-stage cancers, the time has come for oncologists to add this role to their many others in patient care and support.

At this writing, clinical research into the use of such therapies in early prostate cancer and PIN is young. Much more of this kind of research is imperative for the creation of consistent and effective protocols for chemoprevention–not just of prostate cancer, but of other cancers as well. Recommendations for standardization and dosages of herbal medicines are often frustratingly difficult to determine because of the lack of this kind of research. Still, the benefits of herbal and nutritional chemoprevention appear to greatly outweigh any harm that could come to a patient, particularly in the earliest stages of detectable disease, where "watchful waiting" would be the most likely intervention.

References

1. Sonn GA, Aronson W, Litwin MS: Impact of diet on prostate cancer: a review. Prost Cancer Prost Dis 8:304–310, 2005.

2. Shimizu H, Ross RK, Bernstein L, et al: Cancers of the prostate and breast among Japanese and white immigrants in Los Angeles County. Br J Cancer 63:963–966, 1991-.

3. Moradi T, Delfino RJ, Bergstrom SR: Cancer risk among Scandinavian immigrants in the US and Scandinavian residents compared with US whites. Eur J Cancer Prev 7:117–125, 1998 Apr.

4. Ornish D, Weidner G, Fair WR, et al: Intensive lifestyle changes may affect the progression of prostate cancer. J Urol 174:1065–1070, 2005.

5. Blair A, Fraumeni JF: Geographic patterns of prostate cancer in the United States. J Natl Cancer Inst 61:1379–1384, 1978.

6. Rose DP, Boyar AP, Wynder EL: International comparisons of mortality rates for cancer of the breast, ovary, prostate and colon, and per capita food consumption. Cancer 58:2363–2371, 1986.

7. Schuurman AG, van den Brandt PA, Dorant E, et al: Association of energy and fat intake with prostate carcinoma risk: results from The Netherlands Cohort Study. Cancer 86:1019–1027, 1999.

8. Lee MM, Wang RT, Hsing AW, et al: Case-control study of diet and prostate cancer in China. Cancer Causes Control 9:545–552, 1998.

9. West DW, Slattery ML, Robison LM, et al: Adult dietary intake and prostate cancer risk in Utah: a case-control study with special emphasis on aggressive tumors. Cancer Causes Control 2:85–94, 1991.

10. Ngo TH, Barnard RJ, Anton T, et al: Effect of isocaloric low-fat diet on human LAPC-4 prostate cancer xenografts in SCID mice and the IGF axis. Clin Cancer Res 9:2734–2743, 2003.

11. Bosland MC, Dreef-van der Meulen HC, Scherrenberg PM: Effect of dietary fat on rat prostate carcinogenesis induced by N-methyl-N-nitrosurea and testosterone [abstract]. Proc Am Assoc Cancer Res 31:144, 1990.

12. Pour PM, Groot K, Kasakoff K, et al: Effects of high-fat diet on the patterns of prostatic cancer induced in rats by N-nitrosobis(2-oxopropyl)amine and testosterone. Cancer Res 51:4757–4761, 1991.

13. Clinton SK, Palmer SS, Spriggs CE, Visek WJ: Growth of Dunning transplantable prostate adenocarcinomas in rats fed diets with various fat contents. J Nutr 118: 908–914, 1988.

14. Mai V: NCI study presented at Experimental Biology meeting in New Orleans, 2002.

15. Hsieh EA, Chai CM, Hellerstein MK: Effects of caloric restriction on cell proliferation in several tissues in mice: role of intermittent feeding. Am J Physiol Endocrinol Metab 288: E965–972, 2005 May.

16. Heber D: The linkage between obesity and prostate cancer. The Prostate Cancer Research Institute 7. www.prostate-cancer.org/education/nutrprod/Heber_Obesity.html. Accessed 11/24/06.

17. Lew EA, Garfinkel L: Variations in mortality by weight among 750,000 men and women. J Chron Dis 32:563–576, 1979.

18. Tymchuk CN, Tessler SB, Aronson WJ, Barnard RJ: Effects of diet and exercise on insulin, sex hormone-binding globulin, and prostate-specific antigen. Nutr Cancer 31:127–131, 1998.

19. Gong Z, Neuhouser ML, Goodman PJ, et al: Obesity, diabetes, and risk of prostate cancer: results from the prostate cancer prevention trial. Cancer Epidemiol Biomarkers Prev 15:1977–1983, 2006.

20. Kelavkar U, Lin Y, Landsittel D, et al: The yin and yang of 15-lipoxygenase-1 and delta-desaturases: dietary omega-6 linoleic acid metabolic pathway in prostate. J Carcinogenesis 5:9, 2006.

21. Augustson K, Michaud DS, Rimm EB, et al: A prospective study of intake of fish and marine fatty acids and prostate cancer. Cancer Epidemiol Biomarkers Prev 12:64–67, 2003.

22. Colli JL, Colli A: International comparisons of prostate cancer mortality rates with dietary practices and sunlight levels. Urol Oncol 24:184–194, 2006.

23. Colli JL, Colli A: Comparisons of prostate cancer mortality rates with dietary practices in the United States. Urol Oncol 23:390–398, 2005.

24. Golden RJ, Noller KL, Titus-Ernstoff L, et al: Environmental endocrine modulators and human health: an assessment of the biological evidence. Crit Rev Toxicol 28:109–227, 1998.

25. Ramos JG, Varayoud J, Sonnenschein C, et al: Prenatal exposure to low doses of bisphenol A alters the periductal stroma and glandular cell function in the rat ventral prostate. Biol Reprod 65:1271–1277, 2001.

26. Giovannucci E: Nutrition, insulin, insulin-like growth factors, and cancer. Horm Metab Res 35:694–704, 2003.

27. Hebert JR, Hurley TG, Olendzki BC, et al: Nutritional and socioeconomic factors in relation to prostate cancer mortality: a cross-national study. J Natl Cancer Inst 90:1637–1647, 1998.

28. Aronson WJ, Tymchuk CN, Elashoff RM, et al: Decreased growth of human LNCaP tumours in SCID mice fed a low-fat, soy protein diet with isoflavones. Nutr Cancer 35: 130–136, 1999.

29. Mills P, Beeson W, Phillips R, Fraser G: Cohort study of diet, lifestyle and prostate cancer in Adventist men. Cancer 64:598–604, 1989.

30. Ren S, Lien EJ: Natural products and their derivatives as cancer chemopreventive agents. Prog Drug Res 48:147–171, 1997.

31. Stattin P, Bylund A, Biessy C, et al: Prospective study of plasma enterolactone and prostate cancer risk (Sweden). Cancer Causes Control 15:1095–1112, 2004.

32. Demark-Wahnefried W, Robertson CN, Walther PJ, et al: Pilot study of dietary fat restriction and flaxseed supplementation in men with prostate cancer before surgery: exploring the effects of hormonal levels, prostate-specific antigen, and histopathologic features. Urology 58:47–52, 2001.

33. Lin X, Switzer B, Demark-Wahnefried W: Effect of mammalian lignans on the growth of prostate cancer cell lines. Anticancer Res 21: 3995–4000, 2001.

34. Rosenblat M, Hayek T, Aviram M: Anti-oxidative effects of pomegranate juice (PJ) consumption by diabetic patients on serum and on macrophages. Atherosclerosis 187:363–371, 2006.

35. Loren DJ, Seeram NP, Schulman RN, et al: Maternal dietary supplementation with pomegranate juice is neuroprotective in an animal model of neonatal hypoxic-ischemic brain injury. Pediatr Res 57:858–864, 2005.

36. Malik A, Afaq F, Sarfaraz S, et al: Pomegranate fruit juice for chemoprevention and chemotherapy of prostate cancer. Proc Natl Acad Sci USA 102:14813–14818, 2005.

37. Albrecht M, Jiang W, Kumi-Diaka J, et al: Pomegranate extracts potently suppress proliferation, xenograft growth, and invasion of human prostate cancer cells. J Med Food 7:274–283, 2004.

38. Giovannucci E: Tomatoes, tomato-based products, lycopene, and cancer: review of the epidemiologic literature. J Natl Canc Inst 91:317–331, 1999.

39. Etminan M, Takkouche B, Caamano-Isorna F: The role of tomato products and lycopene in the prevention of prostate cancer: a meta-analysis of observational studies. Cancer Epidemiol Biomarkers Prev 13:340–345, 2004.

40. Mascio P, Kaiser S, Sies H: Lycopene as the most efficient biological carotenoid singlet oxygen quencher. Arch Biochem Biophys 274:532–538, 1989.

41. Levy J, Bosin E, Feldman B, et al: Lycopene is a more potent inhibitor of human cancer cell proliferation than either alpha-carotene or beta-carotene. Nutr Cancer 24:257, 1995.

42. Obermuller-Jevic UC, Olano-Martin E, Corbacho AM, et al: Lycopene inhibits the growth of normal human prostate epithelial cells in vitro. J Nutr 133:3356–3360, 2003.

43. Boileau TW, Liao Z, Kim S, et al: Prostate carcinogenesis in N-methyl-N-nitrosourea testosterone treated rats fed tomato powder, lycopene, or energy-restricted diets. J Natl Cancer Inst 95:1578–1586, 2003.

44. Chen L, Staciewicz-Sapuntzakis M, Duncan C, et al: Oxidative DNA damage in prostate cancer patients consuming tomato sauce-based entrees as a whole-food intervention. J Natl Cancer Inst 93:1872–1879, 2001.

45. Bemis DL, Capodice JL, Desai M, et al: A concentrated aglycone isoflavone preparation (GCP) that demonstrates potent anti-prostate cancer activity in vitro and in vivo. Clin Cancer Res 10:5282–5292, 2004.

46. Ghafar MA, Golliday E, Bingham J: Regression of prostate cancer following administration of Genistein Combined Polysaccharide (GCP), a nutritional supplement: case report. J Altern Complement Med 8:493–497, 2002.

47. Sarkar FH, Yiwei L: Indole-3-carbinol and prostate cancer. J Nutr 134(12S):3493S–3498S, 2004.

48. Auborn KJ, Fan S, Rosen EM: Indole-3-carbinol is a negative regulator of estrogen. J Nutr 133(7 Suppl):2470S–2475S, 2003.

49. Brignall MS: Prevention and treatment of cancer with indole-3-carbinol. Altern Med Rev 6:580–589, 2001.

50. Kobayashi N, Barnard RJ, Henning SM, et al: Effect of altering dietary omega-6/omega-3 fat ratios on prostate cancer membrane composition, cyclooxygenase-2, and prostaglandin E2. Clin Cancer Res 12:4662–4670, 2006.

51. Kelavkar UP, Hutzley J, Dhir R, et al: Prostate tumor growth and recurrence can be modulated by the omega-6:omega-3 ration diet: athymic mouse xenograft model simulating radical prostatectomy. Neoplasia 8:112–124, 2006.

52. Norrish AE, Skeaff CM, Arribas GL, et al: Prostate cancer risk and consumption of fish oils: a dietary biomarker-based case-control study. Br J Cancer 81:1238–1242, 1999.

53. Augustsson K, Michaud DS, Rimm EB, et al: A prospective study of intake of fish and marine fatty acids and prostate cancer. Cancer Epidemiol Biomarkers Prev 12:64–67, 2003.

54. Terry P, Liechtenstein P, Feychting M, et al: Fatty fish consumption and risk of prostate cancer. Lancet 357:1764–1766, 2001.

55. Narayanan NK, Narayanan BA, Reddy BS: A combination of docosahexaenoic acid and celecoxib prevents prostate cancer cell growth in vitro and is associated with modulation of nuclear factor-kB and steroid hormone receptors. Int J Oncol 26:785–792, 2005.

56. MacLean CH, Newberry SJ, Mojica WA, et al: Effects of omega-3 fatty acids on cancer risk: a systematic review. JAMA 295:403–415, 2006.

57. Norman HA, Butrum RR, Feldman E, et al: The role of dietary supplements during cancer therapy. J Nutr 133:3794S–3799S, 2003.

58. Study first: over-expression of COX-2 can predict prostate cancer outcome. Medical News Today, www.medicalnewstoday.com/medicalnews.php?newsid=56224, accessed 11/28/06.

59. Nie D, Che M, Grignon D: Role of eicosanoids in prostate cancer progression. Cancer Metastasis Rev 20:195–206, 2001.

60. Myers CE, Ghosh J: Lipoxygenase inhibition in prostate cancer. Eur Urol 35:395–398, 1999.

61. Ghosh J, Myers CE: Inhibition of arachidonate 5-lipoxygenase triggers massive apoptosis in human prostate cancer cells. Proc Natl Acad Sci 95:13182–13187, 1998.

62. Schroeder CP, Yang P, Newman RA, Lotan R: Simultaneous inhibition of COX-2 and 5-LOX activities augments growth arrest and death of premalignant and malignant human lung cell lines. J Exp Ther Oncol 6:183–192, 2007.

63. Bemis DL, Capodice JL, Anastasiadis AG, et al: Zyflamend, a unique herbal preparation with nonselective COX inhibitory activity, induces apoptosis of prostate cancer cells that lack COX-2 expression. Nutr Cancer 52:202–212, 2005.

64. Katz AE, Pierorazio M, Masson T, et al: Results of a phase I trial administering Zyflamend to subjects with high-grade prostatic intraepithelial neoplasia. ASCO Annual Meeting Proceedings, Part I, J Clin Oncol v24 (Suppl):1126, 2006.

65. Dorai T, Gehani N, Katz A: Therapeutic potential of curcumin in human prostate cancer-I. Curcumin induces apoptosis in both androgen-dependent and androgen-independent prostate cancer cells. Prostate Cancer Prostatic Dis 3:84–93, 2000.

66. Nonn L, Duong D, Peehl M: Chemopreventive anti-inflammatory activities of curcumin and other phytochemicals mediated by MAP kinase phosphatase-5 in prostate cells. Carcinogenesis 28:1188–1196, 2007.

67. Chendil D, Ranga RS, Meigooni D, et al: Curcumin confers radiosensitizing effect in prostate cancer cell line PC-3. Oncogene 23:1599–1607, 2004.

68. Dorai T, Cao YC, Dorai B, et al: Therapeutic potential of curcumin in human prostate cancer. III. Curcumin inhibits proliferation, induces apoptosis, and inhibits angiogenesis of LNCaP prostate cancer cells in vivo. Prostate 47:293–303, 2001.

69. Narayanan BA: Chemopreventive agents alter global gene expression pattern: predicting their mode of action and targets. Curr Cancer Drug Targets 6:711–727, 2006.

70. Csiszar A, Smith K, Labinsky N, et al: Resveratrol attenuates TNF-alpha-induced activation of coronary artery endothelial cells: role of NF-kappaB inhibition, Am J Physiol Heart Circ Physiol 291:H1694–1699, 2006.

71. Adhami VM, Ahmad N, Mukhtar H: Molecular targets for green tea in prostate cancer chemoprevention. J Nutr 133(7Suppl):2417S–2424S, 2003.

72. Pezzato E, Sartor L, Dell'Aica I, et al: Prostate carcinoma and green tea. PSA-triggered basement membrane degradation and MMP-2 activation are inhibited by epigallocatechin-3-gallate. Int J Cancer 112:787–792, 2004.

73. Stuart EC, Scandlyn MJ, Rosengren RJ: Role of epigallocatechin gallate (EGCG) in the treatment of breast and prostate cancer. Life Sci 79:2329–2336, 2006.

74. Hussain T, Gupta S, Adhami VM, et al: Green tea constituent epigallocatechin-3-gallate selectively inhibits COX-2 without affecting COX-1 expression in human prostate carcinoma cells. Int J Cancer 113:660–669, 2005.

75. Kuo CL, Chi CW, Liu TY: The anti-inflammatory potential of berberine in vitro and in vivo. Cancer Lett 203:127–137, 2004.

76. Mantena SK, Sharma SD, Katiyar SK: Berberine, a natural product, induces GI-phase cell cycle arrest and caspase-3-dependent apoptosis in human prostate carcinoma cells. Mol Cancer Ther 5:296–308, 2006.

77. Bonham M, Posakony J, Coleman I, et al: Characterization of chemical constituents in *Scutellaria baicalensis* with anti-androgenic and growth-inhibitory activities toward prostate carcinoma. Clin Cancer Res 11:3905–3914, 2005.

78. Huang WH, Lee AR, Yang CH: Antioxidative and anti-inflammatory activities of polyhydroxyflavonoids of *Scutellaria baicalensis* GEORGI. Biosci Biotechnol Biochem 70:2371–2380, 2006.

79. Liu BQ, Fu T, Gong WH, et al: The flavonoid baicalin exhibits anti-inflammatory activity by binding to chemokines. Immunopharmacology 49:295–306, 2000.

80. Singh S: Mechanism of action of anti-inflammatory effect of fixed oil of *Ocimum basilicum Linn.* Indian J Exp Biol 37:248–252, 1999.

81. Shukla Y, Singh M: Cancer preventive properties of ginger: a brief review. Food Chem Toxicol 2006 Nov 12; epub ahead of print: dx.doi.org/10.1016/j.fct.2006.11.002, accessed 12/24/06.

82. Di Silverio F, Monti S, Sciarra A, et al: Effects of long-term treatment with *Serenoa repens* (Permixon) on the concentrations and regional distribution of androgens and epidermal growth factor in benign prostatic hyperplasia. Prostate 37:77–83, 1998.

83. Bemis DL, Capodice JL, Gorrochurn P, et al: Anti-prostate cancer activity of a beta-carboline alkaloid enriched extract from Rauwolfia vomitoria. Int J Oncol 29:1065–1073, 2006.

84. New Survey: Older Americans Abandon Healthy Diets, Turn to Supplements for Lower Cancer Risk." icr.com, http://www.icrsurvey.com/Study.aspx?f=Supplement_survey_release.html, accessed 11/14/06.

85. Virtamo J, Pietinen P, Huttunen J: Incidence of cancer and mortality following alpha-tocopherol and beta-carotene supplementation: a post-intervention follow-up. JAMA 290:476–485, 2003.

86. Weinstein SJ, Wright ME, Pietinen P: Serum alpha-tocopherol and gamma-tocopherol in relation to prostate cancer risk in a prospective study. J Natl Cancer Inst 97:396–399, 2005.

87. Sigounas G, Anagnostou A, Steiner M: DL-alpha tocopherol induces apoptosis in erythroleukemia, prostate, and breast cancer cells. Nutr Cancer 28:30–35, 1997.

88. Clark LC, Combs GF, Jr, Turnbull BW, et al: Effects of selenium supplementation for cancer prevention in patients with carcinoma of the skin. A randomized controlled trial. Nutritional Prevention of Cancer Study Group. JAMA 276:1957–1963, 1996.

89. Clark LC, Marshall JR: Randomized, controlled chemoprevention trials in populations at very high risk for prostate cancer: elevated prostate-specific antigen and high-grade prostatic intraepithelial neoplasia. Urology 57(4 Suppl 1):185–187, 2001.

90. Clark LC, Dalkin B, Krongrad A, et al: Decreased incidence of prostate cancer with selenium supplementation: results of a double-blind cancer prevention trial. Br J Urol 81:730–734, 1998.

91. Redman C, Scott JA, Baines AT, et al: Inhibitory effect of selenomethionine on the growth of three selected human tumor cell lines. Cancer Lett 125:103–110, 1998.

92. Venkateswaran V, Fleshner NE, Klotz LH: Synergistic effect of vitamin E and selenium in human prostate cancer cell lines. Prostate Cancer Prostatic Dis 7:54–56, 2004.

93. Yoshizawa K, Willett WC, Morris SJ, et al: Study of prediagnostic selenium level in toenails and the risk of advanced prostate cancer. J Natl Cancer Inst 90:1219–1224, 1998.

94. Van den Brandt PA, Zeegers MP, Bode P, Goldbohm RA: Toenail selenium levels and the subsequent risk of prostate cancer: a prospective cohort study. Cancer Epidemiol Biomarkers Prev 12:866–871, 2003.

95. Coates RJ, Weiss RS, Daling JR, et al: Serum levels of selenium and retinol and the subsequent risk of cancer. Am J Epidemiol 128:515–523, 1988.

96. Criqui MH, Bangdiwala S, Goodman DS, et al: Selenium, retinol, retinol-binding protein, and uric acid. Associations with cancer mortality in a population-based prospective case-control study. Ann Epidemiol 1:385–393, 1991.

97. Helzlsouer KJ, Huang HY, Alberg AJ, et al: Association between alpha-tocopherol, gamma-tocopherol, selenium, and subsequent prostate cancer. J Natl Cancer Inst 92:2018–2023, 2000.

98. Giovannucci E, Rimm EB, Wolk A, et al: Calcium and fructose intake in relation to risk of prostate cancer. Cancer Res 58:442–447, 1998.

99. Rodriguez C, McCullough ML, Mondul AM, et al: Calcium, dairy products, and risk of prostate cancer in a prospective cohort of United States men. Cancer Epidemiol Biomarkers Prev 12:597–603, 2003.

100. Vucenik I, Shamsuddin AM: Cancer inhibition by inositol hexaphosphate (IP6) and Inositol: from laboratory to clinic. J Nutr 133:3778S–3784S, 2003.

101. Singh RP, Agarwal P: Prostate cancer and inositol hexaphosphate: efficacy and mechanisms. Anticancer Res 25:2891–2903, 2005.

102. Shamsuddin AM, Yang GY: Inositol hexaphosphate strongly inhibits growth and induces differentiation of PC-3 human prostate cancer cells. Carcinogenesis 16:1975–1979, 1995.

103. Baten A, Ullah A, Tomazic VJ, et al: Inositol-phosphate-induced enhancement of natural killer cell activity correlates with tumor suppression. Carcinogenesis 10:1595–1598, 1989.

104. Demark-Wahnefried W, Aziz NM, Rowland JH, Pinto BM: Riding the crest of the teachable moment: promoting long–term health after the diagnosis of cancer. J Clin Oncol 23:5814–5830, 2005.

12

Controversies in Prostate Cancer

Adam W. Levinson

KEY POINTS

- Prostate cancer is the most common nondermatologic cancer and the second most common cause of cancer deaths in men in the United States.
- There are many controversies involving the treatment of clinically localized prostate cancer.
- Men with prostate cancer are ideal candidates for chemoprevention with nutrition because of the disease's long latency, high incidence, and strong correlation with specific dietary factors.
- Finasteride decreases the overall detection rate of prostate cancer, but increases the detection of high-grade, more clinically significant prostate cancer.
- Prostate-specific antigen (PSA) testing has dramatically transformed the diagnosis and treatment of prostate cancer.
- There is insufficient evidence to recommend either for or against routine prostate cancer screening with PSA.
- Radical prostatectomy and radiation therapy—whether by external-beam or brachytherapy—are the two most widely accepted and rigorously assessed therapies for localized prostate cancer.
- External-beam radiation therapy must be given in a total dosage of at least 72 Gy to be sufficient to treat prostate cancer.
- Brachytherapy is best suited as a monotherapy for low-risk, localized prostate cancer.
- All therapeutic modalities for prostate cancer lead to some degree of urinary and sexual dysfunction, though at different temporal evolutions.
- Comparing oncologic outcomes of radiation therapy with outcomes of surgery is challenging because of selection biases, era of treatment, and differing definitions of biochemical failure.
- Radical prostatectomy, brachytherapy, and external-beam radiation therapy have generally equivalent oncologic outcomes when modern dosages (more than 72 Gy) of radiation are used, although a slight advantage to radical prostatectomy may exist.
- Radical retropubic prostatectomy is the gold standard surgical therapy for prostate cancer.
- Minimally invasive prostatectomy—laparoscopic or robot-assisted—has less blood loss and a shorter convalescence than radical retropubic prostatectomy.
- All surgical approaches are likely to have identical oncologic and functional outcomes when surgeons with equivalent experiences are compared.
- The ablative therapies of high-intensity focused ultrasound and cryotherapy are promising, but remain experimental as first-line modalities.

Introduction

Prostate cancer is the most common nondermatologic malignancy of American men and the second leading cause of cancer-related death. In 2008, 186,320 American men will be diagnosed with prostate cancer and 28,660 will die of the disease[1] (Fig. 12-1). One in six men will be diagnosed with prostate cancer during their lifetime, and the true prevalence of prostate cancer is even higher, since autopsy studies demonstrate that more than 40% of men older than 50 and 75% of men older than 80 harbor evidence of the disease.[2-6] Despite the nearly ubiquitous incidence of prostate cancer and the millions of dollars poured into research to study the disease, expert urologic and radiation oncologists still disagree on many issues.

This chapter reviews the major areas of controversy in the field of prostate cancer and attempts to provide a balanced overview of many of the topics presented in this book. We begin with a brief overview of the preventive possibilities for prostate cancer and then tackle

Estimated New Cases*		Estimated Deaths	
Male	**Female**	**Male**	**Female**
Prostate 192,280 (25%)	Breast 192,370 (27%)	Lung and bronchus 88,900 (30%)	Lung and bronchus 70,490 (26%)
Lung and bronchus 116,090 (15%)	Lung and bronchus 103,350 (14%)	Prostate 27,360 (9%)	Breast 40,170 (15%)
Colon and rectum 75,590 (10%)	Colon and rectum 71,380 (10%)	Colon and rectum 25,240 (9%)	Colon and rectum 24,680 (9%)
Urinary bladder 52,810 (7%)	Uterine corpus 42,160 (6%)	Pancreas 18,030 (6%)	Pancreas 17,210 (6%)
Melanoma of the skin 39,080 (5%)	Non-Hodgkin lymphoma 29,990 (4%)	Leukemia 12,590 (4%)	Ovary 14,600 (5%)
Non-Hodgkin lymphoma 35,990 (5%)	Melanoma of the skin 29,640 (4%)	Liver and intrahepatic bile duct 12,090 (4%)	Non-Hodgkin lymphoma 9,670 (4%)
Kidney and renal pelvis 35,430 (5%)	Thyroid 27,200 (4%)	Esophagus 11,490 (4%)	Leukemia 9,280 (3%)
Leukemia 25,630 (3%)	Kidney and renal pelvis 22,330 (3%)	Urinary bladder 10,180 (3%)	Uterine corpus 7,780 (3%)
Oral cavity and pharynx 25,240 (3%)	Ovary 21,550 (3%)	Non-Hodgkin lymphoma 9,830 (3%)	Liver and intrahepatic bile duct 6,070 (2%)
Pancreas 21,050 (3%)	Pancreas 21,420 (3%)	Kidney and renal pelvis 8,160 (3%)	Brain and other nervous system 5,590 (2%)
All sites 766,130 (100%)	All sites 713,220 (100%)	All sites 292,540 (100%)	All sites 269,800 (100%)

*Excludes basal and squamous cell skin cancers and in situ carcinoma except urinary bladder.

Figure 12-1. Leading sites of new cancer cases and deaths, 2009 estimates. (From Cancer Facts and Figures 2009. © 2009, American Cancer Society, Inc. Surveillance Research.)

the larger questions, including the two biggest questions in prostate cancer: Whom do we need to treat, and, if we do treat, what is the best treatment? We conclude with topics of dispute that surround the newer, minimally invasive, therapeutic modalities for the treatment of localized prostate cancer.

Diet

Although family history has long been considered a primary risk factor for the development of prostate cancer, along with race and age, it is only recently that a variety of single-nucleotide polymorphisms have been identified as high-risk inherited factors for the disease, playing a role in as many as 48% of incident cases.[7-10] The influence of diet and environment, however, has not always been as readily appreciated in the pathogenesis of prostate cancer. Nevertheless, there is strong epidemiologic evidence that environmental factors, including diet, play a key role in the transformation and/or progression of latent prostate cancer or high-grade prostatic intraepithelial neoplasia into clinically apparent invasive prostate cancer. Much of this evidence comes from

epidemiologic studies of migrant families. For example, whereas prostate cancer is relatively rare in both native Chinese and Japanese populations, immigration studies revealed an increase in the incidence of prostate cancer among these nationalities one generation after migration to the United States. In fact, the rates become similar to those of American men of either Caucasian or Hispanic ethnicity.[11,12] The opposite is true of Scandinavians, who have a higher rate of prostate cancer in their home country, but whose rate drops to American rates after one generation.[13]

In addition to showing a high incidence in many countries, prostate cancer has a long latency period between histologic evidence of the disease and the development of clinical symptoms or death. *These factors—high incidence, long latency, and strong environmental influence—make prostate cancer an ideal target for chemopreventive approaches, such as dietary modulation.*

However, despite the strong circumstantial and epidemiologic evidence of environmental and dietary factors in the pathogenesis of prostate cancer, little traction has been gained by proponents of dietary modulation in prostate cancer prevention. Although many foods and diets have been studied, only a few have been rigorously examined and even fewer have led conclusively to positive results. The one chemopreventive agent that has been rigorously interrogated and found to have "positive" results—finasteride—has its own issues, which are covered separately in the next section.[14] A few of the most studied dietary modulations are discussed in the following text, and a thorough review of the impact of diet on prostate cancer is available in Chapter 11 of this book.

Lycopene, Selenium, and Vitamin E

Lycopene is the red-orange carotenoid pigment found abundantly in processed tomato products, such as tomato sauce and ketchup (Table 12-1). It is a powerful antioxidant and has been examined as a preventive agent against cancer, prostate disease, and cardiovascular disease. Moreover, there is some epidemiologic and interventional evidence to support the use of lycopene against prostate cancer. A large 1999 review found that 57 of 72 studies revealed inverse associations between cancer risk at various sites and blood lycopene level, and further investigations found protective effects of lycopene against prostate cancer specifically.[15–17] In 2003, Kim and associates published a small interventional trial that found that tomato sauce consumption before prostatectomy decreased serum prostate-specific antigen (PSA) and decreased oxidative DNA damage.[18,19]

Selenium and vitamin E also were studied recently for possible prevention of prostate cancer in the Selenium and Vitamin E Chemo-

prevention Trial (SELECT). SELECT was the largest prevention trial ever undertaken using a drug or nutrient and was slated to yield results in 2012. It was designed to involve 32,400 men aged 55 and older (50 and older for African Americans) at 435 research centers in the United States, Puerto Rico, and Canada. The evidence for selenium derives its origin from the Nutritional Prevention of Cancer Trial, a randomized study of oral selenium in patients with nonmelanoma skin cancer whose primary endpoint was recurrence of skin cancer. Although the study demonstrated no significant effect on skin cancer recurrence, daily supplementation with selenium significantly reduced prostate cancer incidence after a mean follow-up of 7.4 years.[20] In subsequent biomarker-based studies, selenium was associated with either a significantly lower risk of prostate cancer or a trend toward lower risk.[21,22] As for vitamin E, a similarly non–prostate cancer-based study provides much of the impetus for current research. In the Alpha-Tocopherol, Beta-Carotene (ATBC) Study, 29,133 male smokers received daily doses of alpha-tocopherol (a form of vitamin E), beta carotene, both, or a placebo. Although beta carotene had no effect on prostate cancer risk, alpha-tocopherol supplementation reduced the risk of prostate cancer by 32%.[23]

Subjects in the SELECT trial received daily doses of 200 µg of selenium, 400 IU of vitamin E, both nutrients, or two placebo capsules. Caution was taken, however, because a recent randomized controlled trial found that 400 IU or more of vitamin E per day increased all-cause mortality and heart failure incidence.[24]

Unfortunately, the medium-term results of the SELECT trial were so poor that the independent data and safety monitoring committee recommended early termination of the study and published the results ahead of schedule. In the final analysis of 35,533 men, after a median of 5.5 years of follow-up, neither selenium nor vitamin E, alone or in combination, had any preventative effect on the development of prostate cancer. In fact, in absolute numbers, more men who were given either the selenium or vitamin E developed prostate cancer than those given a placebo, and the increase in risk with vitamin E was nearly statistically significant ($P = .06$). In addition, men in the vitamin E group had a dubious trend toward developing type 2 diabetes ($P = .16$). A second large randomized study, the Physicians' Health Study II Randomized Con-

Table 12-1. Lycopene Content of Various Foods

Food	Lycopene Content (mg/100 g)
Tomatoes, raw	0.9–4.2
Tomatoes, cooked	3.7–4.4
Tomato sauce	7.3–18.0
Tomato paste	5.4–55.5
Tomato soup (condensed)	8.0–10.9
Tomato juice	5.0–11.6
Catsup	9.9–13.4
Watermelon, fresh	2.3–7.2
Papaya, fresh	2.0–5.3
Grapefruit, pink/red	0.2–3.4

From Miller EC, Giovannucci EL, Erdman JW, Jr, et al: Tomato products, lycopene, and prostate cancer risk. J Urol Clin N Am 29:88–93, 2002, Table 2.

trolled Trial, looked at the effects of vitamin C and vitamin E on prostate cancer development, and these results were published simultaneously with the SELECT results in JAMA. In this study also, after a mean of 8.0 years of follow-up, no beneficial preventative effect of either vitamin E or vitamin C was identified.[25,26]

Other Dietary Associations

Other less rigorously analyzed possible targets for chemoprevention include pomegranate extract, soy proteins, holy basil, fish oils, mushrooms, green tea, and others; clinical trials are ongoing in all of these areas.[27–31] Time will tell which, if any, will prove to be of benefit.

Obesity and fat intake have unclear associations with prostate cancer. There is, at best, a questionable association between increased dietary fat and prostate cancer, gained mainly from observational studies.[4,32–35] The association of decreased prostate cancer-specific mortality with increasing amounts of omega-3 fatty acids seems more promising.[36]

It is possible that high amounts of dietary calcium and vitamin D actually promote prostate cancer. Current guidelines for calcium intake for osteoporosis prevention recommend that men over 50 take 1200 mg of calcium daily. However, in epidemiologic studies of calcium intake from diet and supplements, men with the highest intake of calcium have significantly elevated risk of prostate cancer.[37,38]

Overall, most of the data for chemoprevention and dietary modulation either has been grossly negative or is promising but immature. However, one chemopreventive—finasteride—has been rigorously studied and found to be "successful" in a controversial randomized trial.

Role of Finasteride in Prevention of Prostate Cancer

The Prostate Cancer Prevention Trial

Is it possible to prevent prostate cancer? This is a complex question that goes to the heart of a raging debate within the urologic oncology community. In 2003, the results of the Prostate Cancer Prevention Trial (PCPT) were published.[14] This was a well-run study that ambitiously went past the persistent unanswered questions surrounding screening and treatment

and attempted to discover whether a chemotherapeutic regimen could prevent the diagnosis of prostate cancer. The therapy of choice was finasteride, a 5α-reductase inhibitor that is known to shrink the size of prostate glands and is more commonly used in the medical management of benign prostatic hypertrophy. 5α-Reductase blocks the conversion of testosterone to the more potent androgen, dihydrotestosterone. The significance of the study findings is hotly debated.

Overview of the Study

A brief overview of the PCPT is necessary to understand the controversy surrounding finasteride: Between January 1994 and May 1997, nearly 19,000 men were randomized to receive daily finasteride ($n = 9459$) or daily placebo ($n = 9423$) for a duration of 7 years (Fig. 12-2). As part of the study design, patients received prostate biopsies either for "cause" (determined by a rise in actual or adjusted PSA or by an abnormal digital rectal examination [DRE]) or at the end of the 7-year study period. Through biopsy, prostate cancer was detected in 803 of 4368 men (18.4%) taking finasteride compared with 1147 of the 4692 men (24.4%) in the

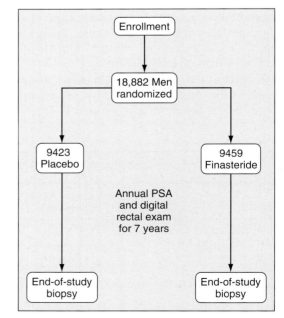

Figure 12-2. Scheme for the Prostate Cancer Prevention Trial. (From Canby-Hagino E, Hernandez J, Brand TC, Thompson I: Looking back at PCPT: looking forward to new paradigms in prostate cancer screening and prevention. Eur Urol 51:27–33, 2007, Figure 1.)

placebo group. This was equivalent to a nearly 25% reduction in the prevalence (or perhaps better stated, detection rate) of prostate cancer in the finasteride group ($P < .001$). As expected, men in the finasteride group had less benign prostatic hypertrophy-related symptoms, but more sexual side effects. They also had glands roughly 25% smaller than the men in the placebo group. These facts are not in dispute.

The controversy begins in regard to patients with high-grade prostate cancer, which is the type that would be more likely to lead to clinically relevant cancer. Although the overall detection rate of prostate cancer was lower in the finasteride group, the prevalence of Gleason grade 7–10 cancers was higher: 6.4% in the finasteride group compared with 5.1% in the placebo group. It could be argued, therefore, that finasteride prevented only the clinically insignificant cancers and either increased the number of clinically significant cancers or, at best, did not decrease them. This finding has dampened the enthusiasm for finasteride as a chemopreventive agent among most urologists.

Significance of the PCPT

In general, the PCPT was significant for various differing findings, many of which have little to do with prostate cancer prevention and many of which were derived from the control arm of the study.

First: There is no absolute cut-off of PSA below which prostate cancer does not occur.

The end-of-study biopsies in the control arm of the PCPT confirmed what many had already suspected. Despite the great stage migration and overall decrease in the death rate from prostate cancer likely due to PSA screening, PSA is not a perfect screening tool. *There is no PSA cut-off level with both a high sensitivity and a high specificity to screen healthy men for prostate cancer.* In the cohort of men with low PSA (less than 4.0 ng/mL) and normal DRE, prostate cancer was found in 15.2% when they underwent a biopsy (not for a specific cause) at the end of the study. However, only 2% of these cancers were high-grade cancers.[39] Cancer was even found in 6.2% of men with PSA lower than 0.5 ng/mL.[39] However, one must wonder how many of these low-PSA, negative-DRE cancers would ever have become clinically significant during that man's lifetime. Nevertheless, pros-

tate cancers, even high-grade prostate cancers, may be found at all PSA levels, although it is true that higher PSA values are correlated with a higher prevalence of high-grade and total prostate cancers.

Second: The prevalence of prostate cancer, including the end-of-study biopsies, was roughly four times the expected prevalence from prior population-based studies (i.e., 24% versus 6%).

A surprising finding in this study was the high prevalence of prostate cancer among men without clinical suspicion for prostate cancer. The study design assumed a 6% prevalence based on prior population and epidemiologic studies.[40] This estimate was deliberately conservative to reduce the risk of underpowering the study. It is interesting that the incidence of prostate cancer detected on the basis of clinical suspicion (i.e., an abnormal prostate examination or elevated PSA) during the study was 6%, which is similar to the rate in prior studies. This suggests that a substantial percentage of prostate cancers detected in end–of-study biopsies might never develop into clinically significant cancers. By extension, this finding questions the significance of many of the lower-grade, lower-stage cancers that we currently diagnose and treat. *Since only 3% of men ever die of prostate cancer, the PCPT reveals the significant number of men who may harbor clinically insignificant disease.* This finding calls into serious question the risks of overdetection and overtreatment, which is further discussed more in the next section.

Overall Summary of PCPT

To date, finasteride is the only agent that is definitively proven in a randomized, placebo-controlled, prospective clinical trial to prevent prostate cancer. Finasteride lowers the diagnosis of prostate cancer by 25%. Unfortunately, it is correlated to the detection of a higher number of high-grade, and therefore perhaps clinically significant, cancers. The general urologic consensus is that these two factors directly offset each other, and therefore most urologists question its true benefit. The authors of the trial, however, have controversially attempted to claim that by decreasing the number of Gleason 6 prostate cancers, treatment with finasteride is actually selecting out clinically relevant cancers and is therefore beneficial.[41,42] To say that this is widely accepted would be a stretch, although other well-respected oncologists seem to agree,[43] and a joint statement from the American Urological Association and the American Society of Clinical Oncology attempts to sway the unconvinced masses.[40,44,45]

Ironically, if there is a theoretical benefit in finasteride chemoprevention, it might not be in the prevention of significant prostate cancer, but rather in the prevention of the diagnosis of *insignificant* prostate cancer. Despite the relative lack of aggressiveness of many Gleason 6 cancers, most men—up to 95% in a recent CaPSURE (Cancer of the Prostate Strategic Urologic Research Endeavor) database review—choose to undergo treatment. This is usually at a cost of not only dollars but also of quality of life.[46] Therefore, from a public health perspective, if finasteride chemoprevention could prevent the burden of diagnosis and subsequent treatment of some cancers that were never likely to produce morbidity or mortality, this in and of itself could be viewed as beneficial.[47,48]

To Screen or Not to Screen

Routine prostate cancer screening consists of an annual DRE and serum PSA test in men with a life expectancy of at least 10 years who are over the age of 50, or younger if they have a high risk of prostate cancer. The American Cancer Society and the American Urological Association recommend offering this routine screening to these appropriately selected patients, yet the American Association of Family Practitioners and the American Medical Association are reluctant to do so. All of these professional organizations, who acknowledge the controversy, recommend that the decision to screen for prostate cancer must be an individualized decision between the patient and the physician.

With the arguments over the merits and necessity of screening and the still somewhat unsettled debate as to whether early intervention in prostate cancer affects survival, it is easy to forget the lethality of the disease. Prostate cancer is the fifth most common cause of death in men over age 45, following heart disease, lung cancer, stroke, and emphysema.[6] As with most other cancers, the risk of being diagnosed with prostate cancer increases with age (Table 12-2). One in 33 men will die of prostate cancer.[1,6] Thankfully, owing to prostate cancer screening, and serum PSA specifically, the death rate from prostate cancer is decreasing. In addition, screen-

Table 12-2. Risk of Being Diagnosed with Prostate Cancer by Age

Age	Risk
45	1 in 2500
50	1 in 476
55	1 in 120
60	1 in 43
65	1 in 21
70	1 in 13
75	1 in 9
Ever	1 in 6

From U.S. Department of Health and Human Services: *Prostate Cancer Screening: A Decision Guide.* Atlanta, GA: Centers for Disease Control and Prevention and National Cancer Institute, 2006.

ing is already prevalent, since most American men over the age of 50 will receive a PSA test and will be screened for prostate cancer.[49] Yet, there is wide disagreement among the major medical organizations over the value of prostate cancer screening. In 2002, the U.S. Preventive Services Task Force (USPSTF), after careful deliberation, determined that insufficient evidence existed to recommend either for or against routine prostate cancer screening with PSA.[50] This statement from the USPSTF places the major points of the debate in context:

> The USPSTF found good evidence that PSA screening can detect early-stage prostate cancer but mixed and inconclusive evidence that early detection improves health outcomes. Screening is associated with important harms, including frequent false-positive results and unnecessary anxiety, biopsies, and potential complications of treatment of some cancers that may never have affected a patient's health. The USPSTF concludes that evidence is insufficient to determine whether the benefits outweigh the harms for a screened population. (U.S. Preventive Services Task Force. Screening for Prostate Cancer. Release Date: December 2002.[50])

Let's examine the statement above on the basis of the facts we know.

PSA early detection programs have transformed the diagnosis and treatment of prostate cancer. The incidence of prostate cancer rose steadily after the introduction of PSA until a peak in 1991 and then reached a plateau (Fig. 12-3). As expected, this more than doubled the incidence of prostate cancer. The lifetime risk

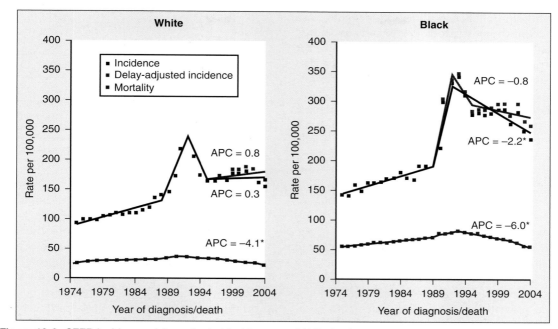

Figure 12-3. SEER incidence, delay adjusted incidence, and U.S. death rates for prostate cancer, by race. APC, annual percentage change for the regression line segments. (From SEER Cancer Statistics Review 1975–2005.)

of being diagnosed with prostate cancer is now 1 in 6. As a result of PSA screening, however, 50% of newly diagnosed prostate cancers are early-stage and localized, and 90% are regional. This represents a considerable downward stage migration and has been driven almost entirely by PSA. Indeed, in 1980, 20% of patients presented with metastases; in 2004, only 5% did.[51,52]

Perhaps the strongest argument for the usefulness of prostate cancer screening has been the concomitant dramatic reduction in prostate cancer-specific mortality that has come with early detection. The annual age-adjusted prostate cancer death rate in the United States has declined steadily and dramatically since the widespread dissemination of PSA screening in the early 1990s[6,52] (see Fig. 4-3).

What is the reason for this decline? Whereas the increase in 5-year survival rates from 69% 25 years ago to nearly 100% at the present time can be mainly explained by lead-time bias, the overall decrease in age-adjusted death rates due to prostate cancer cannot. The reason for this decline is the availability of curative modalities for localized prostate cancer, namely, surgery and radiation. These modalities have now proved to be superior to no treatment, although because of the long natural history of prostate cancer, it took nearly 10 years to see the beneficial effect of therapy.[53]

Prostate-Specific Antigen

What is the chemical at the heart of the debate? PSA was originally discovered in the early 1970s as a criminal forensic adjunct to aid in the examination of cases of rape. Not until the 1980s was its association with prostate cancer noted.[54,55] PSA is a serine protease that serves to liquefy the seminal coagulum after ejaculation. It is mostly confined to the prostate and is produced primarily by epithelial cells that line the prostatic ducts and acini.[54]

Part of the problem is that using PSA is not like using a home pregnancy test. You do not get a "+" or "−" to tell you "yes cancer" or "no cancer."

PSA enters the serum via disruptions of the prostatic cell and basement membranes. When prostate cancer becomes invasive, it disrupts the basement membrane, allowing more PSA to leak into the bloodstream, and serum PSA values subsequently rise. Unfortunately, the PSA elevations suffer from a lack of specificity because these PSA leaks may also occur with a host of benign conditions, such as benign prostatic hypertrophy, prostatitis, urinary tract infections, constipation, urinary catheterization, and other manipulations of the urinary tract.[55] Thus, *high serum PSA concentrations are associated with both benign and cancerous prostates.*

Therefore, PSA is not specific enough for use as a blunt diagnostic tool. Fortunately, in knowledgeable hands with the use of a variety of PSA metrics, we may increase the specificity and sensitivity of screening regimens, thereby preventing unnecessary morbidity and distress.

Before discussing the metrics that increase the specificity and sensitivity of PSA as a prostate cancer screening tool, we must first briefly readdress one element of the "pregnancy test–like" desired myth of PSA, namely, the existence of a rigid cut-off value. *There is no rigid cut-off value to label a PSA value normal or abnormal.*

As already addressed in the discussion of the PCPT, cancer and no cancer alike may be found at all values of PSA. Higher PSA values are associated with a greater likelihood of prostate cancer and with a greater likelihood of high-grade prostate cancer, but no values are absolute. Classically, a value greater than 4.0 ng/mL is considered worrisome, but some have suggested lowering this value to 2.5 ng/mL for greater sensitivity.[49,56] It is important to recognize that even if more cancers are discovered at the lower threshold, there is no evidence that treating the cancers at 2.5 ng/mL leads to any greater survival than waiting until the PSA rises to the 4.0 ng/mL threshold.[39,57–59]

PSA Metrics to Improve Sensitivity and Specificity

Why do rigid cut-off values not work? The answer is because not all prostates or prostate cancers are the same.

Besides the lack of specificity of PSA elevations that we have already discussed, it is important to recognize the distinct lack of homogeneity in populations with similar PSA values. First, we need to understand that larger glands naturally make more PSA, and older men naturally have larger glands. This brings to light two important and easily understandable metrics that increase the specificity of PSA screening, namely, the concept of age-specific PSA and PSA density. A PSA of 4.2 is likely to be completely normal in a 75-year-old man with an 80-g prostate, whereas the same PSA of 4.2 is worrisome in a 45-year-old man with a 20-g prostate and requires a biopsy. Using these principles, investigators have been able to increase the accuracy of PSA in detecting prostate cancer by establishing age-

Table 12-3. Normal PSA Levels by Age Ranges and Race

Age Range	Asian	White	Black
40–49	0–2.0 ng/mL	0–2.5 ng/mL	0–2.0 ng/mL
50–59	0–3.0 ng/mL	0–3.5 ng/mL	0–4.0 ng/mL
60–69	0–4.0 ng/mL	0–4.5 ng/mL	0–4.5 ng/mL
70–79	0–5.0 ng/mL	0–6.5 ng/mL	0–5.5 ng/mL

From The Prostate Specific Antigen (PSA) Blood Test, Prostate Cancer Coalition of North Carolina. Available at http://www.pccnc.org/early-detection/psa. (Originally referenced in Urology Times.)

related PSA and PSA density thresholds[60,61] (Table 12-3).

The next breakthrough in improving the usefulness of PSA as a prostate cancer screening tool was the recognition of the value of PSA kinetics, namely, PSA velocity and PSA doubling-time. It was discovered that benign prostatic hypertrophy does consistently elevate serum PSA values over time, but typically at a slower rate than prostate cancer. Studies have shown that, within a PSA range of 4.0 to 10.0 ng/mL, a rise of more than 0.75 ng/mL per year shows a specificity of cancer detection of 90% and a sensitivity of 79%.[62] For patients with PSA values less than 4.0 ng/mL, a lower-velocity threshold between 0.3 and 0.5 ng/mL is required to improve the sensitivity while maintaining the specificity.[49,63,64]

Free PSA

Finally, a novel isoform of PSA is available to increase the usefulness of PSA screening regimens. Free PSA refers to that proportion of the total PSA that circulates in the blood unbound to protein.[65] The majority of PSA that circulates in the blood—65% to 95%—is complexed to one of several proteins, primarily α_1-antichymotrypsin. The remaining 5% to 35% of circulating PSA is unbound.[66,67] PSA released from prostate cancer cells tends to escape intracellular proteolytic processing, thereby leading to reduced proportions of free PSA in the serum of prostate cancer patients. This characteristic has been used to provide additional specificity for cancer detection.[68–72]

In the future, we will have novel biomarkers superior to PSA to improve the diagnostic accuracy of screening regimens. Although they are beyond the scope of this chapter, tests such as EPCA-2, PCA3, AMACR, and human kallikrein-2 show great promise and may lead to a more simplistic and accurate regimen of prostate cancer screening.[73–78]

Digital Rectal Exam

The other half of the prostate cancer screening regimen is the digital rectal examination (DRE). DRE relies on the recognition that most prostate cancers develop in the peripheral zone of the prostate, and the hope that these cancers may then be palpated before becoming symptomatic and early enough to still be curable. Although DRE has been used for many years, a rigorous interrogation of the modality is lacking. Even in the best hands, DRE is notoriously inaccurate, and its relevance in the PSA era may be decreasing. DRE has a roughly 25% positive predictive value for prostate cancer, and when cancers are found via DRE, it is often too late for cure. Classic studies have found that as few as 20% to 30% of prostate cancers diagnosed via DRE are localized, and as many as 25% of patients with metastatic prostate cancer may still have a normal rectal examination.[79–81] However, case-control studies have found a 20% to 30% reduction in prostate cancer mortality rates when DRE is used and up to 25% of cancers may be found *only* via DRE, even with a normal (below 4.0 ng/mL) PSA.[39,57,58,82,83]

Therefore, because DRE is cheap and easy and may improve overall prostate cancer mortality despite its low positive predictive value, it is still recommended as part of the routine screening regimen.

Are there any randomized controlled trials that assess the value of prostate cancer screening? The answer is yes. But like every other topic related to prostate cancer, the results are contradictory and require a bit of extrapolation. There are actually four large ongoing randomized trials assessing the benefits of prostate cancer screening, and two have recently published (somewhat prematurely) their results in the *New England Journal of Medicine*. These studies are the European Randomized Study of Screening for Prostate Cancer (ERSPC) and the Prostate Lung Colorectal and Ovarian (PLCO) Cancer Screening Trial in the United States.[1,6,84,85] Both are admirable massive undertakings, and both have significant methodological flaws. Let's approach the studies one at a time.

The first, the PLCO trial, is a randomized study of 76,693 men between the ages of 55 and 74 who were recruited between 1993 and 2001 and assigned to either annual prostate cancer screening (DRE and serum PSA) or "usual care" as a control. Though the study was designed to run much longer, the trial results were published after a median 11.5 years of follow-up. *The study found no benefit to prostate cancer screening in overall or prostate cancer specific mortality*. There are many problems with the study, however; we will focus on three of them here.

First, it is important to understand that while an "intent-to-screen" analysis is the correct and valid method for primary analysis of the study, in an analysis of this type researchers do not actually compare patients who were screened against patients who were not. What is compared is the randomized population of patients *who were intended to be screened* against the population of patients *who were intended not to be screened*. Instead of a perfect comparison of a population with 100% screening versus a population of 0% screening, this study was severely contaminated. At least 52% of patients in the nonscreening "control" arm of the study were in fact screened for prostate cancer with at least one PSA and then compared to the "screened" arm of the study, in which only 85% of the patients were actually screened. The overall "contamination" of the nonscreened arm may in fact be much higher, because the 52% number represents only a survey of patients in a single year of the study. Overall, many more patients in the control arm may have been screened at least once during the study period, and the number may very well approximate the 85% of men who actually received a PSA and DRE in the screened arm. In an intent-to-screen analysis, this "contamination" would make it all the more difficult to find a survival benefit in the screened population. Second, nearly half (44%) of patients had already undergone PSA screening prior to study initiation. Because patients with a "positive" test were excluded from the study group, many men who were diagnosed with prostate cancer via screening prior to study initiation, and who then benefited from subsequent treatment, were not included in the analysis, further weakening the study's power to detect a survival benefit in the screening arm. Finally, the study used a rigid "cut-off" value of 4.0 ng/mL to determine a "positive" test, and we have already described limitations of such a protocol. In addition, the study did not make use of any of the other PSA metrics that we have described to increase both the sensitivity and specificity of the test.

In contrast to the findings of the PLCO trial, the ESRPC *did show a 20% reduction in prostate cancer mortality with PSA screening*. This trial involved a much larger cohort, 182,160 men aged 50 to 74, of which 162,387 were in the "core age group" of 55 to 69 years of age. The study is comprised of men from seven countries who were recruited via similar protocols between 1991 and 2003 and were randomly assigned to PSA screening or usual care. Mean and median follow-up were both approximately 9 years. Besides the significantly larger study size and shorter follow-up time, there are several important distinctions between this study and the PLCO. First, no digital rectal examination was used. Second, PSA screening was not annual but was instead scheduled to be done roughly once every four years. Third, the protocol was not uniform between study centers. Fourth, a different rigid PSA cutoff value of 3.0 ng/mL was used. Eighty-two percent of the patients in the study arm received at least one PSA test, and those who received a PSA test did so an average of 2.1 times during the trial. This study therefore suffers from many of the same deficits as the PLCO trial, namely too short a follow-up, incomplete penetration of PSA testing in the study arm, and use of a rigid cutoff value for PSA. In addition, without annual testing, none of the valuable PSA metrics and none of the supplemental information garnered from a DRE could be used. Nevertheless, because of greater overall numbers and likely significantly lower contamination of the control arm by PSA screening, this study was able to identify a statistically significant reduction in prostate cancer mortality, even after the very short follow-up time. Men who were *actually* screened (as opposed to those who were intended to be screened in the intent-to-screen analysis) had an even greater reduction in mortality. Even more promising, patients in the screening arm had a 41% reduction in either positive bone scans or PSA values greater than 100 ng/mL (a surrogate for grossly metastatic disease). These results anticipate even greater reductions in prostate cancer specific mortality to be seen with longer follow-up times.

It cannot be ignored, however, that questions of judicious allocation of resources and quality-of-life cost-benefit analyses were also brought to the forefront of the prostate cancer screening discussion with the publication of these studies. According to calculations of the ERSPC authors, 1410 men must be screened and 48 men treated for prostate cancer to prevent a single prostate cancer death.[84] With longer follow-up times (more deaths in the control arm), improvements in prostate cancer therapies, and improved specificity of screening regimens for clinically significant prostate cancer, these numbers are expected to improve. As they stand, these numbers are similar to those in screening regimens for both colorectal cancer and breast cancer, but with a notable increased morbidity of insignificant diagnoses.[86]

In the end, it is likely that much of what ERSPC proves is what was discarded in the exclusion criteria of the PLCO—namely, the value of even a single PSA test in an asymptomatic man to diagnose clinically relevant prostate cancer. Patients who had already received a "positive" PSA test prior to initiation of the PLCO were ineligible for that study. Both studies are still ongoing, and further results with longer follow-up times are anxiously awaited.

Whom do we need to screen for prostate cancer? Because prostate cancer is generally slow-growing and differences in overall survival with early treatment have been found mainly in those less than 65 years old, it seems reasonable to limit those who are screened.[53] In August 2008, the U.S. Preventive Services Task Force formally recommended against screening for prostate cancer in men age 75 years or older as it found "moderate certainty that the harms of screening for prostate cancer outweigh the benefits" in this population.[87,108]

Generally speaking, only men older than age 50 with a life expectancy of at least 10 years should be screened for prostate cancer with an annual PSA blood test and DRE. For African Americans and men with a family history of prostate cancer, screening should begin at age 40 or 45 years.

Management of Localized Prostate Cancer

To Treat or Not to Treat: Debate Over Expectant Management

There are many controversies related to prostate cancer, but perhaps the largest among these are:

- Which prostate cancers warrant treatment?
- What treatment is best?

There is no simple answer to either question. The simplest answer for the first question is that some men require treatment for prostate cancer and some do not. Prostate cancers are known to encompass a diverse range of natural histories—some destined to aggressive outcomes and most destined to clinically insignificant indolent courses. Whereas autopsy series, as mentioned earlier, reveal that a majority of elderly men will harbor prostate cancer, only 3% of men die of the disease.[2,3,88,89] Because prostate cancer is a common cancer of old age, the median time from diagnosis to death by the disease often exceeds the life expectancy of elderly men. This outcome is often accentuated by the lead-time bias that is inherent in screening regimens. Nevertheless, 30,000 men per year do die of prostate cancer, so there is obviously a population that would benefit from curative treatment. How many must be treated to save a life? For younger patients with high-risk disease, it may be 15 to 20 men. But for patients older than 65, it skyrockets to 330 men who must undergo the morbidity of prostate cancer treatment to save only one life.[53,90–94]

Since the morbidity of treatment of prostate cancer may be severe, regardless of modality, the challenge of determining which cancers need not be treated is important. We must be able to find better ways of focusing our resources while preserving quality of life. In this section, I explore the rationale for withholding immediate treatment in some men with prostate cancer.

Why Not Treat?

The first question to ask is why would some men choose to wait or not be treated at all? What are the risks and morbidities of treating prostate cancer with curative intent? This is the question that the Prostate Cancer Outcomes Study was designed to answer. This large, prospective, population-based study enrolled men with localized prostate cancer diagnosed in 1994 and 1995 and collected follow-up data through 2001. Of the 1291 men undergoing radical prostatectomy, 59.9% were impotent and 8.4% were incontinent within 18 months after surgery. Forty-one percent of the study participants undergoing surgery reported that sexual performance was a moderate to large problem after treatment. Of the 497 patients who received external-beam radiation therapy, 43% of the previously potent men were impotent within 2 years and 5.4% had significant bowel dysfunction.[95] Similar findings have been noted in a large randomized trial in Sweden that compared radical prostatectomy with conservative management.[96]

As mentioned earlier, PSA screening not only detects more cancers but detects cancers earlier (i.e., lead time before symptomatic presentation) and at a less aggressive stage. The lead time is likely to be shorter for aggressive cancers and longer for indolent ones. For men aged 55 to 75 years who are diagnosed by screening, this lead time may be 12 or more years.[97,98] Other studies have shown that the mean time to prostate cancer-specific mortality in patients with PSA-only detected, nonpalpable (pT1) lesions is 17 years. For palpable lesions (pT2 or greater), it is 11.2 years. In the United States in 2004, the average life expectancy for a 65-year-old man was 17.1 years; for a 75-year-old man, 10.7 years.[99,100] It has been estimated that with current screening regimens even in relatively young men, more than half of cases would be expected to be destined to clinically insignificant courses.[101–113]

The long lead time, downward stage migration, and long natural history of prostate cancer make it an excellent disease option for preintervention monitoring (expectant management) or for overall conservative management in patients with short life expectancies.[103] In properly selected cases, there is a long quiescent period during which observation is safe without losing the opportunity for cure. This is the rationale behind expectant management, a rationale bolstered by the not insignificant morbidity associated with all prostate cancer therapeutic modalities.

How Long to Wait Before Intervention

In the population destined to require curative intent, how long is it safe to wait before treatment? Many studies have documented long survival in patients who receive no treatment.[104,105] A recent study from Johns Hopkins provides further pathologic information for patients who eventually undergo treatment. In their study, patients were advised to proceed with definitive treatment in the event of progression of disease on subsequent prostate biopsies (i.e., an increase in the number of positive needle cores demonstrating cancer or an increase in the grade of the cancer). From this study, it appears that over 2 years may pass from diagnosis to treatment in appropriately selected low-risk patients without significantly altering the pathology or prognosis at the time of radical prostatectomy. The researchers concluded that delayed prostate cancer surgery for patients with small, lower-grade prostate cancers followed expectantly does not appear to compromise the surgical curability of these cancers.[106] Therefore, at the very worst, expectant management delays the potential morbidity of surgery in an otherwise low-risk cohort of patients, and these patients are not adversely affected by deferring their treatment.

Evidence of Improved Survival with Early Intervention

Although there is certainly a population of patients with prostate cancer who benefit from conservative or expectant management, this discussion leads us to another of the landmark trials in urology, *the only randomized trial to prove that in some men intervention does improve survival*, albeit marginally. The study in question is the Scandinavian Prostate Cancer Study Group's prospective randomized trial originally published by Holmberg and associates[107] in 2002 and updated by Bill-Axelson and associates[53] in 2005 and again in 2008.[108] This trial compared radical prostatectomy with watchful waiting (followed by palliative rather than curative therapy) in men presenting with clinically localized prostate cancer. It is critical to recognize the difference of the patient population in this study from the typical screened population of today. Namely, these patients had significantly higher-risk disease. The majority of patients presented with palpable disease and a higher PSA than is typical in the current era. *These factors would most likely bias the cohort toward benefiting from therapy with curative intent.* Nevertheless, it was not until the second update of the study in 2005 after a median of 8.2 years of follow-up that a small but significant overall survival benefit to radical prostatectomy, compared with watchful waiting, became apparent (Fig. 12-4). There were also more clearly demonstrated benefits in the radical prostatectomy group in relative risk of prostate cancer-specific mortality 0.56 (95% CI 0.36-0.88), distant metastasis 0.60 (95% CI 0.42-0.86), and local progression 0.33 (95% CI 0.25-0.44). The

2008 update further expands and confirms these findings. Other landmark studies have also revealed the limitations and inferiority of a simple watchful waiting protocol in certain patient populations.[90,91,105] Of note, given the long natural history of prostate cancer, further follow-up may reveal an even greater survival benefit.

However, in the Scandinavian Prostate Cancer Study, the majority of the survival benefit was discovered in patients with relatively advanced disease and who were younger than 65 (see Fig. 4-9). This reinforces the importance of bearing in mind a patient's comorbidities and life expectancy when considering either screening or intervention for localized prostate cancer. The Scandinavian Prostate Cancer Study Group's authors continue to study the cohort to determine what other clinical parameters can predict improved survival with intervention.[109]

Definitive Therapy: Surgery or Radiation

Which is superior, radical surgery or radiation therapy? Only two basic therapies have the long-term oncologic and functional results to be considered first-line therapies with curative intent for localized prostate cancer. These are surgical extirpation via radical prostatectomy and radiation therapy via external-beam radiation or brachytherapy. We have already seen from the results of the Prostate Cancer Outcomes Study[95] that both therapies are accompanied by morbidity and that these morbidities are roughly equal in large population-based studies. Note that all therapies for prostate cancer have associated morbidity, specifically bowel, urinary, and sexual dysfunction, although the temporal evolution of these side effects is different, as are the specific types of dysfunction. Surgery is associated with less bowel but more early urinary and sexual side effects, which tend to improve over time. Radiation therapy causes more bowel problems and worsening urinary and sexual dysfunction over time. Discussing these temporal relationships between treatment and side effects and their relative implications on quality of life is critical when counseling individual patients on treatment alternatives for prostate cancer.

Therefore, if one were to accept that both surgery and radiation therapy have generally similar morbidity profiles (though at different time courses), then the discussion must lead

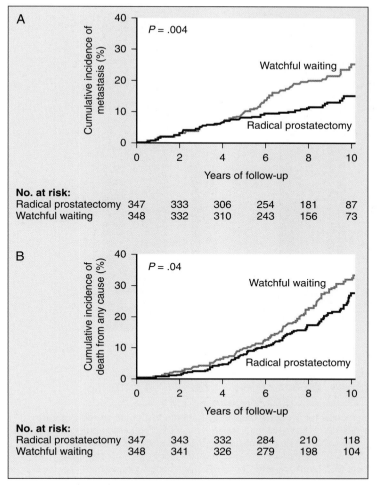

toward discovering which of the modalities has better oncologic outcomes. Unfortunately, this is a question for the ages. There has never been a prospective randomized trial comparing surgery with radiation therapy, and there may never be one. Studies that compare retrospective series and results are plagued by four main problems that make historical interpretations hazardous:

1. Surgery and radiation therapy are not used on similar patient populations.

Compared with patients who elect radical prostatectomy, men treated with radiation are typically older and have more advanced disease, both of which have significant implications with regard to oncologic cure as well as functional (i.e., urinary and sexual) outcomes. In a recent review of men with clinically localized prostate cancer treated with either surgery or radiation,

the average surgical patient was 5 to 7 years younger than the average radiation therapy patient.[110] Men treated with radiation also have higher Gleason scores and pretreatment PSAs. In the 1999 Patterns of Care study for prostate cancer radiation, more than 60% of men treated with external-beam therapy had intermediate- or high-risk disease.[111] Twice as many clinically low-risk patients elect radical prostatectomy than those who elect radiation therapy[51] (Fig. 12-5).

2. The advances in radiation therapy more greatly affect oncologic outcomes than do the changes in surgery.

Although it is true that surgical technique continues to evolve and that cancer-specific outcomes continue to improve for surgery, these changes are not as dramatic as the changes in radiation therapy during the last 25 years. The

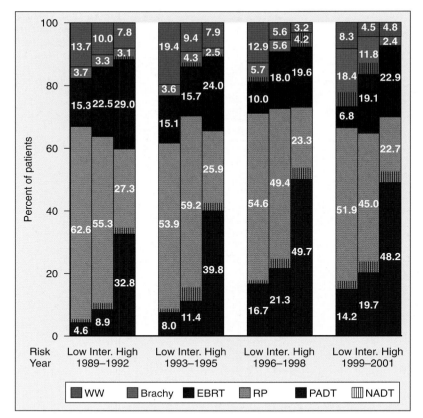

Figure 12-5. Trends in primary treatment selection for prostate cancer by patients in Cancer of the Prostate Strategic Urologic Research Endeavor (CaPSURE). Cross-hatched areas of each bar indicate the proportion of patients receiving prior neoadjuvant androgen deprivation. WW, watchful waiting; Brachy, brachytherapy; EBRT, external beam radiotherapy; RP, radical prostatectormy; PADT, primary androgen-deprivation therapy; NADT, neoadjuvant androgen-deprivation therapy. (From Cooperberg MR, Moul JW, and Carroll PR: The changing face of prostate cancer. J Clin Oncol 23:8146–8151, 2005, Figure 2.)

biggest of these is the recognition that subtherapeutic dosages of radiation were given routinely to the prostate for many years. It is now known that a minimum of 72 Gy must be given to the prostate, and there is a direct correlation of increasing dosages and improved prostate cancer-specific survival. Earlier series that compare surgery with subtherapeutic radiation therapy reveal a clear survival advantage to surgery.[110,112] Of note, there is also a direct correlation of increasing morbidity with increasing radiotherapeutic dosages. The second advance has been the discovery and incorporation of intensity-modulated radiation therapy (IMRT) as a replacement for three-dimensional conformal radiation therapy. This newer modality allows deliverance of increased dosages to the target organ, while permitting rapid dose fall-off, and therefore less risk of injury, to surrounding structures.

3. Surgery and radiation therapy have different definitions of intermediate success and failure.

Forget for a moment that there is a controversy around whether PSA itself is suitable to use as a surrogate for post-treatment prostate cancer survival or any prostate cancer-specific outcomes.[113–116] Such a controversy is beyond the scope of this chapter. Generally, a surgical "success" is an undetectable PSA that remains undetectable (although even this is under debate, since many patients who have a recurrence with a detectable PSA are never likely to present with signs or symptoms of prostate cancer even at long-term follow-up). For radiation therapy, it is more complex, and either the ASTRO (American Society for Therapeutic Radiology and Oncology) or Phoenix (an updated definition by the ASTRO group) definitions are used.[117,118]

The original ASTRO criteria defined biochemical failure as occurring after three consecutive PSA rises after a nadir with the date of failure as the point halfway between the nadir date and the first rise or any rise great enough to provoke initiation of therapy. The Phoenix criteria defined biochemical failure as a rise by 2 ng/mL or more above the nadir PSA and defined the date of failure "at call" (not backdated). Although many groups have compared results between the modalities with both definitions, these comparisons are imperfect.[119] The *only* truly comparable outcome measures are overall and prostate cancer-specific mortality.

4. Androgen deprivation therapy is more commonly used in combination with radiation therapy than with surgery.

Seventy-five percent of all patients who receive external-beam radiation therapy receive androgen deprivation, compared with only 8% of radical prostatectomy patients.[51] There is good rationale for this. Androgen blockade results in apoptosis of hormone-responsive prostate cancer cells and may have a synergistic killing effect when combined with radiation. Multiple randomized trials have shown a survival benefit when androgen deprivation is combined with radiation therapy.[120–122] But these combinations make it difficult to discern which aspect of survival is due to the radiation and which is due to the androgen deprivation. Since androgen deprivation has its own morbidity, this also clouds quality-of-life comparisons between the modalities.

Imperfect Comparisons

I have just mentioned the hazards of retrospective comparisons between surgery and radiation therapy, but I will nonetheless attempt to compare their outcomes here. To determine which treatment is best also depends somewhat on the clinical risk group of the patient. In general, patients with low-risk prostate cancer are candidates for, and will do well with, any therapeutic modality. This includes expectant management, external-beam radiation therapy, brachytherapy, and surgery. The efficacies of these therapies, with the exception of the superiority shown by radical prostatectomy versus watchful waiting,[53] have not been directly compared in randomized controlled trials. The major

retrospective attempts at comparing radiation therapy with surgery suggest that at contemporary doses of radiation more than 72 Gy, radiation therapy and surgery have generally similar overall and disease specific outcomes.[123–126]

Brachytherapy

Brachytherapy is a method of delivering high dosages of radiation directly into the prostate using radiation-laden seed implants. Most commonly, iodine 125 (^{125}I) or palladium 103 (^{103}Pd) seeds are used.[127] Brachytherapy may be used as monotherapy, in combination with external-beam radiation therapy, and is also commonly used with androgen deprivation.

There are a variety of relative contraindications to the use of prostate brachytherapy, including large prostate size (greater than 50 to 60 g), history of transurethral resection of the prostate, colonic disorders, and preexisting severe irritative or obstructive urinary symptoms. These factors predispose the patient to an increased risk of complications.[128,129] Patients with a large prostate are occasionally placed on androgen deprivation before brachytherapy for purposes of decreasing gland size. The androgen deprivation is sometimes continued after the procedure as well. Side-effect profiles of brachytherapy are similar to those of the other modalities, but with more early irritative voiding symptoms (i.e., urinary frequency and urgency) and with impotence occurring later. The use of brachytherapy alone has also not been directly compared with either surgery or external-beam radiation therapy in a randomized trial. At best, we can use the surrogate measure of biochemical (PSA)-free survival. Using the surrogate outcome, 10-year biochemical-free survival rates with brachytherapy (87% to 94%) equivalent to surgery and external-beam radiation therapy have been reported in patients with low-risk disease.[130–134]

Because brachytherapy does not deliver what is felt to be adequate doses to periprostatic tissues, brachytherapy is generally best used as a solo modality only in patients with low-risk disease.[135]

Most studies that have attempted to compare all three modalities of prostatectomy, brachytherapy, and external-beam radiation therapy have generally found equivalence of the surrogate endpoint of biochemical disease-free survival.[136,137]

Radical Prostatectomy

Certainly for low-risk disease, and even with good efficacy in high-risk disease, radical prostatectomy is considered the gold standard.[138] Radical prostatectomy has become the most commonly performed treatment for clinically localized prostate cancer with abundant long-term data confirming its efficacy. Anatomic radical retropubic prostatectomy has become the gold standard surgical treatment for prostate cancer for the past 25 years. Excellent long-term outcomes of open radical retropubic prostatectomy are available for cancer control as well as for the preservation of potency and continence.[139-143] It is believed that radical prostatectomy provides the best chance for cure for men whose tumor is confined to the prostate gland. Some studies have shown survival advantages to radical prostatectomy versus the other primary modalities.[138,144-146]

Which modalities do patients typically choose? Of all patients diagnosed with prostate cancer between 1998 and 2003, an estimated 40% were initially treated with some form of radiation treatment, making it the most common modality.[111] However, among low-risk patients, radical prostatectomy remains the most common therapeutic modality, with over half of these patients electing some form of surgical extirpation.[51] Among the recent trends, of note is the rapid rise in brachytherapy and robot-assisted laparoscopic prostatectomy.

In 1994, only 5% of prostate cancer patients were treated with brachytherapy. In 1999, this number had increased to 36%. As already mentioned, brachytherapy is generally not used as monotherapy for anything other than low-risk disease. In patients with intermediate- and high-risk disease, the American Brachytherapy Society (ABS) has recommended that supplemental external-beam radiation therapy be delivered.[135] As for robot-assisted laparoscopic prostatectomy, according to industry figures, in 2007 more than 50% of all radical prostatectomies in the United States were performed with robotic assistance, and that percentage rose even higher in 2008 (Fig. 12-6). Lastly, for patients with high-risk disease features, a multi-modality approach is often used.

Traditional or Minimally Invasive?

Today there are many methods of surgical extirpation of a cancerous prostate gland, and con-

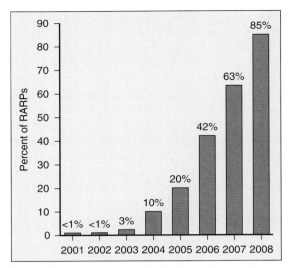

Figure 12-6. Percentage of radical prostatectomies (RPs) performed with robotic assistance in the United States by year. The first robot-assisted radical prostatectomy (RARP) with the da Vinci surgical system was performed in Europe in 2000. Later that year, the first of 36 RARPs was performed in the United States. This number accounted for less than 1% of all radical prostatectomies performed in the United States that year. In 2007, over 50% of all radical prostatectomies were performed with robotic assistance. (Data from Intuitive Surgical Systems Company, Sunnyvale, California.)

troversy exists over the "ideal" method. Four such methods of the radical prostatectomy are used today: two open modalities and two minimally invasive modalities. The classic open surgical modalities are radical perineal prostatectomy and radical retropubic prostatectomy. The minimally invasive modalities are laparoscopic radical prostatectomy and robot-assisted laparoscopic prostatectomy. To understand the differences, we need to describe all four.

Radical Perineal Prostatectomy

Radical perineal prostatectomy (RPP) is the oldest method of surgical extirpation of a cancerous prostate, although it is rarely performed today. RPP has good, long-term oncologic and functional outcomes and has some advantages when compared with the radical retropubic prostatectomy.[147] These include less pain, lower blood loss, and the ability to be performed in morbidly obese men, or men with significant prior pelvic surgery. Several recent case series have supported the feasibility of RPP in morbidly obese patients with a body mass index of more than 40 kg/m.[148,149] One disadvantage is the inability to perform a simultaneous pelvic lymph node dissection through a perineal incision without making a second abdominal incision to access the pelvic nodes. A second disadvantage is the relative difficulty in preserving the cavernous nerves responsible for sexual function during RPP compared with the retropubic approach.

Radical Retropubic Prostatectomy

The open radical retropubic prostatectomy (RRP) is the current gold standard surgical approach and has been since the modernization of the technique in the early 1980s by Dr. Patrick C. Walsh, who popularized an anatomic approach to prostatectomy with prospective preservation of the cavernous nerves (i.e., anatomic nerve-sparing RRP). RRP has been the most widely performed method for the last 20 years. In experienced hands, it is associated with the most well-established long-term oncologic and functional outcomes of any of the modalities.[139,150] Yet, recent research demonstrates inferior cancer-specific results when the procedure is performed by less experienced surgeons.[151] This observation is likely the case for all of the extirpative modalities. Also, in obese men RRP is relatively difficult from a technical standpoint and wrought with more complications.[152]

Laparoscopic Radical Prostatectomy

In the 1990s, the first of the minimally invasive approaches, the laparoscopic radical prostatectomy (LRP), was introduced in an effort to further reduce patient morbidity. LRP has many advantages when compared with RRP. Minimally invasive approaches such as LRP have the lowest blood loss and transfusion rates of all the modalities.[153–155] These approaches are also associated with shorter hospital times and convalescence.[156–158] Although the pain of open RRP is generally tolerable,[159] many studies have shown less pain with the minimally invasive techniques.[157,158,160] LRP may also be performed readily in obese males.[161–163] Centers of excellence have demonstrated equivalent functional and oncologic outcomes when compared with the open technique.[164] However, LRP is considered the most technically challenging of all the surgical modalities; for this reason, expansion of the technique has generally been limited to a few high-volume medical centers.

Robot-Assisted Laparoscopic Prostatectomy

Most recently, great enthusiasm has surrounded the da Vinci surgical system (Intuitive Surgical, Sunnyvale, California) and the robot-assisted laparoscopic prostatectomy (RALP). Potential advantages of RALP are many. First, one gains all the minimally invasive advantages of the LRP, with the added benefit of stereoscopic (i.e., three-dimensional) vision, compared with the two-dimensional view offered by conventional laparoscopy. The surgeon therefore has better depth perception. Second, because of the wrist-like robotic instruments, the surgeon is provided 7 degrees of freedom of motion during the procedure. This essentially allows a surgeon to operate with the facility of miniature human wrists. This feature is especially useful during complex laparoscopic tasks such as laparoscopic suturing of the bladder-urethral anastomosis. Last, there is an ergonomic advantage of RALP over LRP in that the surgeon operates while seated comfortably at a console station compared with LRP, in which the surgeon stands at the patient's bedside. Disadvantages are that despite the relative ease when compared with the LRP, the RALP is still a technically challenging procedure and requires a significant level of expertise.[165,166] Moreover, the exorbitant expense of RALP compared with the other modalities cannot be discounted.[167–169]

Choosing the Best Therapy

Which therapy is the best? In the end, *experience of the surgeon in any single modality is the most important predictive factor for good results.* A patient should primarily consider and select an experienced surgeon over the method of prostatectomy. In addition, a thorough inquiry into the rate of positive margins, the percentage of patients who receive cavernous nerve preservation, and the continence and potency rates should be discussed with the surgeon to weigh options among different surgeons and different techniques.

Ablative Therapies

There are two ablative therapies for prostate cancer, high-intensity focused ultrasound (HIFU), and cryoablation. Significant research and enthusiasm surround both. Both modalities have encouraging results in the field of salvage therapy after radiation failure, but are still relatively unproven as therapies for primary prostate cancer. Simply put, despite popular enthusiasm, neither has available long-term survival outcomes, which are necessary to recommend a therapy, and therefore both should be considered unproven and experimental. For these reasons, I review them only briefly here. Nonetheless, enthusiasm for the modalities persists because they both possess certain advantages over standard therapies. Significant among these is the minimal invasive nature of the procedures. They both may be done as outpatient therapy and, unlike other modalities, they both may be repeated, Both HIFU and cryoablation are evolving, and although their early history was plagued by specific serious morbidities such as gastrointestinal fistula formation and urethral strictures, modern iterations have far less of these risks.[170–173]

High-Intensity Focused Ultrasound

HIFU is very attractive in theory because the technology platform has the theoretical capability to precisely target the tissue in question within a single millimeter of accuracy. Advantages are minimal pain and no blood loss, and no hospitalization is necessary. Retreatment, as mentioned, is possible. However, retreatment is usually associated with an increase in complications.[174] In addition, if the treatment is designed to be curative, then impotence results by definition as a consequence of thermal injury to the cavernous nerves, although experimentation with "partial" treatments is ongoing.[175–177] Early biochemical recurrence data are sparse but promising.[175,177] Other disadvantages of HIFU are a general inability to monitor the treatment while ongoing and limitations to the depth of penetration of the ultrasonic wave. This limits the size of the prostate that can be treated, although some centers have had success with concomitant transurethral resection of the prostates for purposes of cytoreduction.[173,177,178]

Cryoablation of the Prostate

Cryotherapy of the prostate, though still experimental, actually now has a significant advantage in the ablative battle over HIFU, since there is now a randomized trial that has revealed equivalency to radiation therapy after 10 years of follow-up. With endpoints of biochemical recur-

rence and mandatory biopsies 3 years after therapy, a Canadian group has revealed oncologically acceptable results and at least equivalent results to external-beam radiation therapy.[169] It should be mentioned, however, that radiation therapy dosages were subtherapeutic at the beginning of the randomized trial, consistent with standard of care at the time. Of course, no randomized long-term survival data exist yet, but given time, the results may prove to be acceptable for a certain population of patients.[170] Like HIFU, advantages are minimal pain, no blood loss, no hospitalization necessary, and it is possible to retreat. Also like HIFU, if performed correctly, most patients suffer from impotence due to effects on the adjacent cavernous nerves.

Conclusions

Prostate cancer is a field in continuous evolution. With this constant motion come many disagreements and controversy. These give rise to more research and yet more debate. Fortunately, in addition to anticipated updates of the PLCO and ERSPC, there are two more ongoing large randomized clinical trials that may help to answer many of the basic questions. These are the Prostate Cancer Intervention Versus Observation Trial (PIVOT) in the United States and the Prostate Testing for Cancer and Treatment (PROTECT) trial in the United Kingdom (Current Controlled Trials number ISRCTN20141297).[181,182] It is hoped that these ongoing randomized trials will answer questions about screening, the natural history of prostate cancer, overdetection, and other issues. For many of the rest of the conundrums, only time will tell. Until then, we as health care providers must act on the best evidence-based data available.

References

1. American Cancer Society: Cancer Facts and Figures 2008, 2008.
2. Jemal A, Siegel R, Ward E, et al: Cancer statistics 2008. CA Cancer J Clin 58:71–96, 2008.
3. Scardino PT, Weaver R, Hudson MA: Early detection of prostate cancer. Hum Pathol 23:211, 1992.
4. Sonn GA, Aronson W, Litwin MS: Impact of diet on prostate cancer: a review. Prostate Cancer Prostatic Dis 8:304–310, 2005.
5. Sakr WA, Grignon DJ, Crissman JD, et al: High grade prostatic intraepithelial neoplasia (HGPIN) and prostatic adenocarcinoma between the ages of 20–69: an autopsy study of 249 cases. In Vivo 8:439–443, 1994.

6. U.S. Department of Health and Human Services: Prostate Cancer Screening: A Decision Guide. Atlanta, GA: Centers for Disease Control and Prevention and National Cancer Institute, 2006. Available at www.cdc.gov/cancer/prostate/publications/decisionguide/.

7. Zheng SL, Sun J, Wiklund F, et al: Cumulative association of five genetic variants with prostate cancer. N Engl J Med 358:910–919, 2008.

8. Carter BS, Beaty TH, Steinberg GD, et al: Mendelian inheritance of familial prostate cancer. Proc Natl Acad Sci U S A 89:3367–3371, 1992.

9. Ghadirian P, Howe GR, Hislop TG, et al: Family history of prostate cancer: a multi-center case-control study in Canada. Int J Cancer 70:679–681, 1997.

10. Grönberg H, Wiklund F, Damber JE: Age specific risks of familial prostate carcinoma: a basis for screening recommendations in high risk populations. Cancer 86:477–483, 1999.

11. Muir CS, Nectoux J, Staszewski J: The epidemiology of prostatic cancer. Geographical distribution and time-trends. Acta Oncol 30:133–140, 1991.

12. Shimizu H, Ross RK, Bernstein L, et al: Cancers of the prostate and breast among Japanese and white immigrants in Los Angeles County. Br J Cancer 63:963–966, 1991.

13. Moradi T, Delfino RJ, Bergstrom SR: Cancer risk among Scandinavian immigrants in the US and Scandinavian residents compared with US whites. Eur J Cancer Prev 7:117–125, 1998.

14. Thompson IM, Goodman PJ, Tangen CM, et al: The influence of finasteride on the development of prostate cancer. N Engl J Med 349:215–224, 2003.

15. Giovannucci E: Tomatoes, tomato-based products, lycopene, and cancer: review of the epidemiologic literature. J Natl Canc Inst 91:317–331, 1999.

16. Etminan M, Takkouche B, Caamaño-Isorna F: The role of tomato products and lycopene in the prevention of prostate cancer: a meta-analysis of observational studies. Cancer Epidemiol Biomarkers Prev 13:340–345, 2004.

17. Obermuller-Jevic UC, Olano-Martin E, Corbacho AM, et al: Lycopene inhibits the growth of normal human prostate epithelial cells in vitro. J Nutr 133:3356–3360, 2003.

18. Chen L, Stacewicz-Sapuntzakis M, Duncan C, et al: Oxidative DNA damage in prostate cancer patients consuming tomato sauce-based entrees as a whole-food intervention. J Natl Cancer Inst 93:1872–1879, 2001.

19. Kim HS, Bowen P, Chen L, et al: Effects of tomato sauce consumption on apoptotic cell death in prostate benign hyperplasia and carcinoma. Nutr Cancer 47:40–47, 2003.

20. Duffield-Lillico AJ, Dalkin BL, Reid ME, et al: Se supplementation, baseline plasma Se status, and incidence of prostate cancer: an analysis of the complete treatment period of the Nutritional Prevention of Cancer study group. BJU Int 91:608–612, 2003.

21. Yoshizawa K, Willett WC, Morris SJ, et al:. Study of prediagnostic selenium level in toenails and the risk of advanced prostate cancer. J Natl Cancer Inst 90:1219–1224, 1998.

22. Van den Brandt PA, Zeegers MP, Bode P, Goldbohm RA: Toenail selenium levels and the subsequent risk of prostate cancer: a prospective cohort study. Cancer Epidemiol Biomarkers Prevent 12:866–871, 2003.

23. Virtamo J, Pietinen P, Huttunen J: Incidence of cancer and mortality following alpha-tocopherol and beta-carotene supplementation: a post-intervention follow-up. JAMA 290:476–485, 2003.

24. Lonn E, Bosch J, Yusuf S, et al: HOPE and HOPE-TOO Trial Investigators. Effects of long-term vitamin E supplementation on cardiovascular events and cancer: a randomized controlled trial. JAMA 293:1338–1347, 2005.

25. Lippman SM, Klein EA, Goodman PJ, et al: Effect of selenium and vitamin E on risk of prostate cancer and other cancers: the Selenium and Vitamin E Cancer Prevention Trial (SELECT). JAMA 301:39–51, 2009.

26. Gaziano JM, Glynn RJ, Christen WG, et al: Vitamins E and C in the prevention of prostate and total cancer in men: the Physicians' Health Study II randomized controlled trial. JAMA 301:52–62, 2009.

27. Malik A, Afaq F, Sarfaraz S, et al: Pomegranate fruit juice for chemoprevention and chemotherapy of prostate cancer. Proc Natl Acad Sci U S A 102:14813–14818, 2005.

28. Ren S, Lien EJ: Natural products and their derivatives as cancer chemopreventive agents. Prog Drug Res 48:147–171, 1997.

29. Augustson K, Michaud DS, Rimm EB, et al: A prospective study of intake of fish and marine fatty acids and prostate cancer. Cancer Epidemiol Biomarkers Prev 12:64–67, 2003.

30. Barnes S, Peterson TG, Coward L: Rationale for the use of genistein-containing soy matrices in chemoprevention trials for breast and prostate cancer. J Cell Biochem 22:181–187, 1995.

31. Jian L, Xie LP, Lee AH, Binns CW: Protective effect of green tea against prostate cancer: a case-control study in southeast China. Int J Cancer 108:130–135, 2004.

32. Lew EA, Garfinkel L: Variations in mortality by weight among 750,000 men and women. J Chron Dis 32:563–576, 1979.

33. Whittemore AS, Kolonel LH, Wu AH, et al: Prostate cancer in relation to diet, physical activity and body size, in blacks, whites and Asians in the United States and Canada. J Nat Cancer Inst 87:652–661, 1995.

34. Boyle P, Kevi R, Lucchuni F, LaVecchia C: Trends in diet-related cancers in Japan: a conundrum? Lancet 349:752, 1993.

35. Kolonel LN, Hankin JH, Lee J, et al: Nutrient intakes in relation to cancer incidence in Hawaii. Br J Cancer 44:332–339, 1981.

36. Kelavkar UP, Hutzley J, Dhir R, et al: Prostate tumor growth and recurrence can be modulated by the omega-6:omega-3 ratio n diet: athymic mouse xenograft model simulating radical prostatectomy. Neoplasia 8:112–124, 2006.

37. Giovannucci E, Rimm EB, Wolk A, et al: Calcium and fructose intake in relation to risk of prostate cancer. Cancer Res 58:442–447, 1998.

38. Rodriguez C, McCullough ML, Mondul AM, et al: Calcium, dairy products, and risk of prostate cancer in a prospective cohort of United States men. Cancer Epidemiol Biomarkers Prevent 12:597–603, 2003.

39. Thompson IM, Pauler DK, Goodman PJ, et al: Prevalence of prostate cancer among men with a prostate-specific antigen level ≤4.0 ng per milliliter. N Engl J Med 350:2239, 2004.

40. Canby-Hagino E, Hernandez J, Brand TC, Thompson I: Looking back at PCPT: looking forward to new paradigms in prostate cancer screening and prevention. Eur Urol 51:27–33, 2007. Epub 2006 Sep 15. Review.

41. Thompson IM, Tangen CM, Goodman PJ, et al: Finasteride improves the sensitivity of digital rectal examination for prostate cancer detection. J Urol 177:1749–1752, 2007.

42. Thompson IM, Chi C, Ankerst DP, et al: Effect of finasteride on the sensitivity of PSA for detecting prostate cancer. J Natl Cancer Inst 98:1128–1133, 2006.

43. D'Amico AV, Barry MJ: Prostate cancer prevention and finasteride. J Urol 176:2010–2012, 2006; discussion 2012–2013.

44. Kramer BS, Hagerty KL, Justman S, et al: Use of 5-alpha-reductase inhibitors for prostate cancer chemoprevention: American Society of Clinical Oncology/American Urological Association 2008 Clinical Practice Guideline. J Clin Oncol 27:1502–1516, 2009.

45. Kramer BS, Hagerty KL, Justman S, et al: Use of 5-alpha-reductase inhibitors for prostate cancer chemoprevention: American Society of Clinical Oncology/American Urological Association 2008 Clinical Practice Guideline. J Urol 181:1642–1657, 2009.

46. Harlan SR, Cooperberg MR, Elkin EP, et al: Time trends and characteristics of men choosing watchful waiting for initial treatment of localized prostate cancer: results from CaPSURE. J Urol 170:1804–1807, 2003.

47. Goetzl MA, Holzbeierlein JM: Finasteride as a chemopreventive agent in prostate cancer: impact of the PCPT on urologic practice. Nat Clin Pract Urol 3:422–429, 2003. Review.

48. Klein EA, Tangen CM, Goodman PJ, et al: Assessing benefit and risk in the prevention of prostate cancer: the Prostate Cancer Prevention Trial Revisited. J Clin Oncol 23:7460–7466, 2003.

49. Loeb S, Catalona WJ: Prostate-specific antigen in clinical practice. Cancer Lett 249:30–39, 2007. Epub 2007 Jan 26. Review.

50. U.S. Preventive Services Task Force: Screening for prostate cancer: recommendation and rationale. Ann Intern Med 137:915–916, 2002.

51. Cooperberg MR, Lubeck DP, Meng MV, et al: The changing face of low-risk prostate cancer: trends in clinical presentation and primary management. J Clin Oncol 22:2141, 2004.

52. Han M, Partin AW, Chan DY, et al: An evaluation of the decreasing incidence of positive surgical margins in a large retropubic prostatectomy series. J Urol 171:23, 2004.
53. Bill-Axelson A, Holmberg L, Ruutu M, et al: Radical prostatectomy versus watchful waiting in early prostate cancer. N Engl J Med 352:1977–1984, 2005.
54. Lilja H, Laurell CB: Liquefaction of coagulated human semen. Scand J Clin Lab Invest 44:447, 1984.
55. Stamey TA, Yang N, Hay AR, et al: Prostate-specific antigen as a serum marker for adenocarcinoma of the prostate. N Engl J Med 317:909, 1987.
56. Catalona WJ, Smith DS, Ornstein DK: Prostate cancer detection in men with serum PSA concentrations of 2.6 to 4.0 ng/mL and benign prostate examination. Enhancement of specificity with free PSA measurements. JAMA 277:1452, 1997.
57. Schroder FH, Alexander FE, Bangma CH, et al: Screening and early detection of prostate cancer. Prostate 44:255, 2000.
58. Thompson IM, Ankerst DP, Chi C, et al: Assessing prostate cancer risk: results from the Prostate Cancer Prevention Trial. J Natl Cancer Inst 98:529, 2006.
59. Network, NCC: Prostate Cancer, 2006.
60. Benson MC, Olsson CA: Prostate specific antigen and prostate specific antigen density: roles in patient evaluation and management. Cancer 74:1667–1673, 1994.
61. Oesterling JE, Jacobsen SJ, Chute CG, et al: Serum prostate-specific antigen in a community-based population of healthy men: establishment of age-specific reference ranges. JAMA 270:860–864, 1993.
62. Carter HB, Pearson JD, Metter EJ, et al: Longitudinal evaluation of prostate-specific antigen levels in men with and without prostate disease. JAMA 267:2215, 1992.
63. Berger AP, Deibl M, Strasak A, et al: Large-scale study of clinical impact of PSA velocity: long-term PSA kinetics as method of differentiating men with from those without prostate cancer. Urology 69:134–138, 2007.
64. Sun L, Moul JW, Hotaling JM, et al: Prostate-specific antigen (PSA) and PSA velocity for prostate cancer detection in men aged <50 years. BJU Int 99:753–757, 2007. Epub 2007 January 19.
65. Catalona WJ, Smith DS, Wolfert RL, et al: Evaluation of percentage of free serum prostate-specific antigen to improve specificity of prostate cancer screening. JAMA 274:1214–1220, 1995.
66. McCormack RT, Rittenhouse HG, Finlay JA, et al: Molecular forms of prostate-specific antigen and the human kallikrein gene family: a new era. Urology 45:729, 1995.
67. Woodrum DL, Brawer MK, Partin AW, et al: Interpretation of free prostate specific antigen clinical research studies for the detection of prostate cancer. J Urol 159:5, 1998.
68. Stenman UH, Hakama M, Knekt P, et al: Serum concentrations of prostate specific antigen and its complex with alpha 1-antichymotrypsin before diagnosis of prostate cancer. Lancet 344:1594, 1994.
69. Lilja H: Significance of different molecular forms of serum PSA. The free, noncomplexed form of PSA versus that complexed to alpha 1-antichymotrypsin. Urol Clin North Am 20:681, 1993.
70. Leinonen J, Lovgren T, Vornanen T, et al: Double-label time-resolved immunofluorometric assay of prostate-specific antigen and of its complex with alpha 1-antichymotrypsin. Clin Chem 39:2098, 1993.
71. Christensson A, Bjork T, Nilsson O, et al: Serum prostate specific antigen complexed to alpha 1-antichymotrypsin as an indicator of prostate cancer. J Urol 150:100, 1993.
72. Haese A, Graefen M, Noldus J, et al: Prostatic volume and ratio of free-to-total prostate specific antigen in patients with prostatic cancer or benign prostatic hyperplasia. J Urol 158:2188, 1997.
73. Leman ES, Cannon GW, Trock BJ, et al: EPCA-2: a highly specific serum marker for prostate cancer. Urology 69:714–720, 2007.
74. Marks LS, Fradet Y, Deras IL, et al: PCA3 molecular urine assay for prostate cancer in men undergoing repeat biopsy. Urology 69:532–535, 2007.
75. Darson MF, Pacelli A, Roche P, et al: Human glandular kallikrein 2 (hK2) expression in prostatic intraepithelial neoplasia and adenocarcinoma: a novel prostate cancer marker. Urology 49:857, 1997.
76. Kwiatkowski MK, Recker F, Piironen T, et al: In prostatism patients the ratio of human glandular kallikrein to free PSA

77. improves the discrimination between prostate cancer and benign hyperplasia within the diagnostic "gray zone" of total PSA 4 to 10 ng/mL. Urology 52:360, 1998.
77. Luo J, Zha S, Gage WR, et al: Alpha-methylacyl-CoA racemase: a new molecular marker for prostate cancer. Cancer Res 62:2220, 2002.
78. Rubin MA, Zhou M, Dhanasekaran SM, et al: alpha-Methylacyl coenzyme A racemase as a tissue biomarker for prostate cancer. JAMA 287:662, 2002.
79. Chodak GW, Keller P, Schoenberg HW: Assessment of screening for prostate cancer using the digital rectal examination. J Urol 141:1136–1138, 1989.
80. Wajsman Z, Chu TM: Detection and diagnosis of prostatic cancer. In Murphy GP (ed): Prostatic cancer. Littleton, Mass: PSG Publishing Company, 1987, pp 94–99.
81. Thompson IM, Zeidman EJ: Presentation and clinical course of patients ultimately succumbing to carcinoma of the prostate. Scand J Urol Nephrol 25:111–114, 1991.
82. Weinmann S, Richert-Boe K, Glass AG, et al: Prostate cancer screening and mortality: a case-control study (United States). Cancer Causes Control 15:133–138, 2004.
83. Jacobsen SJ, Bergstralh EJ, Katusic SK, et al: Screening digital rectal examination and prostate cancer mortality: a population-based case-control study. Urology 52:173–179, 1998.
84. Schröder FH, Hugosson J, Roobol MJ, et al: Screening and prostate-cancer mortality in a randomized European study. N Engl J Med 2009 Mar 18. [Epub ahead of print]
85. Andriole GL, Grubb RL 3rd, Buys SS, et al: Mortality results from a randomized prostate-cancer screening trial. N Engl J Med 2009 Mar 18. [Epub ahead of print]
86. Barry MJ: Screening for prostate cancer—the controversy that refuses to die. N Engl J Med 2009 Mar 18. [Epub ahead of print]
87. U.S. Preventive Services Task Force. Screening for prostate cancer: U.S. Preventive Services Task Force recommendation statement. Ann Intern Med 149:185–191, 2008. Summary for patients in: Ann Intern Med 149:I37, 2008.
88. Sakr WA, Grignon DJ: Prostate cancer: indicators of aggressiveness. Eur Urol 32(Suppl 3):15, 1997.
89. Minino AM, Heron MP, Smith BL: Deaths: preliminary data for 2004. Natl Vital Stat Rep 54:1, 2006.
90. Albertsen PC, Fryback DG, Storer BE, et al: Long-term survival among men with conservatively treated localized prostate cancer. JAMA 274:626, 1995.
91. Albertsen PC, Hanley JA, Gleason DF, et al: Competing risk analysis of men aged 55 to 74 years at diagnosis managed conservatively for clinically localized prostate cancer. JAMA 280:975, 1998.
92. Bangma CH, Roemeling S, Schroder FH: Overdiagnosis and overtreatment of early detected prostate cancer. World J Urol 25:3–9, 2007. Epub 2007 Feb 14. Review.
93. Choo R, Klotz L, Danjoux C, et al: Feasibility study: watchful waiting for localized low to intermediate grade prostate carcinoma with selective delayed intervention based on prostate specific antigen, histological and/or clinical progression. J Urol 167:1664, 2002.
94. Klotz L: Active surveillance versus radical treatment for favorable-risk localized prostate cancer. Curr Treat Options Oncol 7:355–362, 2006. Review.
95. Hamilton AS, Stanford JL, Gilliland FD, et al: Health outcomes after external beam radiation therapy for clinically localized prostate cancer: results from the Prostate Cancer Outcomes Study. J Clin Oncol 19:2517–2526. 2001.
96. Steineck G, Helgesen F, Adolfsson J, et al: Quality of life after radical prostatectomy or watchful waiting. N Engl J Med 347:790–796, 2002.
97. Auvin A, Maattanen L, Stenman UH, et al: Lead-time in prostate cancer screening (Finland). Cancer Causes Control 13:279–285, 2002.
98. Draisma G, Boer R, Otto SJ, et al: Lead times and overdetection due to prostate-specific antigen screening: estimates from the European randomized study of screening for prostate cancer. J Natl Cancer Inst 95:868–878, 2003.
99. Horan AH, McGehee M: Mean time to cancer-specific death of apparently clinically localized prostate cancer: policy implications for threshold ages in prostate-specific antigen screening and ablative therapy. BJU Int 85:1063, 2000.
100. Arias E: United States life tables, 2000. Natl Vital Stat Rep 51:1–38, 2000.

101. Draisma G, Postma R, Schroder FH, et al: Gleason score, age and screening: modeling dedifferentiation in prostate cancer. Int J Cancer 119:2366–2371, 2006.
102. Albertsen PC: PSA testing: public policy or private penchant? JAMA 296:2371–2373, 2006.
103. Rietbergen JB, Hoedemaeker RF, Kruger AE, et al: The changing pattern of prostate cancer at the time of diagnosis: characteristics of screen detected prostate cancer in a population based screening study. J Urol 161:1192–1198, 1999.
104. Johansson JE, Adami HO, Andersson SO, et al: High 10-year survival rate in patients with early, untreated prostatic cancer. JAMA 267:2191, 1992.
105. Adolfsson J, Ronstrom L, Lowhagen T, et al: Deferred treatment of clinically localized low grade prostate cancer: the experience from a prospective series at the Karolinska Hospital. J Urol 152:1757, 1994.
106. Warlick C, Trock BJ, Landis P, et al: Delayed versus immediate surgical intervention and prostate cancer outcome. J Natl Cancer Inst 98:355, 2006.
107. Holmberg L, Bill-Axelson A, Helgesen F, et al: A randomized trial comparing radical prostatectomy with watchful waiting in early prostate cancer. N Engl J Med 347:781, 2002.
108. Bill-Axelson A, Holmberg L, Filén F, et al: Scandinavian Prostate Cancer Group Study Number 4. Radical prostatectomy versus watchful waiting in localized prostate cancer: the Scandinavian prostate cancer group-4 randomized trial. J Natl Cancer Inst 100:1144–1154, 2008.
109. Holmberg L, Bill-Axelson A, Garmo H, et al: Prognostic markers under watchful waiting and radical prostatectomy. Hematol Oncol Clin North Am 20:845, 2006.
110. Kupelian PA, Potters L, Khuntia D, et al: Radical prostatectomy, external beam radiotherapy <72 Gy, external beam radiotherapy ≥72 Gy, permanent seed implantation, or combined seeds/external beam radiotherapy for stage T1-T2 prostate cancer. Int J Radiat Oncol Biol Phys 58:25–33, 2004.
111. Lee WR, Moughan J, Owen JB, et al: The 1999 patterns of care study of radiotherapy in localized prostate carcinoma: a comprehensive survey of prostate brachytherapy in the United States. Cancer 98:1987–1994, 2003.
112. Kupelian PA, Buchsbaum JC, Elshaikh MA, et al: Improvement in relapse-free survival throughout the PSA era in patients with localized prostate cancer treated with definitive radiotherapy: year of treatment an independent predictor of outcome. Int J Radiat Oncol Biol Phys 57:629–634, 2003.
113. D'Amico AV, Moul JW, Carroll PR, et al: Surrogate end point for prostate cancer-specific mortality after radical prostatectomy or radiation therapy. J Natl Cancer Inst 95:1376–1383, 2003.
114. Petrylak DP, Ankerst DP, Jiang CS, et al: Evaluation of prostate-specific antigen declines for surrogacy in patients treated on SWOG 99-16. J Natl Cancer Inst 98:516–521, 2006.
115. Baker SG: Surrogate endpoints: wishful thinking or reality? J Natl Cancer Inst 98:502–503, 2006.
116. Ruckle HC, Klee GG, Oesterling JE: Prostate-specific antigen: concepts for staging prostate cancer and monitoring response to therapy. Mayo Clin Proc 69:69–79, 1994.
117. Consensus statement: guidelines for PSA following radiation therapy. American Society for Therapeutic Radiology and Oncology Consensus Panel. Int J Radiat Oncol Biol Phys 37:1035–1041, 1997.
118. Roach M, III, Hanks G, Thames H, Jr, et al: Defining biochemical failure following radiotherapy with or without hormonal therapy in men with clinically localized prostate cancer: recommendations of the RTOG-ASTRO Phoenix Consensus Conference. Int J Radiat Oncol Biol Phys 65:965–974, 2006.
119. Kupelian PA, Mahadevan A, Reddy CA, et al: Use of different definitions of biochemical failure after external beam radiotherapy changes conclusions about relative treatment efficacy for localized prostate cancer. Urology 68:593–598, 2006.
120. Bolla M, Gonzalez D, Pierpart M, et al: Improved survival in patients with locally advanced prostate cancer treated with radiotherapy and goserelin. N Engl J Med 337:295–300, 1997.
121. Bolla M, Collette L, Blank L, et al: Long-term results with immediate androgen suppression and external irradiation in patients with locally advanced prostate cancer (an EORTC study): a phase III randomised trial. Lancet 360:103–108, 2002.
122. Pilepich MV, Winter K, Roach M, et al: Phase III Radiation Therapy Oncology Group (RTOG) trial 86-10 of androgen deprivation before and during radiotherapy in locally advanced carcinoma of the prostate. Proc Am Soc Clin Oncol 17:308a, 1998.
123. Fowler JE, Jr, Braswell NT, Pandey P, et al: Experience with radical prostatectomy and radiation therapy for localized prostate cancer at a Veterans Affairs medical center. J Urol 153:1026–1031, 1995.
124. Gibbons RP, Correa RJ, Jr, Brannen GE, et al: Total prostatectomy for localized prostatic cancer. J Urol 131:73–76, 1984.
125. Hanks GE, Asbell S, Krall JM, et al: Outcome for lymph node dissection negative T-1b, T-2 (A-2,B) prostate cancer treated with external beam radiation therapy in RTOG 77-06. Int J Radiat Oncol Biol Phys 21:1099–1103, 1991.
126. Kupelian PA, Elshaikh M, Reddy CA, et al: Comparison of the efficacy of local therapies for localized prostate cancer in the prostate-specific antigen era: a large single-institution experience with radical prostatectomy and external-beam radiotherapy. J Clin Oncol 20:3376–3385, 2002.
127. Lee WR, DeSilvio M, Lawton C, et al: A phase II study of external beam radiotherapy combined with permanent source brachytherapy for intermediate-risk, clinically localized adenocarcinoma of the prostate: preliminary results of RTOG P-0019. Int J Radiat Oncol Biol Phys 64:804–809, 2006.
128. Blasko JC, Ragde H, Grimm PD: Transperineal ultrasound-guided implantation of the prostate: morbidity and complications. Scand J Urol Nephrol Suppl 137:113–118, 1991.
129. Terk MD, Stock RG, Stone NN: Identification of patients at increased risk for prolonged urinary retention following radioactive seed implantation of the prostate. J Urol 160:1379–1382, 1998.
130. Grimm PD, Blasko JC, Sylvester JE, et al: 10-year biochemical (prostate-specific antigen) control of prostate cancer with (125)I brachytherapy. Int J Radiat Oncol Biol Phys 51:31–40, 2001.
131. Blasko JC, Grimm PD, Sylvester JE, et al: The role of external beam radiotherapy with I-125/Pd-103 brachytherapy for prostate carcinoma. Radiother Oncol 57:273–278, 2000.
132. Blasko JC, Grimm PD, Sylvester JE, et al: Palladium-103 brachytherapy for prostate carcinoma. Int J Radiat Oncol Biol Phys 46:839–850, 2000.
133. Zelefsky MJ, Wallner KE, Ling CC, et al: Comparison of the 5-year outcome and morbidity of three-dimensional conformal radiotherapy versus transperineal permanent iodine-125 implantation for early-stage prostatic cancer. J Clin Oncol 17:517–522, 1999.
134. Crook J, Lukka H, Klotz L, et al: Systematic overview of the evidence for brachytherapy in clinically localized prostate cancer. CMAJ 164:975–981, 2001.
135. Nag S, Beyer D, Friedland J, et al: American brachytherapy society (ABS) recommendations for transperineal permanent brachytherapy of prostate cancer. Int J Radiat Oncol Biol Phys 44:789–799, 1999.
136. D'Amico AV, Whittington R, Malkowicz SB, et al: Biochemical outcome after radical prostatectomy, external beam radiation therapy, or interstitial radiation therapy for clinically localized prostate cancer. JAMA 280:969–974, 1998.
137. Gondi V, Deutsch I, Mansukhani M, et al: Intermediate-risk localized prostate cancer in the PSA era: radiotherapeutic alternatives. Urology 69:541–546, 2007.
138. Freedland SJ, Partin AW, Humphreys EB, et al: Radical prostatectomy for clinical stage T3a disease. Cancer 109:1273–1278, 2007.
139. Han M, Partin AW, Pound CR, et al: Long-term biochemical disease-free and cancer-specific survival following anatomic radical retropubic prostatectomy. The 15-year Johns Hopkins experience. Urol Clin North Am 28:555–565, 2001
140. Hull GW, Rabbani F, Abbas F, et al: Cancer control with radical prostatectomy alone in 1,000 consecutive patients. J Urol 167:528–534, 2002.
141. Roehl KA, Han M, Ramos CG, et al: Cancer progression and survival rates following anatomical radical retropubic prostatectomy in 3,478 consecutive patients: long-term results. J. Urol 172:910–914, 2004.
142. Mettlin CJ, Murphy GP, Sylvester J, et al: Results of hospital cancer registry surveys by the American College of Surgeons: outcomes of prostate cancer treatment by radical prostatectomy. Cancer 80:1875–1881, 1997.

143. Kundu SD, Roehl KA, Eggener SE, et al: Potency, continence and complications in 3,477 consecutive radical retropubic prostatectomies. J Urol 172:2227–2231, 2004.

144. Potters L, Klein EA, Kattan MW, et al: Monotherapy for stage T1-T2 prostate cancer: radical prostatectomy, external beam radiotherapy, or permanent seed implantation. Radiother Oncol 71:29–33, 2004.

145. Han M, Partin AW, Piantadosi S, et al: Era specific biochemical recurrence-free survival following radical prostatectomy for clinically localized prostate cancer. J Urol 166:416–419, 2001.

146. Freedland SJ, Humphreys EB, Mangold LA, et al: Risk of prostate cancer-specific mortality following biochemical recurrence after radical prostatectomy. JAMA 294:433–439, 2005.

147. Holzbeierlein JM, Langenstroer P, Porter HJ, et al: Case selection and outcome of radical perineal prostatectomy in localized prostate cancer. Int Braz J Urol 29:291, 2003.

148. Boczko J, Melman A: Radical perineal prostatectomy in obese patients. Urology 62:467, 2003.

149. Dahm P, Yang BK, Salmen CR, et al: Radical perineal prostatectomy for the treatment of localized prostate cancer in morbidly obese patients. J Urol 174:131, 2005.

150. Walsh PC. Radical prostatectomy for localized prostate cancer provides durable cancer control with excellent quality of life: a structured debate. J Urol 163:1802–1807, 2000.

151. Vickers AJ, Bianco FJ, Serio AM, et al: The surgical learning curve for prostate cancer control after radical prostatectomy. J Natl Cancer Inst 99:1171–1177, 2007. Epub 2007 July 24.

152. Chang SS, Duong DT, Wells N, et al: Predicting blood loss and transfusion requirements during radical prostatectomy: the significant negative impact of increasing body mass index. J Urol 171:1861, 2004.

153. Guillonneau B, Vallancien G: Laparoscopic radical prostatectomy: the Montsouris experience. J Urol 163:418, 2000.

154. Basillote JB, Ahlering TE, Skarecky DW, et al: Laparoscopic radical prostatectomy: review and assessment of an emerging technique. Surg Endosc 18:1694, 2004.

155. Ahlering TE, Skarecky D, Lee D, Clayman RV: Successful transfer of open surgical skills to a laparoscopic environment using a robotic interface: initial experience with laparoscopic radical prostatectomy. J Urol 170:1738, 2003.

156. Kaul S, Menon M: Robotic radical prostatectomy: evolution from conventional to VIP. World J Urol 24:152, 2006.

157. Bhayani SB, Pavlovich CP, Hsu TS, et al: Prospective comparison of short-term convalescence: laparoscopic radical prostatectomy versus open radical retropubic prostatectomy. Urology 61:612, 2003.

158. Ghavamian R, Knoll A, Boczko J, Melman A: Comparison of operative and functional outcomes of laparoscopic radical prostatectomy and radical retropubic prostatectomy: single surgeon experience. Urology 67:1241, 2006.

159. Slabaugh TK, Jr, Marshall FF: A comparison of minimally invasive open and laparoscopic radical retropubic prostatectomy. J Urol 172:2545, 2004.

160. Menon M, Tewari, A, Baize B, et al: Prospective comparison of radical retropubic prostatectomy and robot-assisted anatomic prostatectomy: the Vattikuti Urology Institute experience. Urology 60:864, 2002.

161. Mikhail AA, Stockton BR, Orvieto MA, et al: Robotic-assisted laparoscopic prostatectomy in overweight and obese patients. Urology 67:774, 2006.

162. Brown JA, Rodin DM, Lee B, Dahl DM: Laparoscopic radical prostatectomy and body mass index: an assessment of 151 sequential cases. J Urol 173:442, 2005.

163. Link RE: Laparoscopic radical prostatectomy in obese patients: feasible or foolhardy? Rev Urol 7:53, 2005.

164. Touijer K, Kuroiwa K, Eastham JA, et al: Risk-adjusted analysis of positive surgical margins following laparoscopic and retropubic radical prostatectomy. Eur Urol 2006.

165. Raman JD, Dong S, Levinson A, et al: Robotic radical prostatectomy: operative technique, outcomes, and learning curve. JSLS 11:1–7, 2007.

166. Samadi D, Levinson A, Hakimi A, et al: From proficiency to expert, when does the learning curve for robotic-assisted prostatectomies plateau? The Columbia University experience. World J Urol 25:105–110, 2007.

167. Burgess SV, Atug F, Castle EP, et al: Cost analysis of radical retropubic, perineal, and robotic prostatectomy. J Endourol 20:827, 2006.

168. Lotan Y, Cadeddu JA, Gettman MT: The new economics of radical prostatectomy: cost comparison of open, laparoscopic and robot assisted techniques. J Urol 172:1431, 2004.

169. Link RE, Su LM, Bhayani SB, Pavlovich CP: Making ends meet: a cost comparison of laparoscopic and open radical retropubic prostatectomy. J Urol 172:269, 2004.

170. Uchida T, Ohkusa H, Yamashita H, et al: Five-year experience of transrectal high-intensity focused ultrasound using the Sonablate device in the treatment of localized prostate cancer. Int J Urol 13:228–233, 2006.

171. Aus G: Current status of HIFU and cryotherapy in prostate cancers—a review. Eur Urol 50:927–934, 2006.

172. Mouraviev V, Polascik TJ: Update on cryotherapy for prostate cancer 2006. Curr Opin Urol 16:152–156, 2006.

173. Marberger M: Energy-based ablative therapy of prostate cancer: high-intensity focused ultrasound and cryoablation. Curr Opin Urol 17:194–199, 2007. Review.

174. Blana A, Rogenhofer S, Ganzer R, et al: Morbidity associated with repeated transrectal high intensity focused ultrasound treatment of localized prostate cancer. W J Urol 24:585–590, 2006.

175. Onik G: The male lumpectomy: rationale for a cancer targeted approach for prostate cryoablation. A review. Technol Cancer Res Treat 3:365–370, 2004.

176. Madersbacher S, Pedevilla M, Vingers L, et al: Effect of high-intensity focused ultrasound on human prostate cancer in vivo. Cancer Res 55:3346–3351, 1995.

177. Poissonnier L, Chapelon JY, Rouviere O, et al: Control of prostate cancer by transrectal HIFU in 227 patents. Eur Urol 51:381–387, 2007.

178. Chaussy Y, Thuroff S, Bergsdorf T: Local recurrence of prostate cancer after curative therapy. HIFU (Ablatherm) as a treatment option [German]. Urologe 45:1271–1275, 2006.

179. Donnelly BJ, Saliken JC, Brasher P, et al: A randomized trial of external beam radiotherapy versus cryoablation in patients with localized prostate cancer [abstract]. J Urol 177:376, 2007.

180. Katz AE, Prepelica K, McKiernan JM, et al: Salvage cryosurgical ablation of the prostate (TCAP) for patients failing radiation efficacy and tolerability. AUA Annual Meeting Program. J Urol 175:364, 2006.

181. Wilt TJ, Brawer MK, Barry MJ, et al: The Prostate Cancer Intervention Versus Observation Trial: VA/NCI/AHRQ Cooperative Studies Program #407 (PIVOT): design and baseline results of a randomized trial comparing radical prostatectomy to watchful waiting for men with clinically localized prostate cancer. Contemp Clin Trials 30:81–87, 2009.

182. Donovan J, Hamdy F, Neal D, et al: Prostate Testing for Cancer and Treatment (ProtecT) feasibility study. Health Technol Assess 7:1–88, 2003.

Index

Note: Page numbers followed by f indicate figures; those followed by t indicate tables; and those followed by b indicate boxed material.

>Index   255

Extraprostatic extension (EPE), as prognostic factor, 64–65, 64f
Extraprostatic fat invasion, as prognostic factor, 65

F

Fat intake, and prostate cancer, 209, 232
Fatty acids, and prostate cancer risk, 210–213, 212f, 213f
Fecal incontinence, after perineal prostatectomy, 154, 155f
Fiber, dietary, and prostate cancer risk, 213–214, 214f
Fibromuscular bands, in open radical retropubic prostatectomy, 111, 112f
Fibroplasia, mucinous, in prostate cancer, 47f, 48
Fibrosis, periprostatic, after hormonal therapy, 62–63
Finasteride
    for chemoprevention, 232–234, 232f
    and PSA concentration, 4–5, 18
Fine-needle aspiration (FNA), of prostate, 11
Fish, in diet
    for chemoprevention, 218
    and prostate cancer risk, 212–213
Fish oil supplements, for chemoprevention, 213, 218–219
Flat HGPIN, 74, 74f
Flax seed, and prostate cancer risk, 213–214, 214f
Flutamide, and radiation therapy, 165
FNA (fine-needle aspiration), of prostate, 11
Foamy gland adenocarcinoma, 56f, 57–58
Food pyramid, 215f
Free PSA, 5, 236–237
    and deferred treatment, 99
Free-to-total PSA, 5, 5f
Fused glands, 51f, 52

G

Genistein, for chemoprevention, 217
Genistein-combined polysaccharide (GCP), for chemoprevention, 217
German Cancer Study Group trial, on adjuvant radiation, 167–168, 168t
Ginger, for chemoprevention, 222
Gleason, Donald F., 26–27, 50
Gleason grading system, 50–55
Gleason patterns, 50–52, 51f
Gleason score(s), 26–27, 50
    in expectant management, 97, 101
    as prognostic factor, 65
    in prostate needle biopsies, 52–53, 54–55
    and radiation therapy, 163
    in radical prostatectomy specimens, 53–55
    and tumor upgrading between biopsy and prostatectomy, 37–38, 37t
Glomeruloid features, adenocarcinoma with, 56f, 57
Golden root, for chemoprevention, 222
Goserelin, and radiation therapy, 165
Grade, tumor, 26–27, 37–38, 37t
    as prognostic factor, 65, 89, 89f
    PSA and, 48–49, 86–88, 88t
Gray (Gy), 159
Green tea, for chemoprevention, 221–222, 222t
Grossly visible prostate cancer, 45–46, 46f
Guthrie, George, 138

H

Hasson techniques, for laparoscopic radical prostatectomy, 124
HCAs (heterocyclic amines), and prostate cancer risk, 213

HDR (high-dose rate) brachytherapy, 171–172
Health-related quality of life (HRQOL), after perineal prostatectomy, 152–154, 153f–155f, 154t
Hematuria, due to biopsy, 14
Hemostatic suture placement, in neurovascular bundles and prostatic pedicles, in open radical retropubic prostatectomy, 112
Herb(s), for chemoprevention, 209t, 219–223, 220t, 222t
    Chinese goldthread and barberry as, 222
    ginger, 222
    golden root (Scutellaria baicalensis) as, 222
    green tea as, 221–222
    holy basil (Ocimum sanctum) as, 222
    Prostabel as, 223
    resveratrol from hu zhang (Polygonum cuspidatum) as, 221
    saw palmetto as, 222–223
    turmeric (Curcuma longa) as, 221, 221f
    zyflamend as, 220–222, 220t, 222t
5-HETE, and prostate cancer risk, 219
Heterocyclic amines (HCAs), and prostate cancer risk, 213
HIFU. See High-intensity focused ultrasound (HIFU).
High-dose rate (HDR) brachytherapy, 171–172
High-grade prostatic intraepithelial neoplasia (HGPIN), 18, 73–76
    architectural patterns and variants of, 74–75, 74f
    with atypical small acinar proliferation, suspicious for malignancy, 71, 72
    diagnosis of, 73–74
    differential diagnosis of, 75
    epidemiology of, 73
    isolated, 75–76
    location of, 73
    morphology after treatment of, 75
    re-biopsy for, 76
High-intensity focused ultrasound (HIFU), 177–191
    commercially available devices for, 179–182, 179f–181f, 181t
    controversies over, 246
    efficacy of, 184–189
    erectile dysfunction after, 190–191
    follow-up after, 184
    future directions for, 191
    for high-risk patients, 188–189
    historical background of, 178
    indications and contraindications for, 182
    for localized disease, 182, 184–187, 185t–187t
    mechanism of action of, 178–179, 178f
    new strategies for, 184
    patient preparation for, 183
    positioning for, 179, 181f, 183
    postoperative care after, 184
    procedure for, 182–184
    rectourethral fistula after, 190
    safety of, 183, 189–190
    as salvage therapy, 182, 189
    stress incontinence after, 190, 190t
    treatment parameters for, 182–183, 183t
    treatment planning for, 183–184
    TURP prior to, 182, 187–188, 188t, 189
    urinary complications with, 190, 190t
    urinary retention after, 190
High-molecular-weight cytokeratin, 49, 50f
Histologic type(s), 55–61
    adenocarcinoma as
        atrophic, 56f, 57
        ductal, 55–57, 56f
        foamy gland, 56f, 57–58
        with glomeruloid features, 56f, 57